THIRD EDITION

# CASE FILES®
# Pediatrics

Eugene C. Toy, MD
Robert J. Yetman, MD
Rebecca G. Girardet, MD
Mark D. Hormann, MD
Sheela L. Lahoti, MD
Margaret C. McNeese, MD
Mark Jason Sanders, MD

Mc Graw Hill Medical

New York Chicago San Francisco Lisbon London Madrid Mexico City
Milan New Delhi San Juan Seoul Singapore Sydney Toronto

The McGraw-Hill Companies

**Case Files®: Pediatrics, Third Edition**



5 6 7 8 9 0 DOC/DOC 12

ISBN 978-0-07-159867-5
MHID 0-07-159867-7

**Notice**

Medicine is an ever-changing science. As new research and clinical experience broaden our knowledge, changes in treatment and drug therapy are required. The authors and the publisher of this work have checked with sources believed to be reliable in their efforts to provide information that is complete and generally in accord with the standard accepted at the time of publication. However, in view of the possibility of human error or changes in medical sciences, neither the editors nor the publisher nor any other party who has been involved in the preparation or publication of this work warrants that the information contained herein is in every respect accurate or complete, and they disclaim all responsibility for any errors or omissions or for the results obtained from use of the information contained in this work. Readers are encouraged to confirm the information contained herein with other sources. For example and in particular, readers are advised to check the product information sheet included in the package of each drug they plan to administer to be certain that the information contained in this work is accurate and that changes have not been made in the recommended dose or in the contraindications for administration. This recommendation is of particular importance in connection with new or infrequently used drugs.

This book was set in Goudy by International Typesetting and Composition.
The editors were Catherine A. Johnson and Christie Naglieri.
The production supervisor was Catherine H. Saggese.
Project management was provided by Gita Raman, International Typesetting and Composition.
The designer was Janice Bielawa; the cover designer was Aimee Nordin.
RR Donnelley was printer and binder.

This book is printed on acid-free paper.

**Library of Congress Cataloging-in-Publication Data**

Case files. Pediatrics/Eugene C. Toy ... [et al.]—3rd ed.
p. ; cm.
Includes bibliographical references and index.
ISBN-13: 978-0-07-159867-5 (pbk. : alk. paper)
ISBN-10: 0-07-159867-7 (pbk. : alk. paper)
1. Pediatrics—Problems, exercises, etc. 2. Pediatrics—Case studies.
I. Toy, Eugene C. II. Title: Pediatrics.
[DNLM: 1. Pediatrics—Case Reports. 2. Pediatrics—Problems and Exercises. WS 18.2 2009]
RJ48.2.C537 2009
618.92—dc22 2009012379

McGraw-Hill books are available at special quantity discounts to use as premiums and sales promotions, or for use in corporate training programs. To contact a representative please e-mail us at bulksales@mcgraw-hill.com.

International Edition ISBN 978-0-07-163906-4; MHID 0-07-163906-3

# AUTHORS

**Eugene C. Toy, MD**
The John S. Dunn, Senior Academic Chair and Program Director
The Methodist Hospital Ob/Gyn Residency Program
Houston, Texas

Vice Chair of Academic Affairs
Department of Obstetrics and Gynecology
The Methodist Hospital
Houston, Texas

Associate Clinical Professor and Clerkship Director
Department of Obstetrics and Gynecology
University of Texas Medical School at Houston
Houston, Texas

Associate Clinical Professor
Weill Cornell College of Medicine

**Robert J. Yetman, MD**
Professor of Pediatrics
Director, Division of Community and General Pediatrics
Department of Pediatrics
University of Texas Medical School at Houston
Houston, Texas

**Rebecca G. Girardet, MD**
Associate Professor of Pediatrics
Division of Community and General Pediatrics
Department of Pediatrics
University of Texas Medical School at Houston
Houston, Texas

**Mark D. Hormann, MD**
Associate Professor of Pediatrics
Director, Medical Student Education
Division of Community and General Pediatrics
Department of Pediatrics
University of Texas Medical School at Houston
Houston, Texas

**Sheela L. Lahoti, MD**
Associate Professor of Pediatrics
Assistant Dean of Student Affairs
Division of Community And General Pediatrics
Department of Pediatrics
University of Texas Medical School at Houston
Houston, Texas

**Margaret C. McNeese, MD**
Professor of Pediatrics
Associate Dean for Admissions and Student Affairs
Division of Community and General Pediatrics
Department of Pediatrics
University of Texas Medical School at Houston
Houston, Texas

**Mark Jason Sanders, MD**
Assistant Professor of Pediatrics
Division of Community and General Pediatrics
Department of Pediatrics
University of Texas Medical School at Houston
Houston, Texas

# CONTENTS

# DEDICATION

*To my father-in-law, J. Yen (Tommy) Ligh, whose inventive genius and sense of humor are infectious, and in loving memory of Lillie Woo Ligh, my mother-in-law, whose grace and beauty continue to shine.*

**— ECT**

# PREFACE

We appreciate all the kind remarks and suggestions from the many medical students over the past 3 years. Your positive reception has been an incredible encouragement, especially in light of the short life of the *Case Files* series. In this third edition of *Case Files: Pediatrics*, the basic format of the book has been retained. Improvements were made in updating many of the chapters. New cases include VSD/ASD, foreign body aspirated, lead poisoning, infantile spasm, pernicious anemia, and neuroblastoma. We reviewed the clinical scenarios with the intent of improving them; however, their "real-life" presentations patterned after actual clinical experience were accurate and instructive. The multiple-choice questions have been carefully reviewed and rewritten to ensure that they comply with the National Board and USMLE format. Through this third edition, we hope that the reader will continue to enjoy learning diagnosis and management through the simulated clinical cases. It certainly is a privilege to be teachers for so many students, and it is with humility that we present this edition.

*The Authors*

# ACKNOWLEDGMENTS

The clerkship curriculum that evolved into the ideas for this series was inspired by two talented and forthright students, Philbert Yao and Chuck Rosipal, who have since graduated from medical school. It has been a tremendous joy to work with the excellent pediatricians at the University of Texas Medical School at Houston. I am greatly indebted to my editor, Catherine Johnson, whose exuberance, experience, and vision helped to shape this series. I appreciate McGraw-Hill's believing in the concept of teaching through clinical cases. I am also grateful to Catherine Saggese for her excellent production expertise, and Christie Naglieri for her wonderful editing. I cherish the ever-organized and precise Gita Raman, senior project manager, whose friendship and talent I greatly value; she keeps me focused and nurtures each of my books from manuscript to print.

At the University of Texas Medical School at Houston we appreciate Dr Giuseppe N. Colasurdo, MD, Department Chair of Pediatrics, and Dean of the medical school, for his support and dedication to student education. Without my dear colleagues Drs. Konrad Harms, Jeane Holmes, Priti Schachel, and Christopher Hobday, this book could not have been written. At Methodist Hospital, I appreciate Drs. Marc Boom, Dirk Sostman, Judy Paukert, and Alan Kaplan. Ayse McCracken, an excellent administrator, was instrumental to our new home at Methodist. Most of all, I appreciate my ever-loving wife Terri, and my four wonderful children Andy, Michael, Allison, and Christina, for their patience and understanding.

*Eugene C. Toy*

# INTRODUCTION

Mastering the cognitive knowledge within a field such as pediatrics is a formidable task. It is even more difficult to draw on that knowledge, procure and filter through the clinical and laboratory data, develop a differential diagnosis, and finally form a rational treatment plan. To gain these skills, the student often learns best at the bedside, guided and instructed by experienced teachers, and inspired toward self-directed, diligent reading. Clearly, there is no replacement for education at the bedside. Unfortunately, clinical situations usually do not encompass the breadth of the specialty. Perhaps the best alternative is a carefully crafted patient case designed to stimulate the clinical approach and decision making. In an attempt to achieve that goal, we have constructed a collection of clinical vignettes to teach diagnostic or therapeutic approaches relevant to pediatrics. Most importantly, the explanations for the cases emphasize the mechanisms and underlying principles, rather than merely rote questions and answers.

This book is organized for versatility: It allows the student "in a rush" to go quickly through the scenarios and check the corresponding answers, while allowing the student who wants more thought-provoking explanations to go at a more measured pace. The answers are arranged from simple to complex: a summary of the pertinent points, the bare answers, an analysis of the case, an approach to the topic, a comprehension test at the end for reinforcement and emphasis, and a list of resources for further reading. The clinical vignettes are purposely placed in random order to simulate the way that real patients present to the practitioner. A listing of cases is included in Section III to aid the student who desires to test his or her knowledge of a specific area or who wants to review a topic, including basic definitions. Finally, we intentionally did not primarily use a multiple-choice question format in our clinical case scenarios because clues (or distractions) are not available in the real world. Nevertheless, several multiple-choice comprehension questions are included at the end of each case discussion to reinforce concepts or introduce related topics.

## HOW TO GET THE MOST OUT OF THIS BOOK

Each case is designed to simulate a patient encounter with open-ended questions. At times, the patient's complaint is different from the most concerning issue, and sometimes extraneous information is given. The answers are organized into four different parts:

## PART I

1. **Summary:** The salient aspects of the case are identified, filtering out the extraneous information. Students should formulate their summary from the case before looking at the answers. A comparison to the summation in the answer will help to improve their ability to focus on the important data while appropriately discarding the irrelevant information—a fundamental skill in clinical problem solving.
2. A **Straightforward Answer** is given to each open-ended question.
3. The **Analysis of the Case** is composed of two parts:
   a. **Objectives of the Case:** A listing of the two or three main principles that are crucial for a practitioner to manage the patient. Again, the students are challenged to make educated "guesses" about the objectives of the case upon initial review of the case scenario, which helps to sharpen their clinical and analytical skills.
   b. **Considerations:** A discussion of the relevant points and brief approach to the specific patient.

## PART II

**Approach to the Disease Process** consists of two distinct parts:

a. **Definitions:** Terminology pertinent to the disease process.
b. **Clinical Approach:** A discussion of the approach to the clinical problem in general, including tables, figures, and algorithms.

## PART III

**Comprehension Questions:** Each case contains several multiple-choice questions, which reinforce the material or introduce new and related concepts. Questions about material not found in the text have explanations in the answers.

## PART IV

**Clinical Pearls:** Several clinically important points are reiterated as a summation of the text. This allows for easy review, such as before an examination.

SECTION I

# How to Approach Clinical Problems

- Part 1. Approach to the Patient
- Part 2. Approach to Clinical Problem Solving
- Part 3. Approach to Reading

# Part 1. Approach to the Patient

The transition from the textbook or journal article to the clinical situation is perhaps the most challenging in medicine. Retention of information is difficult; organization of the facts and recall of these myriad of data to apply to the patient are crucial. This text aids in the process. The first step is gathering information, otherwise known as establishing the database. This consists of taking the history (asking questions), performing the physical examination, and obtaining selective laboratory and/or imaging tests.

The history is the single most important method of establishing a diagnosis. Depending on the age of the child, the information may be gathered solely from the parent, from both the parent and the child, or solely from the adolescent. The student should remember not to be misled by the diagnosis of another physician or by a family member. A statement such as "Johnnie has pneumonia and needs antibiotics" may or may not be correct; an astute clinician will keep an open mind and consider other possibilities, such as upper respiratory tract infection, aspirated foreign body, reactive airway disease, or even cystic fibrosis. The art of seeking the information in a nonjudgmental, sensitive, and thorough method cannot be overemphasized.

## HISTORY

1. **Basic information:**
   a. **Age, gender, and ethnicity** are important because some childhood illnesses occur with increased regularity at various ages, with higher frequency in one gender or, more commonly, in one ethnic group. For instance, anorexia nervosa is more common in white adolescent females, whereas complications of sickle cell anemia are more common in African American children of both genders.
2. **Chief complaint:** This is usually the response that the patient or the patient's family member gives to the question: "Why are you seeing the doctor today?"
3. **History of present illness:** The onset, duration, and intensity of the primary complaint, as well as associated symptoms, exacerbating and relieving factors, and previous attempts at therapy should be determined. For children, especially adolescents, a hidden agenda must be considered; **it is not uncommon for the adolescent to actually have questions about sexuality when the stated reason for the office visit is totally unrelated.** Both positive findings (the stool was loose, voluminous, and foul-smelling) and negative findings (without blood or mucus) are appropriate.
4. **Past history:**
   a. **Pregnancy and delivery:** The age of the mother, the number of pregnancies, the route of delivery, and the gestational age of the infant can often

provide clues as to the etiology of pediatric conditions. For instance, a large, full-term infant born by cesarean delivery who then develops an increased respiratory rate and streakiness on chest radiograph is more likely to have **transient tachypnea of the newborn** than is an infant born vaginally at 28-week gestation with similar symptoms. Similarly, a history of drug use (including over-the-counter, prescription, and illicit drugs) or infections during pregnancy should be obtained.

b. **Neonatal history:** Any problems identified in the neonatal period, such as severe jaundice, infections, feeding difficulties, and prolonged hospitalization, should be reviewed, especially for the younger pediatric patients in whom residua of these problems may remain.

c. **Surgical history:** When, where, and for what reason the surgery was performed should be explored. Complications should be noted.

d. **Medical history:** Whereas minor illnesses (such as occasional upper respiratory infections) can be reviewed quickly, more serious illnesses (such as diabetes mellitus) should be investigated fully. The age at diagnosis, treatments prescribed, and response to therapies can be reviewed. The number and nature of hospitalizations and complications are often important. For instance, a diabetic patient with frequent hospitalizations for ketoacidosis may indicate a lack of education of the family or underlying psychosocial issues complicating therapy. A child with a history of frequent, serious accidents should alert the physician of possible child abuse.

e. **Developmental history:** For preschool children, a few questions about **language and fine motor, gross motor, and psychosocial skills** will provide good clues about development. For school-aged children, areas of strength and weaknesses are helpful.

5. **Allergies:** Reactions to medications should be recorded, including severity and temporal relationship to medications.
6. **Immunizations:** Dates for primary and booster series of immunizations should be recorded, preferably by reviewing the immunization cards. If the child is in school, a presumption about state laws regarding immunization completion can be made while the immunization card is being retrieved.
7. **Medications:** List the names of current medications, dosages, routes of administration and frequency, and durations of use. Prescription, over-the-counter, and herbal remedies are relevant.

## Clinical Pearl

- The adolescent must be treated with sensitivity, respect, and confidentiality to foster the optimal environment for medical care.

8. **Sexual history of adolescents:** Details of an adolescent's sexual habits, contraceptive use, pregnancies, and sexually transmitted diseases (STDs) should be determined.
9. **Family history:** Because many conditions are inherited, the ages and health of siblings, parents, grandparents, and other family members can provide important diagnostic clues. For instance, an obese child with a family history of adult-onset diabetes is at high risk for developing diabetes; early intervention is warranted.
10. **Social history:** Living arrangements, economic situations, type of insurance, and religious affiliations may provide important clues to a puzzling diagnostic case or suggest important information about the acceptability of therapeutic options.
11. **Review of systems:** A few questions about each of the major body systems allow the practitioner to ensure that no problems are overlooked and to obtain crucial history about related and unrelated medical conditions.

## PHYSICAL EXAMINATION

1. **General appearance:** Well- versus poorly nourished; evidence of toxemia, including lethargy (defined as poor or absent eye contact and refusal to interact with environment), signs of poor perfusion, hypo- or hyperventilation, and cyanosis; or stigmata of syndromes (such as Down or Turner).
2. **Skin:** In smaller children, checking the color of the skin for evidence of pallor, plethora, jaundice, or cyanosis is important. Abnormalities such as capillary hemangiomas (eg, "stork bites" in a newborn), café au lait, pigmented nevi (eg, "mongolian spots"), erythema toxicum, or pustular melanosis can be identified. In older children, macules, papules, vesicles, pustules, wheals, and petechiae or purpura should be described, and evidence of excoriation, crust formation, desquamation, hyperpigmentation, ulceration, scar formation, or atrophy should be identified.
3. **Vital signs:** Temperature, blood pressure (generally begin routine measurement after 3 years), heart rate, respiratory rate, height, weight, and head circumference (generally measured until age 3 years). Measurements are plotted and compared to normals for age.
4. **Head, eyes, ears, nose, mouth, and throat:**
   a. **Head:** For the neonate, the size of fontanelles and presence of overriding sutures, caput succedaneum (superficial edema or hematoma that crosses suture lines, usually located over crown), or cephalohematoma (hematoma that does not cross suture lines) should be noted. For the older child, the size and shape of the head as well as abnormalities such as swellings, depressions, or abnormal hair quality or distribution may be identified.
   b. **Eyes:** For infants, abnormalities in the size, shape, and position of the orbits, the color of the sclera (blue sclera, for instance, may indicate

osteogenesis imperfecta), conjunctival hemorrhages or abnormalities, or the presence of iris defects (such as coloboma) may be found. The visual acuity of older children should be determined.

c. **Ears:** For all children, abnormalities in the size, shape, and position of the ears can provide important diagnostic clues. Whereas tympanic membranes are difficult to assess in newborns, their integrity should be assessed in older children. For all children, the quality and character of discharge from the ear canal should be documented.

d. **Nose:** The size, shape, and position of the nose (in relation to the face and mouth) can provide diagnostic clues for various syndromes, such as a small nose in Down syndrome. Patency of the nostrils, especially in neonates who are obligate nose breathers, is imperative. Abnormalities of the nasal bridge or septum, integrity of the mucosa, and the presence of foreign bodies should be noted. A butterfly rash around the nose can be associated with systemic lupus erythematosus (SLE), and a transverse crease across the anterior portion of the nose is seen with allergic rhinitis.

e. **Mouth and throat:** The size, shape, and position of the mouth and lips in relation to other facial structures should be evaluated. In infants, common findings of the mouth include disruption of the palate (cleft palate syndrome), Epstein pearls (a tiny white papule in the center of the palate), and short frenulum ("tongue-tied"). For all children, the size, shape, and position of the tongue and uvula must be considered. The number and quality of teeth for age should be assessed, and the buccal mucosa and pharynx should be examined for color, rashes, exudate, size of tonsils, and symmetry.

5. **Neck:** The neck in infants usually is short and sometimes hard to evaluate. Nonetheless, the size, shape, and preferred position of the neck can be evaluated for all children. The range of motion can be evaluated by gentle movement. Symmetry of the muscles, thyroid gland, veins, and arteries is important. An abnormal mass, such as a thyroglossal duct cyst (midline above the level of the thyroid) or brachial cleft cyst (along the sternomastoid muscle), or unusual findings, such as webbing in Turner syndrome, can be identified.

6. **Chest:** General examination of the chest should include an evaluation of the size and shape of the structures along with identification of obvious abnormalities (such as supernumerary nipples) or movement with respirations. **Respiratory rate varies according to age** and ranges from 40 to 60 breaths/min in the neonate to 12 to 14 breaths/min in the toddler. **The degree of respiratory distress can be stratified, with increasing distress noted when the child moves from subcostal to intercostal to supraclavicular to suprasternal retractions.** Palpation of the chest should confirm the integrity of the ribs and clavicles and any swelling or tenderness in the joints. Percussion in older children may reveal abnormalities, especially if asymmetry is noted. The chest should be auscultated for air

movement, vocal resonance, rales, rhonchi, wheezes, and rubs. In adolescent girls, symmetry of breast development and presence of masses or nipple discharge should be evaluated.

7. **Cardiovascular:** The precardium should be inspected for abnormal movements. The chest should be palpated for the location and quality of the cardiac impulse and to determine if a thrill is present. The presence and quality of the first and second heart sounds, including splitting with respirations, should be noted. Murmurs, clicks, rubs, and abnormalities in rate (which vary by age) or rhythm should be identified. The peripheral perfusion, pulses, and color should be assessed.
8. **Abdominal examination:** The abdomen should be inspected to determine whether it is flat or protuberant, if masses or lesions such as striae are obvious, or if pulsations are present. In older children, the abdomen usually is flat, but in the neonate a very flat abdomen in conjunction with respiratory distress may indicate diaphragmatic hernia. The umbilicus, especially for neonates, should be evaluated for defects, drainage, or masses; a small umbilical hernia often is present and is normal. In the newborn, one umbilical vein and two umbilical arteries are normal. **In the neonate, palpation of the abdomen may reveal a liver edge about 2 cm below the coastal margin, a spleen tip, and, using deep pressure, kidneys.** In older children, these structures are not usually palpable except in pathology. Depending on the history, other masses must be viewed with suspicion for a variety of conditions. Bowel sounds are usually heard throughout the abdomen except in pathology. In adolescent females, the lower abdomen should be palpated for uterine enlargement (pregnancy).
9. **Genitalia:** Examination of the male for the size and shape of the penis, testicles, and scrotum is important. The position of the urethral opening should be assessed. In newborn girls, the labia majora usually is large and completely encloses the labia minora; the genitalia usually is highly pigmented and swollen with an especially prominent clitoris. A white discharge is usually present in the first days of life, and occasionally a blood-tinged fluid is also seen. In toddlers, examination of the genitalia can be challenging. Placing the toddler in a frog-leg position while the toddler sits in the parent's lap (or on the examination table) often allows successful viewing of external genitalia. In older girls, the knee-chest position affords an excellent view of the external genitalia. In girls outside the newborn period, the labia minora are smaller compared to the remainder of the external genitalia, and the vaginal mucosa is red and appears thin. The hymen, which is just inside the introitus, should be inspected. Abnormalities of the hymen, such as imperforation or tags, vaginal discharge, foreign bodies, and labial adhesions, may be noted. A speculum examination should be performed for sexually active adolescent girls. Tanner staging for pubertal development should be done for both boys and girls. Inguinal hernias should be identified; normalcy of anus should be confirmed.

10. **Extremities:** For all children, the size, shape, and symmetry of the extremities should be considered; muscle strength should be evaluated. Joints may be investigated for range of motion, warmth, tenderness, and redness. Normalcy of gait for age should be reviewed. For infants, recognition of dislocated hips is of critical importance, as lifelong growth abnormalities may result. For adolescents, identification of scoliosis is important to prevent the debilitating complications of that condition. Athletes require evaluation of the integrity of their joints, especially those joints that will be used in sporting activities.
11. **Neurologic:** Neurologic evaluation of the older child is similar to that in adults. Consciousness level and orientation are determined as a starting point. The cranial nerves should be assessed. The motor system should be evaluated (including strength, tone, coordination, and involuntary movements). Superficial and deep sensory systems, and deep tendon reflexes should be reviewed. **In younger infants a variety of normal primitive reflexes (Moro, parachute, suck, grasp) can be found, but ensuring that these reflexes have extinguished by the appropriate age is equally important.**

## LABORATORY ASSESSMENT

The American Academy of Pediatrics recommends a few laboratory screening tests be accomplished for pediatric patients. These tests vary according to the child's age and risk factors.

1. **Newborn metabolic screening** is done in all states, usually after 24 hours of age, but the exact tests performed vary by state. Conditions commonly screened for include hypothyroidism, phenylketonuria, galactosemia, hemoglobin type, and adrenal hyperplasia. Other conditions that may be assessed include maple syrup urine disease, homocystinuria, biotinidase deficiency, cystic fibrosis, tyrosinemia, and toxoplasmosis. Some states require a second newborn screen be performed after 7 days of age.
2. **Hemoglobin or hematocrit levels** are recommended for high-risk infants (especially premature infants and those with low birth weight), at 9 to 12 months of age, and yearly on all menstruating adolescents.
3. **Urinalyses** are recommended at 9 to 12 months of age and at 5 years of age, and dipstick urinalysis for leukocytes annually for sexually active adolescents.
4. **Lead screening** is done, especially in high-risk areas, at 9 to 12 months of age, and again at 2 years of age.
5. **Cholesterol screening** is performed in high-risk patients (those with positive family histories) older than 24 months.
6. **Sexually transmitted disease screening** is performed yearly on all sexually active patients.

Other specialized testing is accomplished depending on the child's age, risk factors, chief complaint, and conditions included in the differential diagnosis.

## IMAGING PROCEDURES

1. **Plain radiographs** offer the advantage of inexpensive testing that reveals global views of the anatomy. Unfortunately, fine organ detail is not revealed sometimes, requiring further radiographic study. Bone films for fracture, chest films for pneumonia, and abdomen films for ileus are common uses of this modality.
2. **Ultrasonography** is a fairly inexpensive modality that requires little or no sedation and has no radiation risks. It offers good organ and anatomic detail, but it can be operator dependent. Not all organs are accessible to sonography. Common examinations include the head for intraventricular hemorrhage in the premature infant, the abdomen for conditions such as pyloric stenosis, and the kidneys for abnormal structure.
3. **Computer tomography (CT)** provides good organ and anatomic detail and is quick, but it is fairly expensive, may require contrast, and does involve radiation. Some children require sedation to complete the procedure. This test is often performed on the abdomen or head in trauma victims.
4. **Magnetic resonance imaging (MRI)** is expensive but does not involve radiation. Because it is a slow procedure, sedation is often needed for younger children, and contrast is sometimes required. It allows for superb tissue contrast in multiple planes, and excellent anatomic and functional imaging. It is frequently used to provide detail on the brain in patients with seizures or developmental delay or to provide tissue detail on a mass located virtually anywhere in the body.
5. **Nuclear scan** is moderately expensive and invasive. It provides functional information (usually organ specific) but provides poor anatomic detail. Radiation is involved. Common uses include bone scans for infection and renal scans for function.

# Part 2. Approach to Clinical Problem Solving

There are generally **four steps** to the systematic solving of clinical problems:

1. Making the diagnosis
2. Assessing the severity of the disease
3. Rendering a treatment based on the stage of the disease
4. Following the response to the treatment

## MAKING THE DIAGNOSIS

This is achieved with careful sifting of the database, analysis based on the risk factors present, and development of a list of possibilities (the differential diagnosis). The process includes knowing which pieces of information are more meaningful and which can be discarded. Experience and knowledge from reading help to guide the physician to key in on the most important concerns.

**A good clinician also knows how to ask the same question in several different ways and using different terminology,** because patients at times will deny having been treated for asthma but will answer affirmatively to being hospitalized for wheezing. A diagnosis can be reached by systematically reviewing each possible cause and reading about each disease. The patient's presentation is then matched up against each of these possibilities and either placed higher up on the list as a potential etiology or lower down because of the disease frequency, the patient's presentation, or other clues. A patient's risk factors may influence the probability of a diagnosis. Usually a long list of possible diagnoses can be pared down to two or three top suspicions, based on key laboratory or imaging tests. For example, an adolescent presenting with a fever as the chief complaint can have an extensive differential diagnosis reduced to far fewer possibilities when the history reveals an uncle in the home with cough, weight loss, and night sweats, and the physical examination shows an increased respiratory rate, lymphadenopathy, and right lower lobe lung crackles. In this case, the patient likely has tuberculosis.

## ASSESSING THE SEVERITY OF THE DISEASE

The next step is to characterize the severity of the disease process. In asthma, this is done formally based on guidelines promulgated by the National Heart, Lung, and Blood Institute (NHLBI). Asthma categories range from mild intermittent (least severe) to severe persistent (most severe). For some conditions, such as syphilis, the staging depends on the length of time and follows along the natural history of the infection (ie, primary, secondary, or tertiary syphilis).

## RENDERING TREATMENT BASED ON THE STAGE OF THE DISEASE

Many illnesses are stratified according to severity because prognosis and treatment vary based on the severity. If neither the prognosis nor the treatment was affected by the stage of the disease process, it would not make much sense to subcategorize something as mild or severe. As an example, mild intermittent asthma poses less danger than does severe persistent asthma (particularly if the patient has been intubated for asthma in the past). Accordingly, with mild intermittent asthma, the management would be intermittent short-acting β-agonist therapy while watching for any worsening of the disease into more serious categories (more severe disease). In contrast, a patient with severe persistent asthma would generally require short-acting β-agonist medications as well as long-acting β-agonists, inhaled steroids, and potentially oral steroids.

Group A β-hemolytic streptococcal pharyngeal infection ("strep throat") is associated with complications, including poststreptococcal glomerulonephritis and rheumatic fever. The presence of group A β-hemolytic *Streptococcus* confers an increased risk of problems, but neither the prognosis nor the treatment is affected by "more" group A β-hemolytic *Streptococcus* or "less" group A β-hemolytic *Streptococcus*. Hence, **the student should approach new disease by learning the mechanism, clinical presentation, how it is staged, and how the treatment varies based on stage.**

## FOLLOWING THE RESPONSE TO TREATMENT

The final step in the approach to disease is to follow the patient's response to the therapy. **Whatever the "measure" of response, it should be recorded and monitored.** Some responses are clinical, such as a change in the patient's pain level or temperature, or results of pulmonary examination. Obviously the student must work on being more skilled in eliciting the data in an unbiased and standardized manner. Other patients may be followed by imaging, such as computerized tomographic (CT) scan of a retroperitoneal node size in a patient receiving chemotherapy for neuroblastoma, or a marker such as the platelet count in a patient recovering from Kawasaki syndrome. For syphilis, it may be the nonspecific treponemal antibody test rapid plasma reagin (RPR) titer every month. The student must know what to do if the measured marker does not respond according to the expected. Is the next step to treat further, or to repeat the metastatic workup, or to follow up with another more specific test?

# Part 3. Approach to Reading

The student must approach reading differently than the classic "systematic" review of a particular disease entity. Patients rarely present with a clear diagnosis; hence, the student must become skilled in applying the textbook information to the clinical setting. Everyone retains more when the reading is performed with a purpose. Experience teaches that with reading, there are several crucial questions to consider **thinking clinically.** They are the following:

1. What is the most likely diagnosis?
2. What should be your next step?
3. What is the most likely mechanism for this process?
4. What are the risk factors for this condition?
5. What are the complications associated with this disease?
6. What is the best therapy?

## WHAT IS THE MOST LIKELY DIAGNOSIS?

Establishing the diagnosis was discussed in the previous section. This is a difficult task to give to the medical student; however, it is the basic problem that will confront clinicians for the rest of their careers. One way of attacking this problem is to develop standard "approaches" to common clinical problems. It is helpful to memorize the most common causes of various presentations, such as "the most common cause of mild respiratory distress in a term infant born by cesarean section is retained amniotic fluid (transient tachypnea of the newborn)."

The clinical scenario would entail something such as:

"A 3-hour-old infant is noted to have a mildly increased respiratory rate and slight subcostal retractions. The infant is term, large for gestation age, and was born by repeat cesarean section. The pregnancy was uncomplicated. What is the most likely diagnosis?"

With no other information to go on, the student would note that this baby has respiratory distress. Using the "most common cause" information, the student would guess transient tachypnea of the newborn. If, instead, the gestational age "term" is changed to "preterm at 30 weeks' gestation," a phrase can be added, such as:

"The mother did not receive prophylactic steroids prior to birth."

Now, the student would use the "most common cause of respiratory distress in a preterm child whose mother did not receive prenatal steroids" is surfactant deficiency (respiratory distress syndrome).

## WHAT SHOULD BE YOUR NEXT STEP?

This question in many ways is even more difficult than the most likely diagnosis, because insufficient information may be available to make a diagnosis and the next step may be to pursue more diagnostic information. Another possibility is that the diagnosis is clear, but the next step is the staging of the disease. Finally, the next step may be to treat. Hence, from clinical data a judgment needs to be rendered regarding how far along one is on the road of:

**Make diagnosis → Stage disease →**
**Treat based on the stage → Follow response**

In particular, the student is accustomed to regurgitating the same information that someone has written about a particular disease but is not skilled at giving the next step. This talent is optimally learned at the bedside, in a supportive environment, with freedom to take educated guesses, and with constructive feedback. The student in assessing a child in the hospital should go through the following thinking process:

1. Based on the information I have, I believe that CJ (a 3-month-old child with a positive respiratory syncytial virus nasal washing) has bronchiolitis.
2. I don't believe that this is severe disease (such as significant oxygen requirement, severe retractions, or carbon dioxide retention on blood gas analysis). A chest radiograph shows no lobar consolidation (I believe this is important because a lobar consolidation would suggest a bacterial etiology).
3. Therefore, the treatment is supportive care with supplemental oxygen and intravenous (IV) fluids as needed.

4. I want to follow the treatment by assessing the child's respiratory status (I will follow the oxygen saturation and degree of retractions), his temperature, and his ability to maintain his hydration orally without intravenous fluids. Also, if in the next few days he does not get better or if he worsens, I think he will need a repeat chest radiograph to assess whether he has an evolving bacterial pneumonia.

In a similar patient, when the clinical presentation is not so clear, perhaps the best "next step" may be diagnostic in nature such as blood cultures to determine if bacteremia is present. This information is sometimes tested by the dictum, "the gold standard for the diagnosis and treatment of a bacterial infection is a culture."

Sometimes the next step is therapeutic.

## WHAT IS THE LIKELY MECHANISM FOR THIS PROCESS?

This question goes further than requiring the student to make the diagnosis; it also requires the student to understand the underlying mechanism for the process. For example, a clinical scenario may describe a 5-year-old child with Henoch-Schönlein purpura (HSP) who develops abdominal pain and heme-positive stools 1 week after diagnosis. The student first must diagnose the heme-positive stools associated with Henoch-Schönlein purpura, which occur in approximately 50% of patients. Then, the student must understand that the edema and damage to the vasculature of the gastrointestinal (GI) tract can cause bleeding along with colicky abdominal pain, sometimes progressing to intussusception. The mechanism of the pain and bleeding is, therefore, vasculitis causing enlarged mesenteric lymph nodes, bowel edema, and hemorrhage into the bowel. Answers that a student may speculate, but would not be as likely, include appendicitis, bacterial gastroenteritis, or volvulus.

The student is advised to learn the mechanisms for each disease process and not merely to memorize a constellation of symptoms. In other words, rather than trying to commit to memory the classic presentation of Henoch Schönlein purpura (typical rash, abdominal pain, and arthritis), the student should also understand that vasculitis of the small vessels is the culprit. The vasculitis causes edema, mainly in the dependent areas, that precedes the palpable purpura. This vasculitis is responsible not only for edema in the joints (mainly in dependent areas such as the knees and ankles) causing the arthritis found in approximately two-thirds of patients, but also for damage to the vasculature of the GI tract leading to the intermittent, colicky abdominal pain that can manifest as heme-positive stools or even intussusception.

## WHAT ARE THE RISK FACTORS FOR THIS CONDITION?

Understanding the risk factors helps to establish the diagnosis and interpret test results. For example, understanding the risk factor analysis may help to manage a 1-year-old child with anemia found on routine screening. If the child had no risk factors for lead poisoning or thalassemia, the practitioner may choose to treat with supplemental iron because the likelihood for more serious pathology is low. On the other hand, if the same 1-year-old child were a recent immigrant from an endemic area, lived in an older home with peeling paint, had a father who worked at a battery smelting plant, and ate meals from unglazed pottery, a practitioner should presumptively diagnose lead poisoning until proven otherwise. The physician may want to obtain a serum lead level, a complete blood count (CBC) with differential (looking for basophilic stippling), and thoroughly evaluate the child for developmental delay. Thus, the number of risk factors helps to categorize the likelihood of a disease process.

## WHAT ARE THE COMPLICATIONS ASSOCIATED WITH THIS DISEASE?

A clinician must understand the complications of a disease so that the patient can be monitored. Sometimes, the student will have to make the diagnosis from clinical clues and then apply his or her knowledge of the sequelae of the pathologic process. For example, a child diagnosed with high fever, rash, lymphadenopathy, and oral and conjunctival changes is diagnosed with Kawasaki syndrome. Complications of this condition include arthritis, vasculitis of the medium-sized arteries, hydrops of the gallbladder, urethritis, and aseptic meningitis. Understanding the types of complications helps the clinician to assess the patient. For example, one life-threatening complication of Kawasaki syndrome is coronary artery aneurysm and thrombosis. **The clinical presentation in the subacute phase is desquamation, thrombocytosis, and the development of coronary aneurysms with a high risk of sudden death.** The appropriate therapy is intravenous immunoglobulin in the acute phase and high-dose aspirin as soon as possible after the diagnosis is made. Nonrecognition of the risk of coronary artery aneurysm and appropriate therapy for thrombosis can lead to the patient's death. Students apply this information when they see on rounds a patient with Kawasaki syndrome and monitor for new murmurs, thrombocytosis, myocarditis, and development of coronary artery aneurysms. The clinician communicates to the team to watch the patient for any of these signs or symptoms so that appropriate therapy can be considered.

## WHAT IS THE BEST THERAPY?

This is perhaps the most difficult question, not only because the clinician needs to reach the correct diagnosis and assess the severity of the condition, but also because he or she must weigh the situation to reach the appropriate intervention. The student does not necessarily need to memorize exact dosages, but the medication, the route of delivery, and possible complications are important. It is important for the student to verbalize the diagnosis and the rationale for the therapy. A common error is for the student to "jump to a treatment," almost like a random guess, and therefore be given a "right or wrong" feedback. In fact, the student's guess may be correct but for the wrong reason; conversely, the answer may be a very reasonable one, with only one small error in thinking. It is crucial instead to give the steps so that feedback can be given for each step.

For example, what is the best therapy for a 15-year-old sexually active adolescent female with severe, cystic acne? The incorrect manner of response is for the clinician to blurt out "Accutane." Rather, the student should reason it as follows:

"Severe, cystic acne can be treated with a variety of modalities. Side effects of the medications must be considered in a sexually active teenager who is statistically at high risk for pregnancy. Accutane causes severe birth defects and is absolutely contraindicated in pregnancy. Therefore, the best treatment for this adolescent may be a combination of oral antibiotics and topical medications that present a much lower chance of devastating side effects."

## REFERENCES

Athreya BH, Silverman BK. *Pediatric Physical Diagnosis*. Norwalk, CT: Appleton-Century-Crofts; 1985.

Barness LA. *Manual of Pediatric Physical Diagnosis*. St. Louis, MO: Mosby-Year Book; 1991.

Barness LA. Pediatric history and physical examination. In: McMillan JA, DeAngelis CD, Feigin RD, Warshaw JB, eds. *Oski's Pediatrics: Principles and Practice*. 4th ed. Philadelphia, PA: Lippincott, Williams & Wilkins; 2006:39-51.

Haller JO, Slovis TL. *Pediatric Radiology*. Berlin, Germany: Springer; 1995.

SECTION II

# Clinical Cases

# Case 1

A mother brings her 12-month-old child, a new patient for your clinic, for a well-child visit. The infant appears to be small for her age. Her weight is below the 5th percentile on standardized growth curves (50th percentile for an 8-month-old), her length is at the 25th percentile, and her head circumference is at the 50th percentile. Her vital signs and her examination otherwise are normal.

- What is the next step in the management of this patient?
- What is the most likely diagnosis?
- What is the next step in the evaluation?

# ANSWERS TO CASE 1:

## Failure to Thrive

*Summary:* A 12-month-old girl has poor weight gain, but no etiology is found on examination.

- **Next step:** Gather more information, including birth, past medical, family, social, and developmental histories. A dietary history is especially important.
- **Most likely diagnosis:** Failure to thrive (FTT), most likely "nonorganic" in etiology.
- **Next step in evaluation:** Limited screening laboratory testing to identify organic causes of FTT, dietary counseling, and frequent office visits to assess weight gain.

## ANALYSIS

### Objectives

1. Know the historical clues necessary to recognize organic and nonorganic FTT.
2. Understand the appropriate use of the laboratory in a healthy child with FTT.
3. Appreciate the treatment and follow-up of a child with nonorganic FTT.

### Considerations

This patient's growth pattern (inadequate weight gain, potentially modest length retardation, and head circumference sparing) suggests FTT, most likely nonorganic given that the examination is normal. A nonorganic FTT diagnosis is made after organic etiologies are excluded, and, after adequate nutrition and an adequate environment is assured, growth resumes normally after catch-up growth is demonstrated. Diagnostic and therapeutic maneuvers aimed at organic causes are appropriate when supported by the history (prematurity, maternal infection) or examination (enlarged spleen, significant developmental delay). Although organic and nonorganic FTT can occur simultaneously, attempts to differentiate the two forms are helpful because the evaluation, treatment, and follow-up may be very different.

*Note:* Had the same practitioner followed this patient since birth or had previous records from the previous health-care provider, earlier detection of FTT and its potential etiology with rapid intervention might have occurred. For instance, patients with poor caloric intake usually fail to gain weight but maintain length and head circumference. As nutrition remains poor, length becomes affected next and then ultimately head circumference.

# APPROACH TO
## Failure to Thrive

## DEFINITIONS

**FAILURE TO THRIVE (FTT):** A physical sign, not a final diagnosis. It is suspected when growth is below the third or fifth percentile or crosses more than two major growth percentiles in a short time frame. Usually seen in children younger than 5 years whose physical growth is significantly less than that of their peers.

**NONORGANIC (PSYCHOSOCIAL) FTT:** Poor growth without a medical etiology. Nonorganic FTT often is related to poverty or poor caregiver–child interaction. It constitutes one-third to one-half of FTT cases identified in tertiary care settings and nearly all cases in primary care settings.

**ORGANIC FTT:** Poor growth caused by an underlying medical condition, such as inflammatory bowel disease, renal disease, or congenital heart conditions.

## CLINICAL APPROACH

The goals of the history, physical examination, and laboratory testing are to establish whether the child's caregiver is supplying enough calories, whether the child is consuming enough calories, and whether the child is able to use the calories for growth. Identification of which factor is the likely source of problem helps guide management.

### Diagnosis

The history and physical examination are the most important tools in an FTT evaluation. A dietary history can offer important clues to identify an etiology. The type of milk (breast or bottle) and frequency and quality of feeding, voiding, vomiting, and stooling should be recorded. The milk used (commercial or homemade formula) and the mixing process (to ensure appropriate dilution) should be reviewed (adding too much water to powdered formula results in inadequate nutrition). The amount and type of juices and solid foods should be noted for older children. Significant food aversions might suggest gastric distress of malabsorption. A two-week food diary (the parent notes all foods offered and taken by the child) and any associated symptoms of sweating, choking, cyanosis, difficulty sucking, and the like can be useful.

Pregnancy and early neonatal histories may reveal maternal infection, depression, drug use, intrauterine growth retardation, prematurity, or other chronic neonatal conditions. When children suspected of having FTT are seen in families whose members are genetically small or with a slow growth history (constitutional delay), affected children are usually normal and do not require an exhaustive evaluation. In contrast, a family history of inheritable disease associated with poor growth (cystic fibrosis) should be evaluated more extensively. Because nonorganic FTT is more commonly associated with poverty, a social history is often useful. The child's living arrangements, including primary and secondary caregivers, housing type, caregiver's financial and employment status, the family's social supports, and unusual stresses (such as spousal abuse) should be reviewed. While gathering the history, the clinician can observe for unusual caregiver–child interactions.

All body organ systems potentially harbor a cause for organic FTT (Table 1–1). **The developmental status (possibly delayed in organic and nonorganic FTT) needs evaluation.** Children with nonorganic FTT may demonstrate an occipital bald spot from lying in a bed and failure to attain appropriate developmental milestones resulting from lack of parental stimulation; may be disinterested in their environment; may avoid eye contact, smiling, or vocalization; and may not respond well to maternal attempts of comforting. Children with some types of organic FTT (renal tubular acidosis) and most nonorganic FTT show "catch-up" in developmental milestones with successful therapy. During the examination (especially of younger infants) **the clinician can observe a feeding, which may give clues to maternal–child interaction bonding issues or to physical problems** (cerebral palsy, oral motor or swallowing difficulties, velum cleft palate).

The history or examination suggestive of organic FTT directs the laboratory and radiologic evaluation. In most cases, results of the newborn state

**Table 1–1 MAJOR CAUSES OF INADEQUATE WEIGHT GAIN**

Inadequate Caloric Intake
- Lack of appetite: depression, chronic disease
- Ingestion difficulties: feeding disorders, neurologic disorders (cerebral palsy), craniofacial anomalies, genetic syndromes, tracheoesophageal fistula
- Unavailability of food: neglect, inappropriate food for age, insufficient volume of food

Altered Growth Potential
- Prenatal insult, chromosomal anomalies, endocrine disorders

Caloric Wasting
- Emesis: intestinal tract disorders, drugs, toxins, CNS pathology
- Malabsorption: GI disease (biliary atresia, celiac disease), inflammatory bowel disease, infections, toxins
- Renal losses: diabetes, renal tubular acidosis

Increased Caloric Requirements
- Increased metabolism: congenital heart disease, chronic respiratory disease, neoplasms, chronic infection, hyperthyroidism
- Defective use of calories: metabolic disorders, renal tubular acidosis

Abbreviations: CNS, central nervous system; GI, gastrointestinal.

screen are critical. A child with cystic fibrosis in the family requires sweat chloride or genetic testing. A child with a loud, harsh systolic murmur and bounding pulses deserves a chest radiograph, an electrocardiogram (ECG), and perhaps an echocardiogram and cardiology consult. Most FTT children have few or no signs. Thus, laboratory evaluation is usually limited to a few screening tests: a complete blood count (CBC), lead level (especially for patients in lower socioeconomic classes or in cities with a high lead prevalence), urinalysis and culture, and serum electrolyte levels (including calcium, blood urea nitrogen [BUN], and creatinine). A tuberculosis skin test and human immunodeficiency virus testing may also be indicated. Abnormalities in screening tests are pursued more extensively.

## Treatment and Follow-up

The treatment and follow-up for organic FTT is disease specific. Patients with nonorganic FTT are managed with improved dietary intake, close follow-up, and attention to psychosocial issues.

**Healthy infants in the first year of life require approximately 120 kcal/kg/d of nutrition and about 100 kcal/kg/d thereafter; FTT children require an additional 50% to 100% to ensure adequate catch-up growth.** A mealtime routine is important. Families should eat together in a nondistracting environment (television off!), with meals lasting between 20 and 30 minutes. Solid foods are offered before liquids; children are not force-fed. Low-calorie drinks, juices, and water are limited; age-appropriate high-calorie foods (whole milk, cheese, dried fruits, peanut butter) are encouraged. Formulas containing more than the standard 20 cal/oz may be necessary for smaller children, and high-calorie supplementation (PediaSure or Ensure) may be required for larger children. Frequent office or home health visits are indicated to ensure weight gain. In some instances, hospitalization of an FTT child is required; such infants often have rapid weight gain, supporting the diagnosis of nonorganic FTT.

Nonorganic FTT treatment requires not only the provision of increased calories but also attention to contributing psychosocial issues. Referral to community services (Women, Infants, and Children [WIC] Program, Food Stamp Program, and local food banks) may be required. Caregiver help in the form of job training, substance and physical abuse prevention, parenting classes, and psychotherapy may be available through community programs. Older children and their families may benefit from early childhood intervention and Head Start programs.

Some children with organic FTT also have nonorganic FTT. For instance, a poorly growing special-needs premature infant is at increased risk for superimposed nonorganic FTT because of psychosocial issues, such as poor bonding with the family during a prolonged hospital stay. In such cases, care for the organic causes is coordinated with attempts to preclude nonorganic FTT.

## Comprehension Questions

1.1 Parents bring their 6-month-old son to see you. He is symmetrically less than the fifth percentile for height, weight, and head circumference. He was born at 30 weeks' gestation and weighed 1000 g. He was a planned pregnancy, and his mother's prenatal course was uneventful until an automobile accident initiated the labor. He was ventilated for 3 days in the intensive care unit (ICU) but otherwise did well without ongoing problems. He was discharged at 8 weeks of life. Which of the following is the mostly likely explanation for his small size?

A. Chromosomal abnormality
B. Protein-calorie malnutrition
C. Normal ex-premie infant growth
D. Malabsorption secondary to short gut syndrome
E. Congenital hypothyroidism

1.2 A 13-month-old child is noted to be at the 25th percentile for weight, the 10th percentile for height, and less than the 5th percentile for head circumference. She was born at term. She was noted to have a small head at birth, to be developmentally delayed throughout her life, and to have required cataract surgery shortly after birth. She currently takes phenobarbital for seizures. Which of the following would most likely explain this child's small size?

A. Congenital cytomegalovirus (CMV) infection
B. Down syndrome
C. Glycogen storage disease type II
D. Congenital hypothyroidism
E. Craniopharyngioma

1.3 A 2-year-old boy had been slightly less than the 50th percentile for weight, height, and head circumference, but in the last 6 months he has fallen to slightly less than the 25th percentile for weight. The pregnancy was normal, his development is as expected, and the family reports no psychosocial problems. The mother says that he is now a finicky eater (wants only macaroni and cheese at all meals), but she insists that he eat a variety of foods. The meals are marked by much frustration for everyone. His examination is normal. Which of the following is the best next step in his care?

A. Sweat chloride testing
B. Examination of the eyes for retinal hemorrhages
C. Reassurance and counseling for family about childhood normal developmental stage
D. Testing of stool for parasites
E. Magnetic resonance imaging (MRI) of the brain

1.4 A 4-month-old child has poor weight gain. Her current weight is less than the 5th percentile, height about the 10th percentile, and head circumference at the 50th percentile. The planned pregnancy resulted in a normal, spontaneous, vaginal delivery; mother and child were discharged after a 48-hour hospitalization. Feeding is via breast and bottle; the quantity seems sufficient. The child has had no illness. The examination is unremarkable except for the child's small size. Screening laboratory shows the hemoglobin and hematocrit are 11 mg/dL and 33%, respectively, with a platelet count of 198,000/mm$^3$. Serum electrolyte levels are sodium 140, chloride 105, potassium 3.5, bicarbonate 17, blood urea nitrogen 15, and creatinine 0.3. Liver function tests are normal. Urinalysis reveals a pH of 8 with occasional epithelial cells but no white blood cells, bacteria, protein, ketones, or reducing substances. Which of the following is the most appropriate therapy for this child?

A. Transfusion with packed red blood cells (PRBCs)
B. Intravenous (IV) infusion of potassium chloride
C. Sweat chloride analysis
D. Growth hormone determination
E. Oral supplementation with bicarbonate

## ANSWERS

1.1 **C.** The expected weight versus age must be modified for a preterm infant. Similarly, growth for children with Down or Turner syndrome varies from that for other children. Thus, use of an appropriate growth curve is paramount. For the child in the question, weight gain should follow or exceed that of term infants. For this premature infant, when his parameters are plotted on a "premie growth chart," normal growth is revealed.

1.2 **A.** The developmental delay, intrauterine growth retardation (including microcephaly), cataracts, seizures, hepatosplenomegaly, prolonged neonatal jaundice, and purpura at birth are consistent with a congenital cytomegalovirus (CMV) or toxoplasmosis infection. Calcified brain densities of CMV typically are found in a periventricular pattern; in toxoplasmosis, they are found scattered throughout the cortex.

1.3 **C.** Between 18 and 30 months of age children often become "picky eaters." Their growth rate can slow, and the period can be distressing for families. Calm counseling of parents to provide nutrition, avoid "force-feeding," and avoid providing snacks is usually effective. Close follow-up is required.

1.4 **E.** The patient has evidence of renal tubular acidosis (probably distal tubular), a well-described cause of FTT. Upon confirmation of the findings, oral bicarbonate supplementation would be expected to correct the elevated chloride level, the low bicarbonate and potassium levels (although potassium supplements may be required), and poor growth.

## Clinical Pearls

- In the United States, psychosocial failure to thrive is more common than organic failure to thrive; it often is associated with poverty or poor parent–child interaction.
- Inexpensive laboratory screening tests, dietary counseling, and close observation of weight changes are appropriate first steps for most healthy-appearing infants with failure to thrive.
- Organic failure to thrive can be associated with abnormalities of any organ system. Clues in history, examination, or screening laboratory tests help identify affected organ systems.
- Up to one-third of patients with psychosocial failure to thrive have developmental delay as well as social and emotional problems.
- Patients with renal tubular acidosis, a common cause of organic failure to thrive, can have proximal tubule defects (type 2) caused by impaired tubular bicarbonate reabsorption or distal tubule defects (type 1) caused by impaired hydrogen ion secretion. Type 4 is also a distal tubule problem associated with impaired ammoniagenesis.

## REFERENCES

Bauchner H. Failure to thrive. In: Kleigman RM, Behrman RE, Jenson HB, Stanton BF, eds. *Nelson Textbook of Pediatrics*. 18th ed. Philadelphia, PA: WB Saunders; 2007:184-187.

Chiang ML, Hill LL. Renal tubular acidosis. In: McMillan JA, Feigin RD, DeAngelis CD, Jones MD, eds. *Oski's Pediatrics: Principles and Practice*. 4th ed. Philadelphia, PA: Lippincott Williams & Wilkins; 2006:1886-1892.

Dell KM, Avner ED. Renal tubular acidosis. In: Kleigman RM, Behrman RE, Jenson HB, Stanton BF, eds. *Nelson Textbook of Pediatrics*. 18th ed. Philadelphia, PA: WB Saunders; 2007:2197-2202.

Kirkland RT. Failure to thrive. In: McMillan JA, Feigin RD, DeAngelis CD, Jones MD, eds. *Oski's Pediatrics: Principles and Practice*. 4th ed. Philadelphia, PA: Lippincott Williams & Wilkins; 2006:900-906.

Leleiko NS, Horowitz M. Nutritional deficiency states. In: Rudolph CD, Rudolph AM, Hostetter MK, Lister G, Siegel NJ, eds. *Rudolph's Pediatrics*. 21st ed. New York, NY: McGraw-Hill; 2003:1336-1337.

McLeod R, Remington JS. Toxoplasmosis *(Toxoplasma gondii)*. In: Kleigman RM, Behrman RE, Jenson HB, Stanton BF, eds. *Nelson Textbook of Pediatrics*. 18th ed. Philadelphia, PA: WB Saunders; 2007:1486-1495.

Overby KJ. Pediatric health supervision. In: Rudolph CD, Rudolph AM, Hostetter MK, Lister G, Siegel NJ, eds. *Rudolph's Pediatrics*. 21st ed. New York, NY: McGraw-Hill, 2003:7-12.

Raszka WV. Neonatal toxoplasmosis. In: McMillan JA, Feigin RD, DeAngelis CD, Jones MD, eds. *Oski's Pediatrics: Principles and Practice*. 4th ed. Philadelphia, PA: Lippincott Williams & Wilkins, 2006:530-532.

Sanchez PJ, Siegel JD. Cytomegalovirus. In: McMillan JA, Feigin RD, DeAngelis CD, Jones MD, eds. *Oski's Pediatrics: Principles and Practice*. 4th ed. Philadelphia, PA: Lippincott Williams & Wilkins; 2006:511-516.

Stagno S. Cytomegalovirus. In: Kleigman RM, Behrman RE, Jenson HB, Stanton BF, eds. *Nelson Textbook of Pediatrics*. 18th ed. Philadelphia, PA: WB Saunders; 2007: 1377-1379.

# Case 2

A healthy 16-year-old adolescent male arrives at your office with his parents, who are concerned about his several months' history of erratic behavior. At times he has a great deal more energy, decreased appetite, and less sleep requirement than usual; at other times he sleeps incessantly and is lethargic. He is doing poorly in school. Last evening he appeared flushed and agitated, he had dilated pupils, and he complained "people were out to get him." The family notes that he has been skipping school occasionally, and they reluctantly report that he was arrested for burglary 2 weeks previously. You know he is in good health and he previously has been an excellent student. Today he appears normal.

- What is the most likely diagnosis?
- What is the next step in the evaluation?
- What is the long-term evaluation and therapy?

# ANSWERS TO CASE 2:
# Adolescent Substance Abuse

*Summary:* A 16-year-old previously healthy adolescent with recent behavior changes and declining school performance.

- **Most likely diagnosis:** Drug abuse (probably cocaine, possibly amphetamines).
- **Next steps in evaluation:** History, examination, urine drug screen, and screening for other commonly associated drug abuse consequences (sexually transmitted infections [STIs], hepatitis).
- **Long-term evaluation and therapy:** Threefold approach: (1) detoxification program, (2) follow-up with developmentally appropriate psychosocial support systems, and (3) possible long-term assistance with a professional trained in substance abuse management.

## ANALYSIS

### Objectives

1. Learn the pattern of behavior found among drug-abusing adolescents.
2. Know the signs and symptoms of the more common drugs of abuse.
3. Understand the general approach to therapy for an adolescent abusing drugs.

### Considerations

Rarely, a brain tumor could explain an adolescent with new onset of behavior changes. **In general, however, an adolescent's new-onset truant behavior, depression, or declining grades is more commonly associated with substance abuse.** A previously undiagnosed psychiatric history (mania or bipolar disease), too, must be considered. A history, family history, physical examination (especially the neurologic and psychological portions), and screening laboratory will help provide clarity. Information can come from the patient, his family, or from other interested parties (teachers, coaches, and friends). Direct questioning of the adolescent alone about substance abuse is appropriate during routine health visits or when signs and symptoms are suggestive of abuse.

# APPROACH TO
# The Substance-Abusing Adolescent

## DEFINITIONS

**SUBSTANCE ABUSE:** Alcohol or other drug use leading to impairment or distress, causing failure of school or work obligations, physical harm, substance-related legal problems, or continued use despite social or interpersonal consequences resulting from the drug's effects.

**SUBSTANCE DEPENDENCE:** Alcohol and other drug use, causing loss of control with continued use (tolerance requiring higher doses or withdrawal when terminated), compulsion to obtain and use the drug, and continued use despite persistent or recurrent negative consequences.

## CLINICAL APPROACH

Experimentation with alcohol and other drugs is common among adolescents; some consider this experimentation "normal." Others argue it is to be avoided because substance abuse is often a cause of adolescent morbidity and mortality (homicide, suicide, and unintentional injuries). In all cases, a health-care provider is responsible for discussing facts about alcohol and drugs in an attempt to reduce the adolescent's risk of harm and for identifying those requiring intervention.

Children at risk for drug use include those with significant behavior problems, learning difficulties, and impaired family functioning. Cigarettes and alcohol are the most commonly used drugs; marijuana is the most commonly used illicit drug. Some adolescents abuse common household products (inhalation of glue or aerosols); others abuse a sibling's medications (methylphenidate, which is often snorted with cocaine).

Pediatricians can ask about alcohol or drug use during the adolescent's annual health examination or when an adolescent presents with evidence of substance abuse. Direct questions can identify drug or alcohol use and their effect on school performance, family relations, and peer interactions. Should problems be identified, an interview to determine the degree of drug use (experimentation, abuse, or dependency) is warranted.

**Historical clues to drug abuse include significant behavioral changes at home, a decline in school or work performance, or involvement with the law.** An increased incidence of **intentional or accidental injuries** may be alcohol or drug related. Risk-taking activities (trading sex for drugs, driving while impaired) can be particularly serious and may suggest serious drug problems. Alcohol or other drugs users usually have a normal examination, especially if the use was not recent. Needle marks and nasal mucosal injuries are rarely found.

An adolescent with recent alcohol or drug use can present with a variety of findings (Table 2–1). A urine drug screen (UDS) can be helpful to evaluate the

**Table 2–1 CLINICAL FEATURES OF SUBSTANCE ABUSE**

| AGENT | SIGNS AND SYMPTOMS | RETENTION TIME FOR URINE SCREENING PURPOSES |
|---|---|---|
| Alcohol | Euphoria, grogginess, impaired short-term memory, talkativeness, vasodilation, and at high serum levels, respiratory depression | 7-10 h (blood) or 10-13 h (urine) |
| Marijuana | Elation and euphoria, impaired short-term memory, distortion of time perception, poor performance of tasks requiring concentration (such as driving), and loss of judgment | 3-10 d for occasional users or up to 2 mo for chronic users |
| Cocaine | Euphoria, increased motor activity, decreased fatigability, dilated pupils, tachycardia, hypertension and hyperthermia; sometimes associated with paranoid ideation; physical findings might include changes in nasal mucosa | 2-4 d |
| Methamphetamine and methylenedioxymetham phetamine (ecstasy) | Euphoria, increased sensual awareness, increased psychic and emotional energy, nausea, teeth grinding, blurred vision, jaw clenching, anxiety, panic attacks, and psychosis | 2 d |
| Opiates including heroin, morphine, and codeine | Euphoria, decreased pain sensation, pinpoint pupils, hypothermia, vasodilation, and possible respiratory depression; physical findings might include needle marks over veins | 2 d |
| Phencyclidine (PCP) | Euphoria, nystagmus, ataxia, and emotional lability; hallucinations affecting body image that can result in panic reactions, disorientation, hypersalivation, and abusive language | 8 d |

| Table 2–1 CLINICAL FEATURES OF SUBSTANCE ABUSE (CONTINUED) | | |
|---|---|---|
| AGENT | SIGNS AND SYMPTOMS | RETENTION TIME FOR URINE SCREENING PURPOSES |
| Barbiturates | Sedation, pinpoint pupils, hypotension, bradycardia, hypothermia, hyporeflexia, as well as central nervous system and respiratory depression | 1 d for short-acting agents; 2-3 wk for long-acting agents |

adolescent who (1) presents with psychiatric symptoms, (2) has signs and symptoms commonly attributed to drugs or alcohol, (3) is in a serious accident, or (4) is part of a recovery monitoring program. **An attempt to obtain the adolescent's permission and maintain confidentiality is paramount.**

Treatment of life-threatening acute problems related to alcohol or drug use follows the **ABCs** of emergency care: manage the **A**irway, control **B**reathing, and assess the **C**irculation. Treatment then is directed at the offending agent (if known). After stabilization, a treatment plan is devised. For some, inpatient programs that disrupt drug use allow for continued outpatient therapy. For others, an intensive outpatient therapy program can be initiated to help develop a drug-free lifestyle. The expertise necessary to assist an adolescent through these changes is often beyond a general pediatrician's expertise. Assistance with this chronic problem by qualified health professionals in a developmentally appropriate setting can maximize outcome. Primary care providers can, however, assist families to find suitable community resources.

## Comprehension Questions

2.1 A 14-year-old has ataxia. He is brought to the local emergency department, where he appears euphoric, emotionally labile, and a bit disoriented. He has nystagmus and hypersalivation. Many notice his abusive language. Which of the following agents is most likely responsible for his condition?

A. Alcohol
B. Amphetamines
C. Barbiturates
D. Cocaine
E. Phencyclidine (PCP)

2.2 Parents bring their 16-year-old daughter for a "well-child" checkup. She looks normal on examination. As part of your routine care you plan a urinalysis. The father pulls you aside and asks you to secretly run a urine drug screen (UDS) on his daughter. Which of the following is the most appropriate course of action?

A. Explore the reasons for the request with the parents and the adolescent, and perform a UDS with the adolescent's permission if the history warrants.
B. Perform the UDS as requested, but have the family and the girl return for the results.
C. Perform the UDS in the manner requested.
D. Refer the adolescent to a psychiatrist for further evaluation.
E. Tell the family to bring the adolescent back for a UDS when she is exhibiting signs or symptoms such as euphoria or ataxia.

2.3 A previously healthy adolescent male has a 3-month history of increasing headaches, blurred vision, and personality changes. Previously he admitted to marijuana experimentation more than 1 year ago. On examination he is a healthy, athletic-appearing 17-year-old with decreased extraocular range of motion and left eye visual acuity. Which of the following is the best next step in his management?

A. Acetaminophen and ophthalmology referral
B. Glucose measurement
C. Neuroimaging
D. Trial of methysergide (Sansert) for migraine
E. Urine drug screen

2.4 An 11-year-old girl has dizziness, pupillary dilatation, nausea, fever, tachycardia, and facial flushing. She says she can "see" sound and "hear" colors. The agent likely to be responsible is which of the following?

A. Alcohol
B. Amphetamines
C. Ecstasy
D. Lysergic acid diethylamide (LSD)
E. PCP

## ANSWERS

2.1 **E.** PCP is associated with hyperactivity, hallucinations, abusive language, and nystagmus.

2.2 **A.** The adolescent's permission should be obtained before drug testing. Testing "secretly" in this situation destroys the doctor–patient relationship.

2.3 **C.** Despite previous drug experimentation, his current symptoms and physical findings make drug use a less likely etiology. Evaluation for possible brain tumor is warranted.

2.4 **D.** LSD is associated with symptoms that begin 30 to 60 minutes after ingestion, peak 2 to 4 hours later, and resolve by 10 to 12 hours, including delusional ideation, body distortion, and paranoia. "Bad trips" result in the user becoming terrified or panicked; treatment usually is reassurance of the user in a controlled, safe environment.

## Clinical Pearls

- Cigarettes and alcohol are the most commonly used drugs in adolescence.
- Marijuana is the most common illicit drug used in adolescence.
- Substance abuse behaviors include drug dealing, prostitution, burglary, unprotected sex, automobile accidents, and physical violence.
- Children at risk for drug use include those with significant behavior problems, learning difficulties, and impaired family functioning.

## REFERENCES

Heyman RB. Adolescent substance abuse and other high-risk behaviors. In: McMillan JA, Feigin RD, DeAngelis CD, Jones MD, eds. *Oski's Pediatrics: Principles and Practice*. 4th ed. Philadelphia, PA: Lippincott Williams & Wilkins; 2006:579-584.

Jenkins RR, Adger H. Substance abuse. In: Kleigman RM, Behrman RE, Jenson HB, Stanton BF, eds. *Nelson Textbook of Pediatrics*. 18th ed. Philadelphia, PA: WB Saunders; 2007:824-834.

Marcell AV, Irwin CE. Substance use and abuse. In: Rudolph CD, Rudolph AM, Hostetter MK, Lister G, Siegel NJ, eds. *Rudolph's Pediatrics*. 21st ed. New York, NY: McGraw-Hill; 2003:226-231.

# Case 3

A 36-year-old woman with little prenatal care delivers a 3900-g girl. The infant has decreased tone, upslanting palpebral fissures, epicanthal folds, redundant nuchal skin, fifth finger clinodactyly and brachydactyly, and a single transverse palmar crease.

- What is the most likely diagnosis?
- What is the next step in the evaluation?

# ANSWERS TO CASE 3: Down Syndrome

*Summary:* A newborn with dysmorphic features is born to a woman of advanced maternal age.

- **Most likely diagnosis:** Down syndrome (trisomy 21).
- **Next step in evaluation:** Infant chromosomal evaluation to confirm diagnosis, evaluation for other features of the syndrome, counseling, and family support.

## ANALYSIS

### Objectives

1. Know the physical features and problems associated with Down syndrome (DS) and other common trisomy conditions.
2. Understand the evaluation of a child with dysmorphic features consistent with DS.
3. Appreciate the counseling and support required by a family with a special-needs child.

### Considerations

This newborn has many DS features; confirmation is made with a chromosome evaluation. Upon identification of a child with possible DS, the health-care provider attempts to identify potentially life-threatening features, including cardiac or gastrointestinal (GI) anomalies. A thorough evaluation of the family's psychosocial environment is warranted; these children can be physically, emotionally, and financially challenging.

*Note:* This woman of advanced maternal age had limited prenatal care but was at high risk for pregnancy complications. Adequate care may have included a serum triple screen between the 15th and 20th weeks of pregnancy, which could have demonstrated a DS pattern. Further evaluation (amniocentesis for chromosomal analysis) then could have been offered.

# APPROACH TO
## The Dysmorphic Child

## DEFINITIONS

**ADVANCED MATERNAL AGE:** The incidence of DS increases each year beyond age 35 years. At 35 years, the incidence is 1 in 378 liveborn infants, increasing to 1 in 106 by age 40 and to 1 in 11 by age 49.

**BRACHYDACTYLY:** Excessive shortening of hand and foot tubular bones resulting in a boxlike appearance.

**CLINODACTYLY:** Incurving of one of the digits (in DS the fifth digit curves toward the fourth digit due to midphalanx dysplasia).

**DYSMORPHIC CHILD:** A child with problems of generalized growth or body structure formation. These children can have a *syndrome* (a constellation of features from a common cause; ie, DS features caused by extra chromosome 21 material); an *association* (two or more features of unknown cause occurring together more commonly than expected; ie, **VATER** [**V**ertebral problems, **A**nal anomalies, **T**rachea problems, **E**sophageal abnormalities, and **R**adius or **r**enal anomalies]), or a *sequence* (a single defect that leads to subsequent abnormalities; ie, Potter disease's lack of normal infant kidney function, causing reduced urine output, oligohydramnios, and constraint deformities; common facial features include wide-set eyes, flattened palpebral fissures, prominent epicanthus, flattened nasal bridge, mandibular micrognathia, and large, low-set, cartilage-deficient ears).

**SERUM TRISOMY SCREENING:** Measurements of α-fetoprotein (AFP), human chorionic gonadotropin (hCG), and estriol levels, usually performed at 15 to 20 weeks' gestation. These tests screen for a variety of genetic problems. Approximately 60% of DS babies and 80% to 90% of the babies with neural tube defects will be identified by this testing.

## CLINICAL APPROACH

The first newborn evaluation occurs in the delivery room where attempts are made to successfully transition the infant from an intrauterine to an extrauterine environment; it focuses primarily on the **ABCs** of medicine—**A**irway, **B**reathing, and **C**irculation. The infant is then evaluated for possible abnormalities, including those that might fit into a pattern such as DS.

The prenatal history and course provide some important clues in the evaluation of a dysmorphic child. The parents' age (increased chromosomal abnormalities with increased maternal and sometimes paternal age), degree of fetal movement, maternal drug or teratogen exposure, family history of dysmorphia, and prenatal testing results, including triple screening and chorioamnionic or chorionic villous testing, may prove helpful. For instance, an older mother with a low AFP on her triple screen is at higher risk for having a DS child.

The physical examination is critical to the diagnosis of a dysmorphic child. For DS, a distinctive pattern can lead to a presumptive diagnosis; more than 90% of such children have features, including upslanting palpebral fissures, Brushfield spots (white or grey spots in the periphery of the iris), flat facial profile; small and rounded ears; excess nuchal skin, widespread nipples, pelvic dysplasia, joint hyperflexibility, fifth finger clinodactyly, a single transverse palmar (simian) crease, hypotonia, and a poor Moro reflex. Other features include brachycephaly (disproportionate shortness of the head), epicanthal folds, brachydactyly, wide spacing between first and second toes, and short stature.

In newborns with suspected DS, at least two potentially life-threatening conditions must be addressed. **Approximately 50% of DS infants have cardiac defects—most commonly an endocardial cushion defect (60%)**, ventricular septal defect (VSD, 32%), and tetralogy of Fallot (6%). A cardiology consultation and echocardiogram usually are indicated. **Approximately 12% of DS infants have intestinal (usually duodenal) atresia**, some presenting with a history of polyhydramnios. All DS infants have hypotonia and sometimes slower feeding. Should an infant with presumed DS develop persistent vomiting after feeds (especially if bilious), an upper GI study likely will reveal the characteristic **"double-bubble" pattern of duodenal atresia;** surgical intervention is warranted.

Confirmation of DS requires chromosomal analysis. A complete, extra chromosome 21 (nondysjunction, ie, failure to segregate during meiosis) occurs in almost 95% of cases. Two percent of cases are caused by translocations (breakage and removal of a large DNA segment from one chromosome and attachment to a different one), and 3% are mosaics (more than one cell type; usually described as an abnormal cell percentage). Parents of translocation-caused DS are evaluated for chromosomal aberrations; the recurrence risk can approach 100% in some cases.

Other newborn conditions associated with DS include hearing loss, strabismus, cataracts, nystagmus, and congenital hypothyroidism. Hearing is evaluated by age 3 months. An ophthalmologist evaluates the eyes by age 6 months, and thyroid function is assessed as part of the routine newborn screening program. Longer-term DS consequences include a higher leukemia risk, acquired hypothyroidism, atlantoaxial (cervical spine) instability, and premature aging with an increased risk of Alzheimer disease. All DS children are mentally retarded, but the intelligence quotients vary widely (mosaics can exhibit near-normal intelligence).

"Well-child care" takes on special meaning for DS children. In addition to providing routine care based on the American Academy of Pediatrics (AAP) guidelines for health supervision that apply to all children, the AAP has promulgated DS-specific guidelines (see www.aap.org). Periodic objective thyroid, hearing, and vision screenings are focal points of concern. Equally important in successful DS management is appropriate psychosocial intervention. Proper home or environmental, educational, and vocational interventions can improve the DS child's functioning level, facilitating his or her transition to adulthood. Providing family support and assisting with financial and medical support program applications are within the pediatrician's realm.

## Comprehension Questions

3.1 A small-for-gestational age infant is born to a 35-year-old woman. He has low-set and malformed ears, microcephaly, rocker-bottom feet, inguinal hernias, cleft lip or palate, and micrognathia. Chromosomal analysis is likely to reveal which of the following?

A. Down syndrome (trisomy 21)
B. Edwards syndrome (trisomy 18)
C. Holt-Oram syndrome
D. Patau syndrome (trisomy 13)
E. Turner syndrome

3.2 A 15-day-old infant has respiratory distress. A quick observation suggests she has slight cyanosis, hepatosplenomegaly, and features consistent with DS. The cardiac examination demonstrates a loud first heart sound, a wide and fixed split second heart sound, a low-pitched, mid-diastolic murmur at the lower left sternal border, and a harsh apical holosystolic murmur in the mitral area. An echocardiogram is likely to demonstrate which of the following?

A. Complete atrioventricular (AV) canal (endocardial cushion defect)
B. Hypoplastic left heart
C. Total anomalous venous return
D. Transposition of the great vessels
E. Tricuspid atresia

3.3 A small-for-gestational age, dysmorphic newborn infant has microcephaly and sloping forehead, cutis aplasia (missing portion of the skin and hair) of the scalp, polydactyly, microphthalmia, and omphalocele. Which of the following is the most likely diagnosis?

A. Down syndrome (trisomy 21)
B. Edwards syndrome (trisomy 18)
C. Holt-Oram syndrome
D. Patau syndrome (trisomy 13)
E. Turner syndrome

3.4 The parents of an 8-year-old DS boy arrive for his annual well-child visit. He wants to participate in sports, including the Special Olympics. Until further evaluation can be completed, which of the following sports would you suggest as being safe?

A. Diving
B. Football
C. Tennis
D. Tumbling
E. Wrestling

## ANSWERS

3.1 **B.** The child has trisomy 18. Other features include clenched hands with overlapping digits, small palpebral fissures, prominent occiput, short sternum, and cardiac defects (ventricular septal defect [VSD], atrial septal defect [ASD], patent ductus arteriosus [PDA], or coarctation of the aorta).

3.2 **A.** Although VSDs are common in DS, the most characteristic lesion is endocardial cushion defect (or atrioventricular [AV] canal defect). Slight cyanosis occurs because of the mixing of deoxygenated with oxygenated blood. In the AV canal, a range of defects involving the atrial septum, the ventricular septum, and one or both of the AV valves can be seen. A complete AV canal includes ASDs and VSDs with a common AV valve. A partial AV canal includes defects of the atrial septum and separate mitral and tricuspid valve orifices.

3.3 **D.** The appearance of cutis aplasia and polydactyly suggests trisomy 13. Other common features include holoprosencephaly (failure of growth of the forebrain), cleft lip or palate, postaxial polydactyly, flexed and overlapping fingers, coloboma, and cardiac defects (VSD, ASD, PDA, dextrocardia).

3.4 **C.** Until lateral cervical flexion–extension films confirm normal anatomy, contact sports and other activities that may result in forceful flexion of the neck should be avoided.

## Clinical Pearls

- Down syndrome is the most common autosomal chromosome abnormality in liveborn infants, increasing in incidence with advanced maternal age.
- The most common neonatal Down syndrome features are hypotonia with poor Moro reflex, flat faces, slanted palpebral fissures, laxity of joints, and excessive skin on the back of the neck.
- Common problems associated with Down syndrome include cardiac defects and duodenal atresia.
- Common features of trisomy 18 (Edwards) syndrome include weak cry, single umbilical artery, micrognathia with small mouth and high arched palate, clenched hand with overlapping of index finger over the third finger, simian crease, rocker-bottom feet, small pelvis, and short sternum.
- Common features of trisomy 13 (Patau) syndrome include microcephaly and sloping forehead, deafness, scalp cutis aplasia, microphthalmia, coloboma, cardiac defect (especially ventricular septal defect), omphalocele, single umbilical artery, and hypersensitivity to agents containing atropine and pilocarpine

## REFERENCES


American Academy of Pediatrics. Health supervision for children with Down syndrome. *Pediatrics*. 2001;107:442-449.

Bernstein D. Atrioventricular septal defects (ostium primum and atrioventricular canal or endocardial cushion defects). In: Kleigman RM, Behrman RE, Jenson HB, Stanton BF, eds. *Nelson Textbook of Pediatrics*. 18th ed. Philadelphia, PA: WB Saunders; 2007:1886-1888.

Carey JC. Chromosome disorders. In: Rudolph CD, Rudolph AM, Hostetter MK, Lister G, Siegel NJ, eds. *Rudolph's Pediatrics*. 21st ed. New York, NY: McGraw-Hill; 2003:731-742.

Chen Z, Carey JC. Human cytogenetics. In: Rudolph CD, Rudolph AM, Hostetter MK, Lister G, Siegel NJ, eds. *Rudolph's Pediatrics*. 21st ed. New York, NY: McGraw-Hill; 2003:727-731.

Descartes M, Carroll AJ. Cytogenetics. In: Kleigman RM, Behrman RE, Jenson HB, Stanton BF, eds. *Nelson Textbook of Pediatrics*. 18th ed. Philadelphia, PA: WB Saunders; 2007:502-517.

Lewanda AF, Boyadjiev SA, Jabs EW. Dysmorphology: genetic syndromes and associations. In: McMillan JA, Feigin RD, DeAngelis CD, Jones MD, eds. *Oski's Pediatrics: Principles and Practice*. 4th ed. Philadelphia, PA: Lippincott Williams & Wilkins; 2006:2629-2630.

Sponseller PD. Cervical spine. In: McMillan JA, Feigin RD, DeAngelis CD, Jones MD, eds. *Oski's Pediatrics: Principles and Practice*. 4th ed. Philadelphia, PA: Lippincott Williams & Wilkins; 2006:2491.

Vick GW, Bezoild LI. Defects of the atrial septum, including the atrioventricular canal. In: McMillan JA, Feigin RD, DeAngelis CD, Jones MD, eds. *Oski's Pediatrics: Principles and Practice*. 4th ed. Philadelphia, PA: Lippincott Williams & Wilkins; 2006:1565-1574.

# Case 4

An 8-year-old boy presents to your clinic with a 3-day history of a "white coating" in his mouth. He denies having a sore throat, upper respiratory infection symptoms, gastrointestinal (GI) distress, change in appetite, or fever. His immunizations are current, he has no significant past medical history, and he has been developing normally per his mother. His weight, however, has fallen from the 25th percentile to the 5th percentile, and he has been hospitalized on three occasions in the last year with pneumonia or dehydration. His family history is remarkable only for maternal hepatitis C infection related to past intravenous (IV) drug use. The patient is afebrile today, but his examination is notable for severe gingivitis, bilateral cervical and axillary lymphadenopathy, exudates on his buccal mucosa, and hepatomegaly.

- ➤ What is the most likely diagnosis?
- ➤ What is the next step in evaluation?

# ANSWERS TO CASE 4: Immunodeficiency

*Summary:* A child with lymphadenopathy, organomegaly, weight loss, recurring infection, and oral lesions consistent with candidiasis.

- **Most likely diagnosis:** Immunodeficiency.
- **Next step in evaluation:** Gather additional history, including birth history, details of hospitalizations, dietary history, and patient and family histories of recurring or atypical infection. Consider testing for human immunodeficiency virus (HIV) and obtaining a complete blood count (CBC) and comprehensive metabolic panel to assess cell counts, organ function, and nutritional status.

## ANALYSIS

### Objectives

1. Differentiate between primary and secondary immunodeficiency.
2. Understand selected etiologies of pediatric immunodeficiency.
3. Identify and manage pediatric HIV disease.

### Considerations

Recurring infections in this patient presenting with oral lesions, weight loss, and lymphadenopathy is concerning for immune system dysfunction. He may have a primary immunodeficiency due to an inheritable defect or an acquired (secondary) immunodeficiency related to HIV infection, malignancy, malnutrition, or other disorder. The maternal history of IV drug use makes pediatric HIV infection a strong likelihood, probably due to vertical transmission. Additional patient and family histories and selected initial laboratory tests will aid in diagnosis and help guide management.

APPROACH TO
## The Child with Immunodeficiency

### DEFINITIONS

**HIV ANTIBODY ELISA:** Enzyme-linked immunosorbent assay (ELISA) screening for HIV-1 immunoglobulin G (IgG); initially detectable 2 weeks to 6 months after exposure; sensitivity and specificity greater than 99%; false-positive rate less than 5 in 100,000 assays; false-negative results may occur after immunization or in hepatic disease, autoimmune disease, or advanced acquired immunodeficiency syndrome (AIDS).

**WESTERN BLOT:** Direct visualization of antibodies to virion proteins; used to confirm screening antibody assay; results can be indeterminate and require repeat testing.

**CD4 (T HELPER) CELL:** Essential for humoral (B-cell) and cellular (T-cell) immunity; binds to antigens presented by B cells, prompting antibody production, and to antigens presented by phagocytes, prompting lymphokine release; rendered dysfunctional in HIV infection.

### CLINICAL APPROACH

Evaluation of patients with recurring or atypical infection starts with a comprehensive history and systems review. Clinicians should inquire about perinatal history, growth and development, and past illnesses. **Immunosuppression** is suggested by **failure to thrive (FTT)** or **atypical** or **difficult-to-eradicate infections** (recurring otitis refractory to multiple antimicrobials). Family history includes parental health concerns (unexplained weight loss, growth failure, or developmental delay in siblings) and recurring or atypical infection in immediate family members. A focused physical examination should then be performed to identify signs consistent with immunosuppression (wasting, generalized lymphadenopathy, and organomegaly).

**Primary** (syndromic) **immunodeficiency** is due to a genetic defect, either inherited or related to gene mutation; most are humoral in origin or characterized by both humoral and cellular dysfunction (severe combined immunodeficiency). Other primary immunodeficiencies include phagocytic cell deficiency (chronic granulomatous disease due to defective macrophages) and complement deficiency (autoimmune disease or serious bacterial infection due to C2 deficiency). Patients with **secondary immunodeficiency** have normal immune function at birth, but subsequently develop an illness or metabolic abnormality that disrupts immune cell production or function. Conditions adversely affecting a patient's immune status include HIV infection, diabetes mellitus, malnutrition, hepatic disease, autoimmune disease (scleroderma), aging, and stress.

HIV is a global epidemic, with approximately 33 million people presumably infected worldwide. Unprotected sexual intercourse and needle sharing with IV drug use are known means of transmission. Prior to the mid-1980s, blood transfusion was also a risk factor. In the **pediatric** population, **HIV is typically acquired through vertical transmission.** Approximately 80% of pediatric cases involve intrapartum transfer, but HIV can also be acquired from infected secretions at delivery and from breast milk. It is important to know the HIV status of the pregnant female, so that antiretroviral therapy can be administered during pregnancy to decrease viral replication and diminish the potential for transfer to the neonate. An infected mother has a 25% chance of transmitting the virus to her newborn if antiretroviral therapy is not received during pregnancy. **Zidovudine**, when started by the mother during the second trimester and given to the baby through age 6 weeks, reduces the risk of HIV transmission to less than 10%.

HIV infection gives rise to **dysfunctional CD4 cells** resulting in overall immune system compromise and eventual opportunistic infection. Approximately 75% of pediatric patients who acquire HIV vertically follow a course similar to adults, with an extended period of disease inactivity; a patient will often remain asymptomatic for a decade or more until the CD4 count falls to a critical level. The remaining 25% of pediatric HIV patients progress rapidly during the first several months of life. Therefore, early determination of maternal HIV status and measures to decrease transmission is critical (avoiding breast-feeding, aggressive and appropriate neonatal HIV testing, early antiretroviral therapy).

Verification of HIV infection is made in the patient older than 18 months by performing an HIV antibody ELISA and subsequent Western blot for confirmation. Because of placental transfer of maternal antibodies, **diagnosis in younger patients is made by HIV DNA PCR testing.** Two assays are performed on separate occasions to confirm the diagnosis. Subsequently, HIV RNA activity, CD4 cell count, and clinical findings are used to determine disease status. Centers for Disease Control and Prevention (CDC) classification of HIV status is based on the presence and severity of signs or symptoms and degree of immunosuppression. For example, a patient with *Pneumocystis jiroveci (carinii)* pneumonia (PCP), an AIDS-defining opportunistic infection, is classified with "severe" disease (category C). Degree of immunosuppression is based on an age-adjusted CD4 count. For the patient in this case, a normal CD4 count would be more than or equal to 500 or 25%. Severe suppression is denoted by a CD4 count less than 200 or 15%.

Neonates born to HIV-positive women are tested at birth and at selected intervals through approximately 6 months of age. Traditionally, the exposed neonate receives 6 weeks of antiretroviral therapy in the form of zidovudine starting in the first few hours of life. **PCP prophylaxis** in the form of **trimethoprim–sulfamethoxazole** commences at approximately 6 weeks of age for HIV-positive infants. CD4 levels are followed in quarterly intervals in the patient who becomes HIV-positive. HIV RNA activity is followed and typically correlates with disease progression; RNA activity of more than 100,000 copies/mL has been associated with advanced progression and early death.

Treatment for HIV-positive patients is started early to diminish viral replication before mutation and antiretroviral resistance occur. The **three major classes of antiretrovirals** are **nucleoside reverse transcriptase inhibitors** (didanosine, stavudine, zidovudine), **nonnucleoside reverse transcriptase inhibitors** (efavirenz, nevirapine), and **protease inhibitors** (indinavir, nelfinavir). Combination retroviral therapy in children has led to a marked decline in child mortality. Common adverse effects for all include headache, emesis, abdominal pain, and diarrhea. Osteopenia and drug rash can also be seen. Possible other abnormalities include anemia, neutropenia, elevated transaminases, hyperglycemia, and hyperlipidemia.

The current pediatric antiretroviral therapy recommendation consists of three drugs: two nucleoside reverse transcriptase inhibitors and one protease inhibitor. An existing treatment regimen is altered when toxicity becomes an issue or disease progression occurs. Ultimately, HIV treatment requires a multidisciplinary approach with input from nutritionists, social workers, and pediatric HIV and mental health specialists. In addition to periodic monitoring of viral activity and prophylaxis against opportunistic infection, close monitoring of growth, development, and emotional health is important in pediatric HIV disease management. **Immunizations** should be kept current, with all vaccines administered per the recommended pediatric schedule, often excluding live vaccines such as measles-mumps-rubella (MMR) and varicella.

## Comprehension Questions

4.1 A 15-year-old adolescent female has a 1-month history of urinary frequency without dysuria and recent onset of an itchy rash beneath both breasts. She has been gaining weight over the past year and regularly complains of fatigue. She is afebrile with a weight greater than the 99th percentile and has an erythematous, macular rash beneath both breasts characterized by satellite lesions. Urinalysis is significant for 2+ glucosuria, but no pyuria. Which of the following is the most likely diagnosis?

A. Diabetes mellitus
B. Fanconi syndrome
C. Human immunodeficiency virus
D. Occult malignancy
E. Severe combined immunodeficiency (SCID)

4.2 A mother notes her 6-week-old son's umbilical cord is still attached. His activity and intake are normal; there has been no illness or fever. Delivery was at term without problems. His examination is notable for a cord without evidence of separation and a shallow, 0.5-cm ulceration at the occiput without discharge or surrounding erythema. Mother declares that the "sore," caused by a scalp probe, has been slowly healing since birth and was deemed unremarkable at his 2-week checkup. Which of the following is consistent with this child's likely diagnosis?

A. Defective humoral response
B. Functional leukocyte adherence glycoproteins
C. Marked neutrophilia
D. Normal wound healing
E. Purulent abscess formation

4.3 A 6-month-old girl is seen after an emergency room visit for decreased intake, emesis, and watery diarrhea for the past 3 days. She was diagnosed yesterday with "stomach flu" and given IV fluids. She is doing better today with improved intake and resolution of her emesis and diarrhea. The father is concerned about her thrush since birth (despite multiple courses of an oral antifungal) and that she has been hospitalized twice for pneumonia over the past 4 months. Her weight has dropped from the 50th percentile on her 4-month visit to the 5th percentile today. She has no findings consistent with dehydration, but she does appear to have some extremity muscle wasting. Her examination is remarkable for buccal mucosal exudates and hyperactive bowel sounds. Vital signs and the remainder of her examination are normal. You suspect severe combined immunodeficiency (SCID). Which of the following is consistent with the diagnosis?

A. Autosomal dominant inheritance
B. Persistent lymphocytosis
C. Defective cellular immunity
D. Normal vaccine immune response
E. No curative therapy

4.4 You are called urgently to examine a term, 2-hour-old newborn who has had temperature instability, difficulty with feeding, and a suspected seizure. He has atypical facies (wide-set eyes, a prominent nose, and a small mandible), a cleft palate, and a holosystolic murmur. Stat laboratory tests and chest radiograph reveal marked hypocalcemia, a boot-shaped heart, and no apparent thymus. Which of the following is the most likely diagnosis?

A. Ataxia–telangiectasia
B. DiGeorge syndrome
C. Hyper-IgE syndrome
D. SCID
E. Wiskott-Aldrich syndrome

## ANSWERS

4.1 **A.** The obese adolescent in this case has findings of diabetes mellitus. Her cutaneous candidiasis is likely an indication of secondary immunosuppression related to hyperglycemia. In diabetes, hyperglycemia promotes neutrophil dysfunction, and circulatory insufficiency contributes to ineffective neutrophil chemotaxis during infection. HIV infection is possible and antibody testing might be reasonable, but this scenario is most consistent with hyperglycemia.

4.2 **C.** You suspect leukocyte adhesion deficiency (LAD) as the etiology of this child's problem. LAD is an inheritable disorder of leukocyte chemotaxis and adherence characterized by recurring sinopulmonary, oropharyngeal, and cutaneous infections with delayed wound healing. Neutrophilia is common with WBC counts of typically more than 50,000 cells/$mm^3$. Severe, life-threatening infection is possible with *Staphylococcus* species, *Enterobacteriaceae*, and *Candida* species. Good skin and oral hygiene are important; broad-spectrum antimicrobials and surgical debridement are early considerations with infection.

4.3 **C.** SCID is an autosomal recessive or X-linked disorder of both humoral and cellular immunity. Serum immunoglobulins and T cells are often markedly diminished or absent. Thymic dysgenesis is also seen. Recurring cutaneous, gastrointestinal, or pulmonary infections occur with opportunistic organisms such as cytomegalovirus (CMV) and PCP. Death typically occurs in the first 12 to 24 months of life unless bone marrow transplantation is performed.

4.4 **B.** DiGeorge syndrome is caused by a 22q11 microdeletion. This syndromic immunodeficiency is characterized by decreased T-cell production and recurring infection. Findings include characteristic facies and velocardiofacial defects such as ventricular septal defect and tetralogy of Fallot. Thymic or parathyroid dysgenesis can occur, accompanied by hypocalcemia and seizures. Developmental and speech delay are common in older patients.

## Clinical Pearls

- Primary immunodeficiency is an inheritable disorder characterized by weakened immunity and recurring, serious infection early in life.
- A variety of illnesses can provoke secondary immunodeficiency; malignancy, malnutrition, hepatic disease, and human immunodeficiency virus (HIV) infection are known to adversely influence both humoral and cellular immunity.
- Pediatric HIV disease can be deterred by appropriate testing and treatment of pregnant females and judicious antiretroviral prophylaxis in the exposed neonate. Exposed patients should be closely followed by clinicians and a team approach used in the management of active disease.

## REFERENCES


Borkowsky W. Acquired immunodeficiency syndrome and human immunodeficiency virus. In: Katz SL, Hotez PJ, Gerson AA, eds. *Krugman's Infectious Diseases of Children*. 11th ed. Philadelphia, PA: Mosby; 2004:1-26.

Buckley RH. Evaluation of suspected immunodeficiency. In: Kliegman RM, Behrman RE, Jenson HB, Stanton BF, eds. *Nelson Textbook of Pediatrics*. 18th ed. Philadelphia, PA: WB Saunders; 2007:867-873.

Church JA. Human immunodeficiency virus infection. In: Osborn LM, DeWitt TG, First LR, Zenel JA, eds. *Pediatrics*. 1st ed. Philadelphia, PA: Elsevier-Mosby; 2005:1132-1139.

Lewis DB, Insel RA, Cleary AM. Disorders of lymphocyte function. In: Hoffman R, Benz EJ, Shattil SJ, et al, eds. *Hematology: Basic Principles and Practice*. 4th ed. Philadelphia, PA: Churchill Livingstone; 2005:831-854.

Yogev R, Chadwick EG. Acquired immunodeficiency syndrome (human immunodeficiency virus). In: Kliegman RM, Behrman RE, Jenson HB, Stanton BF, eds. *Nelson Textbook of Pediatrics*. 18th ed. Philadelphia, PA: WB Saunders; 2007:1427-1443.

# Case 5

A somewhat tall-for-his-age 13-year-old adolescent male arrives for routine care. His mother reports that he seems to be much more immature and insecure than her older son was at the same age. His school performance is below average, and this year he has begun to receive special education for language-based classes. On physical examination you note that his extremities are longer than expected and that he is embarrassed by his gynecomastia. He is Tanner stage 1 with small gonads.

➤ What is the most likely diagnosis?

➤ What is the best test to diagnose this condition?

# ANSWERS TO CASE 5: Klinefelter Syndrome

*Summary:* An immature and insecure 13-year-old adolescent male with hypogonadism, long limbs, gynecomastia, and developmental delay.

- **Most likely diagnosis:** Klinefelter syndrome, a trisomy syndrome often due to paternal rather than maternal nondisjunction, affecting 1 in 600 to 800 male infants.
- **Best diagnostic test:** Chromosomal analysis.

## ANALYSIS

### Objectives

1. Understand the signs and symptoms of Klinefelter syndrome.
2. Appreciate the variety of causes of childhood mental retardation (MR).
3. Learn the signs and symptoms of syndromes involving missing or duplicate sex chromosomes.

### Considerations

This child's mother has identified this adolescent's development and behavior to be different from her other children. The school recently has identified his need for special education, especially in the language-based classes. A thorough history (including all school performance and behavioral problems) and physical examination can provide diagnostic clues. The etiology of his condition impacts his psychosocial outcome, his future medical therapy, and his parent's family planning decisions.

# APPROACH TO Klinefelter Syndrome

## DEFINITIONS

**KLINEFELTER SYNDROME:** A specific syndrome associated with behavioral problems (immaturity, insecurity), developmental delay (speech, language, lower IQ), and physical findings (gynecomastia, hypogonadism, long limbs) caused by an extra X chromosome in boys and men.

**MENTAL RETARDATION (MR):** A clinically and socially important impairment of measured intelligence and adaptive behavior that is diagnosed before 18 years of age.

## CLINICAL APPROACH

Causes of MR include **preconceptual and early embryonic disruptions** (teratogens, chromosomal abnormalities, placental dysfunction, congenital central nervous system [CNS] malformations); **fetal brain insults** (infections, toxins, placental problems); **perinatal difficulties** (prematurity, metabolic disorders, infections); **postnatal brain injuries** (infections, trauma, metabolic disorders, toxins, poor nutrition); and miscellaneous **postnatal family difficulties** (poverty, poor caregiver–child interaction, parental mental illness). A category of "unknown etiology" includes children with MR who do not fit into the above categories.

The history of a child with possible MR includes an evaluation of the child's psychosocial skills and a review of school reports. The ultimate diagnosis may require formal testing to determine if the IQ falls below some set point, such as 80. A determination of whether formal testing should be performed is based on physical examination findings, developmental and school histories, and concerns of the family and teachers. Males with Klinefelter syndrome often have developmental delay, especially in verbal cognitive areas where they underachieve in reading, spelling, and mathematics; their full IQ may be normal, but their verbal IQ usually is somewhat decreased. In variants with multiple X chromosomes, the incidence and severity of MR increases. **Boys with Klinefelter syndrome often go unidentified until puberty because of the subtleness of the clinical findings. The diagnosis should be considered for all boys (regardless of age) who have been identified as having mental retardation, or psychosocial, school, or adjustment problems.**

Physical findings to be considered in patients with nonspecific MR include the size of the occiput, unusual hair color or distribution, distinctive eyes, malformed ears or nose, and abnormalities in jaw size, mouth shape, or palate height. The hands and feet may have short metacarpals or metatarsals, overlapping or supernumerary digits, and abnormal creases or nails. The skin may have café au lait spots or depigmented nevi, and the genitalia may be abnormally sized or ambiguous. Patients with MR caused by Klinefelter syndrome typically are tall, slim, and thin with long extremities. Their testes and sometimes the phallus are small for age, but these latter findings may not become apparent until puberty. As adults, males with Klinefelter syndrome develop gynecomastia, sparse facial hair, and azoospermia. The incidence of breast cancer (as well as some hematologic cancers as well) is elevated in Klinefelter syndrome.

Laboratory testing of a child with MR is based on the clinical findings and developmental milestones. A chromosomal analysis is often included in the evaluation of a child with mental retardation; for Klinefelter syndrome such an analysis will demonstrate the extra X chromosome material. Other MR testing may include urine and serum amino and organic acids, serum levels of various compounds including ammonia, lead, zinc, and copper, and serum titers for congenital infections. Radiologic evaluation may include cranial computed tomography (CT), magnetic resonance imaging (MRI), or electroencephalogram (EEG).

Management of children with MR includes specialized educational services, early childhood interventions, social services, vocational training, and psychiatric interventions. Further interventions for children with specific underlying etiologies may include diet modification, genetic counseling, or reviewing the natural disease course with the family.

## Comprehension Questions

Match the following genetic disorders (A-E) to the clinical description [questions 5.1-5.3]:

A. Fragile X syndrome
B. Klinefelter syndrome (XXY)
C. Turner syndrome (XO)
D. XXX syndrome
E. XYY male

5.1 An institutionalized male juvenile delinquent upon close examination has severe nodulocystic acne, mild pectus excavatum, large teeth, prominent glabella, and relatively long face and fingers. His family says he has poor fine motor skills (such as penmanship), an explosive temper, and a low–normal IQ.

5.2 A tall, thin 14-year-old adolescent male has no signs of puberty. He was delayed in his speech development and always has done less well in school than his siblings. He is shy, and teachers report his activity is immature. Physical examination reveals breast development, and long limbs with a decreased upper segment–lower segment ratio. He has small testes and phallus.

5.3 A 15-year-old adolescent female with primary amenorrhea is noted to be well below the fifth percentile for height. She has hypertension, a low posterior hairline, prominent and low-set ears, and excessive nuchal skin.

5.4 A 7-year-old boy with MR was born at home at 26 weeks' gestation to a 28-year-old mother who had received no prenatal care. An evaluation is likely to suggest his MR is related to which of the following?

A. Brain tumor
B. Chromosomal aberration
C. Complications of prematurity
D. Congenital infection with cytomegalovirus
E. Elevated serum lead levels

## ANSWERS

5.1 **E.** XYY-affected males often have explosive tempers. Other findings include long and asymmetrical ears, increased length versus breadth for the hands, feet, and cranium, and mild pectus excavatum. By age 5 to 6 years, they tend to be taller than their peers and begin displaying aggressive or defiant behavior.

5.2 **B.** With Klinefelter syndrome, testosterone replacement allows for more normal adolescent male development, although azoospermia is the rule; the breast cancer incidence approaches that of women.

5.3 **C.** Turner syndrome also includes widely spaced nipples and broad chest; cubitus valgus (increased carrying angle of arms); edema of the hands and feet in the newborn period; congenital heart disease (coarctation of the aorta or bicuspid aortic valve); horseshoe kidney; short fourth metacarpal and metatarsal; hypothyroidism; and decreased hearing. Mental development usually is normal.

5.4 **C.** Prematurity, especially when earlier than 28 weeks' gestation, is associated with complications (such as intraventricular hemorrhage) that can result in developmental delay and low IQ.

## Clinical Pearls

- Males with Klinefelter syndrome (XXY) have mild mental delay, eunuchoid habitus, gynecomastia, long arms and legs, and hypogonadism.
- XYY males have explosive (often antisocial) behavior, weakness with poor fine motor control, accelerated growth in mid-childhood, large teeth, prominent glabella and asymmetrical ears, and severe acne at puberty.
- Girls with Turner syndrome (45, XO) have short stature, amenorrhea, excessive nuchal skin, low posterior hairline, broad chests with widely spaced nipples, cubitus valgus, and coarctation of the aorta. Hypertension is common, possibly due to renal abnormalities (horseshoe kidney).
- Fragile X syndrome, the most common form of inherited mental retardation, is seen primarily in boys and can be diagnosed in patients with mental retardation (particularly boys) who have macrocephaly, long face, high arched palate, large ears, and macroorchidism after puberty.

## REFERENCES


Accardo PJ, Accardo JA, Capute AJ. Mental retardation. In: McMillan JA, Feigin RD, DeAngelis CD, Jones MD, eds. *Oski's Pediatrics: Principles and Practice*. 4th ed. Philadelphia, PA: Lippincott Williams & Wilkins; 2006:608-614.

Carey JC. Chromosome disorders. In: Rudolph CD, Rudolph AM, Hostetter MK, Lister G, Siegel NJ, eds. *Rudolph's Pediatrics*. 21st ed. New York, NY: McGraw-Hill; 2003:731-742.

Chen Z, Carey JC. Human cytogenetics. In: Rudolph CD, Rudolph AM, Hostetter MK, Lister G, Siegel NJ, eds. *Rudolph's Pediatrics*. 21st ed. New York, NY: McGraw-Hill; 2003:727-731.

Descartes M, Carroll AJ. Cytogenetics. In: Kleigman RM, Behrman RE, Jenson HB, Stanton BF, eds. *Nelson Textbook of Pediatrics*. 18th ed. Philadelphia, PA: WB Saunders; 2007:502-517.

Lewanda AF, Boyadjiev SA, Jaabs EW. Dysmorphology: genetic syndromes and associations. In: McMillan JA, Feigin RD, DeAngelis CD, Jones MD, eds. *Oski's Pediatrics: Principles and Practice*. 4th ed. Philadelphia, PA: Lippincott Williams & Wilkins; 2006:2629-2670.

Rapaport R. Hypofunction of the testes. In: Kleigman RM, Behrman RE, Jenson HB, Stanton BF, eds. *Nelson Textbook of Pediatrics*. 18th ed. Philadelphia, PA: WB Saunders; 2007:2379-2384.

Shapiro BK, Batshaw ML. Mental retardation. In: Kleigman RM, Behrman RE, Jenson HB, Stanton BF, eds. *Nelson Textbook of Pediatrics*. 18th ed. Philadelphia, PA: WB Saunders; 2007:191-197.

# Case 6

A 6-month-old child arrives for a well-child examination. His family recently moved to the United States from Turkey. His medical and family histories are unremarkable except that his sole source of nutrition is goat's milk. He appears to be healthy on examination.

➤ What hematologic problem is most likely to develop?

➤ What nonhematologic concerns are considered in an infant fed goat's milk?

# ANSWERS TO CASE 6: Megaloblastic Anemia

*Summary*: This is a 6-month-old child exclusively fed goat's milk.

- **Likely complication:** Megaloblastic anemia from folate or $B_{12}$ deficiency.
- **Other concerns:** Brucellosis if milk is unpasteurized.

## ANALYSIS

### Objectives

1. Appreciate the benefits of breast-feeding.
2. Know the nutritional supplements recommended for breast-feeding mothers.
3. Understand the special needs of infants and toddlers fed goat's milk or vegan diets.
4. Appreciate the clinical syndromes resulting from vitamin excesses and deficiencies.

### Considerations

A variety of feeding regimens exist for infants and toddlers—breast-feeding, goat's milk, other types of nonformula milk, and commercial or handmade foods. Health care providers can educate parents about the benefits and potential dangers of various diet choices.

# APPROACH TO Infant Nutrition

## DEFINITIONS

**LACTOVEGETARIAN:** Diet devoid of animal products but includes milk.

**OMNIVORE:** Diet includes both animal and vegetable products.

**OVOVEGETARIAN:** Diet devoid of animal products but includes eggs.

**VEGAN:** Vegetarian diet devoid of all animal products.

## CLINICAL APPROACH

Infant formulas containing goat's milk are not routinely available in the United States, but they are available elsewhere. Goat's milk has lower sodium levels but more potassium, chloride, linoleic acid, and arachidonic acid than does cow's milk. It is low in vitamin D, iron, folate, and vitamin $B_{12}$; infants receiving **goat's milk** as a primary nutrition source are given **folate** and **vitamin $B_{12}$** (to prevent megaloblastic anemia) and **iron** (to prevent iron deficiency anemia). **Goat's milk** is boiled before ingestion; goats are particularly susceptible to **brucellosis**.

Breast milk is considered the ideal human infant food because it contains complete nutrition (with the possible exception of vitamin D and fluoride), has antimicrobial properties, and offers psychological advantages to mothers and infants. In developing countries, it is associated with lower infant morbidity and mortality, not only due to a reduction in diarrhea associated with contaminated water used in formula preparation but also because it contains **high concentrations of immunoglobulin A (IgA),**which reduces viruses and bacteria intestinal wall adherence, and macrophages, which inhibit *Escherichia coli* growth. **Disadvantages** include potential **HIV** (and other virus) transmission, **jaundice exacerbation** due to increased unconjugated bilirubinemia levels (resolved with a 12- to 24-hour breast-feeding interruption) and its association with **low vitamin K** levels, contributing to hemorrhagic disease of the newborn (prevented by vitamin K administration at birth).

Formula feeding is substituted for breast-feeding for a variety of reasons. Commercial formula manufacturers strive to provide products similar to human milk. Infant growth rates with cow's milk formula are similar to those in infants receiving breast milk. Improved sterilization procedures and refrigeration in developing countries have reduced to some degree the gastrointestinal (GI) infections noted with formula feedings.

Formulas are available for special-needs infants. Infants with phenylketonuria require formulas low in phenylalanine, and those unable to digest protein require nitrogen in the form of amino acid mixtures. Cow's milk allergies sometimes respond to soybean-based formulas.

Vegan diets supply all necessary nutrients if a variety of vegetables is selected. Some evidence suggests that high-fiber vegetarian diets lead to faster gastrointestinal transit time, resulting in reduced serum cholesterol levels, less diverticulitis, and a lower appendicitis incidence. Breast-feeding vegan mothers are given vitamin $B_{12}$ to prevent the infant's developing methylmalonic acidemia (an amino acid metabolism disorder involving a defect in the conversion of methylmalonyl-coenzyme A to succinyl-CoA); patients can present with failure to thrive, seizure, encephalopathy, stroke, or other neurologic manifestations. Toddlers on a vegan diet are given vitamin $B_{12}$ and, because of the high fiber content and rapid gastrointestinal transit time, are given trace minerals that can be depleted.

**Table 6–1 EFFECTS OF VITAMIN AND MINERAL DEFICIENCY OR EXCESS**

| | DEFICIENCY | EXCESS |
|---|---|---|
| Vitamin A | Night blindness, xerophthalmia, keratomalacia, conjunctivitis, poor growth, impaired resistance to infection, abnormal tooth enamel development. | Increased intracranial pressure (ICP), anorexia, carotenemia, hyperostosis (pain and swelling of long bones), alopecia, hepatomegaly, poor growth. |
| Vitamin D | Rickets (with elevated serum phosphatase levels appearing before bone deformities), osteomalacia, infantile tetany. | Hypercalcemia, azotemia, poor growth, nausea and vomiting, diarrhea, calcinosis of a variety of tissues including kidney, heart, bronchi, stomach. |
| Vitamin E | Hemolytic anemia in premature infants. | Unknown. |
| Ascorbic acid (vitamin C) | Scurvy and poor wound healing. | May predispose to kidney stones. |
| Thiamine (vitamin $B_1$) | Beriberi (neuritis, edema, cardiac failure), hoarseness, anorexia, restlessness, aphonia. | Unknown. |
| Riboflavin (vitamin $B_2$) | Photophobia, cheilosis, glossitis, corneal vascularization, poor growth. | Unknown. |
| Niacin | Pellagra (dementia, dermatitis, diarrhea). | Nicotinic acid causes flushing, pruritus. |
| Pyridoxine (vitamin $B_6$) | In infants, irritability, convulsions, anemia; in older patients (on isoniazid), dermatitis, glossitis cheilosis, peripheral neuritis. | Sensory neuropathy. |
| Folate | Megaloblastic anemia, glossitis pharyngeal ulcers, impaired cellular immunity. | Usually none. |
| Cobalamin (vitamin $B_{12}$) | Pernicious anemia, neurologic deterioration, methylmalonic acidemia. | Unknown. |
| Pantothenic acid | Rarely depression, hypotension, muscle weakness, abdominal pain. | Unknown. |
| Biotin | Dermatitis, seborrhea, anorexia, muscle pain, pallor, alopecia. | Unknown. |
| Vitamin K | Hemorrhagic manifestations. | Water-soluble forms can cause hyperbilirubinemia. |

Vitamin deficiencies and excesses can result in a variety of clinical syndromes. Although rare, these syndromes usually can be averted with appropriate nutrition (Table 6–1).

## Comprehension Questions

6.1 A 2-day-old infant has significant nasal and rectal bleeding. He was delivered by a midwife at home; the pregnancy was without complications. His Apgar scores were 9 at 1 minute and 9 at 5 minutes. He has breast-fed well and has not required a health-care professional visit since birth. Which of the following vitamin deficiencies might explain his condition?

A. Vitamin A
B. Vitamin $B_1$
C. Vitamin C
D. Vitamin D
E. Vitamin K

6.2 A 6-month-old infant has been growing poorly. His parents have changed his formula three times without success. His examination is remarkable for a pale, emaciated child with little subcutaneous fat and anterior fontanelle fullness. His laboratory test results are notable for a hemolytic anemia and prolonged bleeding times. Which of the following is the most appropriate next step?

A. Gather urine for pH and electrolytes.
B. Measure serum factor IX levels.
C. Measure serum immunoglobulins.
D. Obtain a sweat chloride concentration.
E. Perform a hemoglobin electrophoresis.

6.3 An exclusively breast-fed infant with poor routine care is switched at 6 months of age to whole milk and table foods. Screening laboratories at 9 months of age demonstrate the hemoglobin and hematocrit to be 8 mg/dL and 25%, respectively, and the lead level to be less than 2 μg/dL. A follow-up complete blood count (CBC) 2 weeks later shows the hemoglobin to be at 7.8 mg/dL, the hematocrit 25%, the mean corpuscular volume (MCV) 62%, and the platelet count to be 750,000/mm$^3$. Which of the following would be the next step in the management of this child?

A. Order a hemoglobin electrophoresis.
B. Obtain a bone marrow aspiration.
C. Initiate iron supplementation.
D. Refer to a pediatric hematologist.
E. Initiate soybean-based formula.

6.4 A 3-week-old is admitted for failure to thrive, diarrhea, and a sepsis-like picture. He does well on intravenous fluids; when begun on routine infant formula with iron, his symptoms return. It is Saturday and the state health department laboratory is closed. You should begin feeds with which of the following?

A. Amino acid–based formula (Nutramigen or Pregestimil)
B. Low-phenylalanine formula (Lofenalac or Phenex-1)
C. Low-iron, routine infant formula (Similac with low iron or Enfamil with low iron)
D. Low-isoleucine, low-leucine, low-valine infant formula (Ketonex-1 or MSUD 1)
E. Soy-based formula (ProSobee or Isomil)

## ANSWERS

6.1 **E.** Newborn infants have a relative vitamin K deficiency, especially if they are breast-fed; most infants are given vitamin K at birth to prevent deficiency-related bleeding complications.

6.2 **D.** The patient appears to have failure to thrive, with deficiencies of vitamin K (bleeding problems), vitamin A (fontanelle fullness), and vitamin E (hemolytic anemia). Cystic fibrosis (associated with vitamin malabsorption) would explain the condition.

6.3 **C.** The child in the question likely did not get iron (or vitamin D) supplementation in the first 6 months of life while exclusively breastfeeding and was switched to whole milk (low in iron) and to table foods (not supplemented with iron as are baby foods) at too young an age. All of the laboratory data are consistent with iron deficiency anemia; iron supplementation in this child with a resultant brisk erythrocyte response is both diagnostic and therapeutic. Failure of the child to respond to the iron therapy would require further evaluation.

6.4 **E.** This patient appears to have galactosemia; uridyl transferase deficiency is the cause and the condition results in features of jaundice, hepatosplenomegaly, vomiting, hypoglycemia, seizures, lethargy, irritability, poor feeding and failure to thrive, aminoaciduria, liver failure, mental retardation, and an increased risk of *E coli* sepsis. Children with galactosemia are managed with a lactose-free formula. The low-phenylalanine formulas are for infants with phenylketonuria; low-iron formulas serve no purpose other than causing iron deficiency anemia; the low-isoleucine, low-leucine, low-valine infant formulas are useful for patients with maple syrup urine disease (MSUD); and the amino acid–based formulas are excellent for children with malabsorption syndromes.

## Clinical Pearls

- Breast-feeding is associated with lower morbidity and mortality (especially in developing countries) mostly because of a reduction in enteric pathogens and diarrhea associated with contaminated water used in formula preparation.
- Breast-feeding provides all of the nutrients necessary for infant growth with the possible exceptions of vitamin D and fluoride, which usually are supplemented.
- A breast-feeding vegan should supplement her infant's diet with vitamin $B_{12}$ to prevent methylmalonic acidemia and supplement her toddler's diet with vitamin $B_{12}$ and trace minerals.

## REFERENCES


Boat TF, Acton JD. Cystic fibrosis. In: Kleigman RM, Behrman RE, Jenson HB, Stanton BF, eds. *Nelson Textbook of Pediatrics*. 18th ed. Philadelphia, PA: WB Saunders; 2007:1803-1817.

Chenoweth WL. Vitamin B complex deficiency and excess. In: Kleigman RM, Behrman RE, Jenson HB, Stanton BF, eds. *Nelson Textbook of Pediatrics*. 18th ed. Philadelphia, PA: WB Saunders; 2007:246-251.

Finberg L. Feeding the healthy child. In: McMillan JA, Feigin RD, DeAngelis CD, Jones MD, eds. *Oski's Pediatrics: Principles and Practice*. 4th ed. Philadelphia, PA: Lippincott Williams & Wilkins; 1006:109-118.

Glader B. Iron-deficiency anemia. In: Kleigman RM, Behrman RE, Jenson HB, Stanton BF, eds. *Nelson Textbook of Pediatrics*. 18th ed. Philadelphia, PA: WB Saunders; 2007:2014-2017.

Greenbaum LA. Rickets and hypervitaminosis D. In: Kleigman RM, Behrman RE, Jenson HB, Stanton BF, eds. *Nelson Textbook of Pediatrics*. 18th ed. Philadelphia, PA: WB Saunders; 2007:253-263.

Greenbaum LA. Vitamin E deficiency. In: Kleigman RM, Behrman RE, Jenson HB, Stanton BF, eds. *Nelson Textbook of Pediatrics*. 18th ed. Philadelphia, PA: WB Saunders; 2007:263-264.

Greenbaum LA. Vitamin K deficiency. In: Kleigman RM, Behrman RE, Jenson HB, Stanton BF, eds. *Nelson Textbook of Pediatrics*. 18th ed. Philadelphia, PA: WB Saunders; 2007:264-265.

Heird WC. The feeding of infants and children. In: Kleigman RM, Behrman RE, Jenson HB, Stanton BF, eds. *Nelson Textbook of Pediatrics*. 18th ed. Philadelphia, PA: WB Saunders; 2007:214-225.

Kishnani PS, Chen Y-T. Defects in galactose metabolism. In: Kleigman RM, Behrman RE, Jenson HB, Stanton BF, eds. *Nelson Textbook of Pediatrics*. 18th ed. Philadelphia, PA: WB Saunders; 2007:609-610.

LeLeiko NS, Horowitz M. Formulas and nutritional supplements. In: Rudolph CD, Rudolph AM, Hostetter MK, Lister G, Siegel NJ, eds. *Rudolph's Pediatrics*. 21st ed. New York, NY: McGraw-Hill; 2003:1322-1334.

Martin PL. Nutritional anemias. In: McMillan JA, Feigin RD, DeAngelis CD, Jones MD, eds. *Oski's Pediatrics: Principles and Practice*. 4th ed. Philadelphia, PA: Lippincott Williams & Wilkins; 1006:1692-1696.

Orenstein DM. Cystic fibrosis. In: Rudolph CD, Rudolph AM, Hostetter MK, Lister G, Siegel NJ, eds. *Rudolph's Pediatrics*. 21st ed. New York, NY: McGraw-Hill; 2003: 1967-1980.

Rosenstein BJ. Cystic fibrosis. In: McMillan JA, Feigin RD, DeAngelis CD, Jones MD, eds. *Oski's Pediatrics: Principles and Practice*. 4th ed. Philadelphia, PA: Lippincott Williams & Wilkins; 2006:1425-1438.

Stuchy FJ, Shneider BL. Disorders of carbohydrate metabolism. In: Rudolph CD, Rudolph AM, Hostetter MK, Lister G, Siegel NJ, eds. *Rudolph's Pediatrics*. 21st ed. New York: McGraw-Hill; 2003:1486.

Wappner RS. Disorders of carbohydrate metabolism. In: McMillan JA, Feigin RD, DeAngelis CD, Jones MD, eds. *Oski's Pediatrics: Principles and Practice*. 4th ed. Philadelphia, PA: Lippincott Williams & Wilkins; 2006:2181-2192.

Zile M. Vitamin A deficiencies and excess. In: Kleigman RM, Behrman RE, Jenson HB, Stanton BF, eds. *Nelson Textbook of Pediatrics*. 18th ed. Philadelphia, PA: WB Saunders; 2007:242-245.

Zile M, Chenoweth WL. Vitamin C (ascorbic acid). In: Kleigman RM, Behrman RE, Jenson HB, Stanton BF, eds. *Nelson Textbook of Pediatrics*. 18th ed. Philadelphia, PA: WB Saunders; 2007:251-253.

# Case 7

An 8-month-old child has a 24-hour history of increased crying when she moves her right leg. She has a prominent bulge over the mid-right thigh where she had received an immunization yesterday. She has not had fever nor change in appetite, and she seems upset only when the leg is disturbed. The child underwent a failed Kasai procedure for biliary atresia and is awaiting a liver transplant. A radiograph of the leg demonstrates a mid-shaft fracture and poor mineralization.

- What is the mechanism for this condition?
- What are the best diagnostic tests to diagnose this condition?

# ANSWERS TO CASE 7:
# Rickets

*Summary:* An 8-month-old child with a chronic medical condition, including biliary atresia, poor bone mineralization, and a fracture.

- **Mechanism:** Malabsorption of vitamin D (among other fat-soluble vitamins) due to lack of intestinal secretion of bile salts, resulting in rickets.
- **Best diagnostic tests:** Serum 25(OH)D, calcium, phosphorus, and alkaline phosphatase levels. Radiographs demonstrate poor bone mineralization.

## ANALYSIS

### Objectives

1. Become familiar with the clinical presentation of rickets.
2. Understand the pathophysiology behind nutritional and nonnutritional rickets.
3. Appreciate some of the other metabolic causes of childhood fractures.

### Considerations

This child has biliary atresia and underwent a failed Kasai procedure. Metabolic aberrations are expected while this child awaits liver transplantation. A review of her medications and compliance in receiving them is warranted. Because of the brittle nature of her bones, her leg was fractured while receiving immunizations.

# APPROACH TO
# The Child with Possible Rickets

## DEFINITIONS

**BILIARY ATRESIA:** A congenital condition affecting approximately 1 in 16,000 live births in which the liver's bile ducts become blocked and fibrotic, resulting in reduced bile flow into the bowel.

**GENU VALGUM:** "Knock" knees.

**GENU VARUM:** "Bowed" legs.

**KASAI PROCEDURE:** An operative procedure in which a bowel loop forms a duct to allow bile to drain from a liver with biliary atresia.

**RICKETS:** Poor mineralization of growing bone or of osteoid tissue.

## CLINICAL APPROACH

A patient with **liver failure** has **poor bile salt secretion**, resulting in **poor fat-soluble vitamin absorption**, including **vitamin D.** The **poor vitamin D absorption** causes low serum 25(OH)D, occasionally **reduced serum calcium levels**, markedly **elevated serum alkaline phosphatase, poor bone mineralization**, and an increased risk of **fractures**. Children with liver failure and ascites are treated with loop diuretics, which often cause urinary calcium losses. Treatment, aimed at restoring normal bone mineralization, consists of high vitamin D doses and calcium supplementation.

**Nutritional rickets**, resulting from **inadequate dietary vitamin D** or a lack of sunlight exposure (Figure 7–1), is rare in industrialized countries in healthy children. It is occasionally seen in dark-skinned infants who do not receive vitamin D supplementation or in breast-fed infants not exposed to sunlight. More common causes of rickets are liver or renal failure and a variety of biochemical abnormalities in calcium or phosphorus metabolism (Table 7–1).

The **most common form of nonnutritional rickets is familial, primary hypophosphatemia** (X-linked dominant) in which phosphate reabsorption is defective, and conversion of 25(OH)D to $1,25(OH)_2D$ in the proximal tubules of the kidneys is abnormal. Low serum $1,25(OH)_2D$, low–normal serum calcium, moderately low serum phosphate, and elevated serum alkaline phosphatase levels, hyperphosphaturia, and no evidence of hyperparathyroidism results. Children at the age of walking present with smooth lower-extremity bowing (as compared to angular bowing of calcium-deficient rickets), a waddling gait, genu varum, genu valgum, coxa vara, and short stature. Other findings of calcium-deficient rickets (myopathy, rachitic rosary, pectus deformities, tetany) usually are not seen. Familial hypophosphatemia can cause intraglobular dentin deformities, whereas calcium-deficient rickets causes enamel defects. Radiologic findings include coarse-appearing trabecular bone and widening, fraying, and cupping of the metaphysis of the proximal and distal tibia, distal femur radius, and ulna.

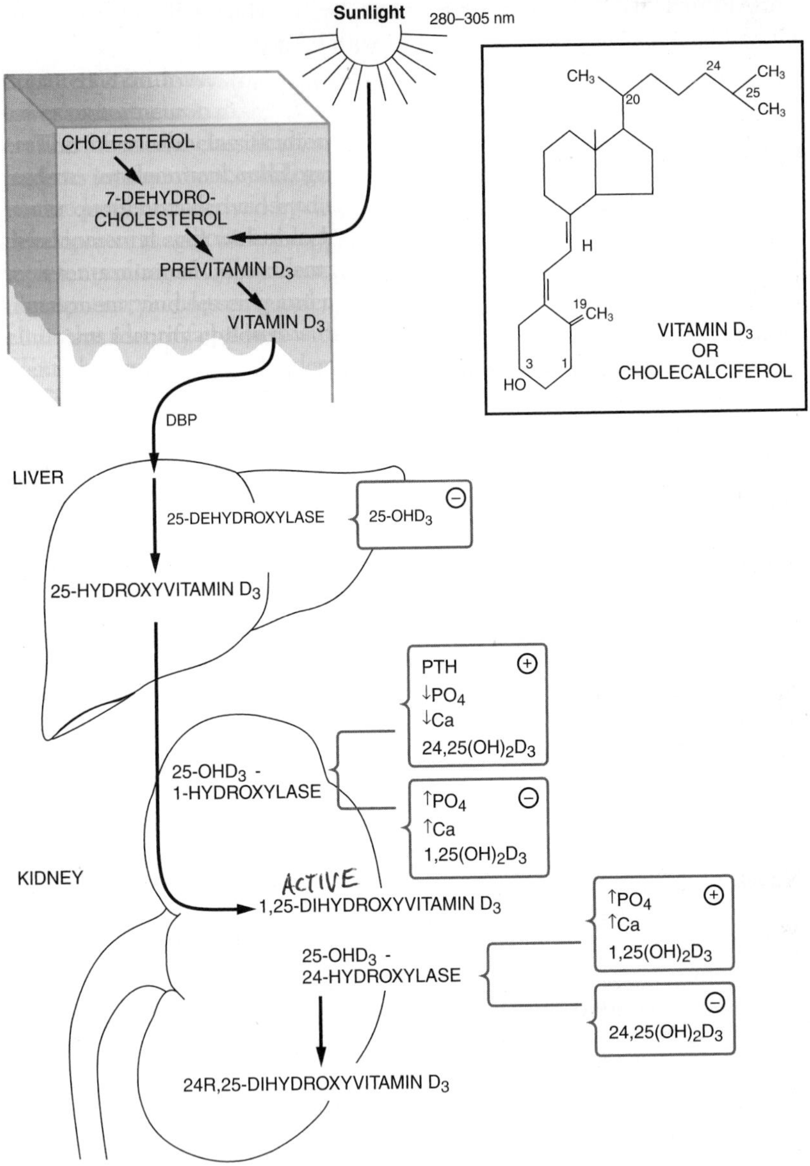


**Figure 7–1.** Vitamin D metabolism.

**Table 7–1 COMMON CAUSES OF ABNORMAL METABOLISM OF CALCIUM AND PHOSPHORUS**

| | SERUM CALCIUM | SERUM PHOSPHORUS | SERUM ALKALINE PHOSPHATASE | URINE AMINO ACIDS | COMMENTS |
|---|---|---|---|---|---|
| Calcium deficiency with secondary hyperparathyroidism [vitamin D deficiency or low 25 (OH) D without stimulation of 1,25$(OH)_2$D production] | | | | | |
| Lack of vitamin D (lack of exposure to sunlight; dietary deficiency vitamin D, congenital) | N or ↓ | ↓ | ↑ | ↑ | Unusual except in dark-skinned infants without vitamin D supplementation, or in exclusively breast-fed infants without exposure to sunlight. |
| Malabsorption of vitamin D | N or ↓ | ↓ | ↑ | ↑ | Such as in celiac disease, cystic fibrosis, or steatorrhea. |
| Hepatic disease | N or ↓ | ↓ | ↑ | ↑ | See discussion of case. |
| Anticonvulsive drugs | N or ↓ | ↓ | ↑ | ↑ | Usually phenobarbital and phenytoin; patients have reduced 25(OH)D levels, possibly as a result of increased cytochrome P450 activity; treatment is with vitamin $D_2$ and adequate dietary calcium. |

(*Continued*)

**Table 7–1 COMMON CAUSES OF ABNORMAL METABOLISM OF CALCIUM AND PHOSPHORUS (CONTINUED)**

| | SERUM CALCIUM | SERUM PHOSPHORUS | SERUM ALKALINE PHOSPHATASE | URINE AMINO ACIDS | COMMENTS |
|---|---|---|---|---|---|
| Renal osteodystrophy | N or ↓ | ↑ | ↑ | Variable | Hypophosphaturia results in hypocalcemia that then stimulates parathyroid secretion and enhanced bone turnover. Additionally, diminished conversion of 25(OH)D to $1,25(OH)_2D$ occurs as renal damage progresses. |
| Vitamin D-dependent type I | ↓ | N or ↓ | ↑ | ↑ | Autosomal recessive; believed to be reduced activity of 25 $(OH)D_1$, α-hydroxylase; responds to massive doses of vitamin $D_2$ or low-dose $1,25(OH)_2D$. |
| **Phosphate deficiency without secondary hyperparathyroidism** | | | | | |
| Genetic primary hypophosphatemia | N | ↓ | ↑ | N | X-linked dominant; most common form of nonnutritional rickets (see text). |
| Fanconi syndrome | N | ↓ | ↑ | ↑ | Includes cystinosis, tyrosinosis, Lowe syndrome, and acquired forms. Cystinosis and tyrosinosis are autosomal recessive, Lowe syndrome X-linked recessive. |

| | | | | | |
|---|---|---|---|---|---|
| Renal tubular acidosis, type II (proximal)<br>↓$H^+$ secretion → acidemia → loss of bone $Ca^{2+}HCO_3$ to neutralize | N | ↓ | ↑ | N | Bicarbonaturia, hyperkaluria, hypercalciuria, hypophosphatemia, and phospha turia are common. Rickets may result from leaching of bone calcium bicarbonate in an attempt to buffer retained hydrogen ions seen in this condition. |
| Oncogenic hypophosphatemia | N | ↓ | ↑ | Usually N | Caused by tumor section of a phosphate-regulating gene product (PEX), which results in phosphaturia and impaired conversion of 25(OH)D to 1,25$(OH)_2$D. The tumors are often hard to detect but are found in the small bones of the hands and feet, abdominal sheath, nasal antrum, and pharynx. Resolution occurs after tumor removal. |
| Phosphate deficiency or malabsorption | N | ↓ | ↑ | N | Caused by parenteral hyperalimentation or low- phosphate intake. |
| **End-organ resistance to 1,25$(OH)_2D_3$** | | | | | |
| Vitamin D-dependent type II<br>Receptor resistance | ↓ | ↓or N | ↑ | ↑ | Autosomal recessive; very high serum levels of 1,25$(OH)_2$D; may result from 1,25$(OH)_2$D receptor-binding disorder. |

## Comprehension Questions

7.1 A 14-month-old child has lower-extremity bowing, a waddling gait, genu varum, and is at the fifth percentile for height. Laboratory data include low–normal serum calcium, moderately low serum phosphate, and elevated serum alkaline phosphatase levels, hyperphosphaturia, and normal parathyroid levels. Which of the following is the most likely diagnosis?

A. Fanconi syndrome
B. Genetic primary hypophosphatemia
C. Malabsorption of vitamin D
D. Phosphate malabsorption
E. Renal osteodystrophy

7.2 An 8-month-old African-American baby arrives to the emergency department with his mother with the complaint of decreased left arm movement. He is the product of a normal term pregnancy, has had no medical problems, and was in good health when his mother dropped him off at the day care center. Upper arm radiographs show a left humerus spiral fracture. Which of the following is the most appropriate next step in management?

A. Admit the child and call child protective services.
B. Obtain serum $1,25(OH)_2D$ levels.
C. Order serum alkaline phosphatase levels.
D. Obtain stool for analysis for fat-soluble vitamins.
E. Send chromosome sample for osteogenesis imperfecti analysis.

7.3 The diet of a 3-year-old child with cystic fibrosis should be supplemented with which of the following?

A. Folate
B. Sodium
C. Vitamin C
D. Vitamin $B_{12}$
E. Vitamin D

7.4 A 5-year-old girl is somewhat short and has mild leg bowing. Her medical history is significant only for well-controlled seizure disorder. Serum calcium, phosphorus, and alkaline phosphatase levels and urinary amino acid concentration are normal. A bone age is notable for abnormal distal radius and ulna mineralization. Which of the following is the most likely diagnosis?

A. Cystic fibrosis
B. Fanconi syndrome
C. Genetic primary hypophosphatemia
D. Rickets associated with anticonvulsive drug use
E. Schmid metaphyseal dysplasia

## ANSWERS

7.1 **B.** Lower-extremity bowing, low–normal calcium and phosphate levels, and normal parathyroid hormone levels suggest familial primary hypophosphatemia.

7.2 **A.** A spiral fracture of the humerus is suspicious but not diagnostic for child abuse. While further laboratory testing is appropriate, the next step in the management of this child is to provide a safe environment until more data are available.

7.3 **E.** In addition to pancreatic enzyme replacement therapy, supplementation with fat-soluble vitamins (A, D, E, and K), often iron, and sometimes zinc is recommended.

7.4 **E.** All of the rickets syndromes present with elevated alkaline phosphatase levels. Schmid metaphyseal dysplasia, an autosomal dominant condition, presents in a similar way with short stature, leg bowing, and waddling gait. Radiographs show irregular long bone mineralization. Biochemically, Schmid-type metaphyseal dysostosis presents with normal serum calcium, phosphorus, and alkaline phosphatase activity and normal urinary amino acid levels.

### Clinical Pearls

- Nutritional rickets (inadequate dietary vitamin D or sunlight exposure) is rare in healthy children in industrialized countries. Medical conditions (liver or renal failure) or abnormalities in calcium and phosphorus metabolism usually are responsible.
- Primary hypophosphatemia (X-linked dominant) is the most common cause of nonnutritional rickets; proximal kidney tubule defects in phosphate reabsorption and conversion of 25(OH)D to $1,25(OH)_2D$ are seen. Findings include low–normal serum calcium, moderately low serum phosphate, elevated serum alkaline phosphatase, and low serum $1,25(OH)_2D$ levels, hyperphosphaturia, and no evidence of hyperparathyroidism.

## REFERENCES

Boat TF, Acton JD. Cystic fibrosis. In: Kleigman RM, Behrman RE, Jenson HB, Stanton BF, eds. *Nelson Textbook of Pediatrics*. 18th ed. Philadelphia, PA: WB Saunders; 2006:1803-1817.

Brewer ED. Pan-proximal tubular dysfunction (Fanconi syndrome). In: McMillan JA, Feigin RD, DeAngelis CD, Jones MD, eds. *Oski's Pediatrics: Principles and Practice*. 4th ed. Philadelphia, PA: Lippincott Williams & Wilkins; 2006:1892-1897.

Chesney RW. Metabolic bone disease. In: Kleigman RM, Behrman RE, Jenson HB, Stanton BF, eds. *Nelson Textbook of Pediatrics*. 18th ed. Philadelphia, PA: WB Saunders; 2006:2893-2898.

Chiang ML. Disorders of renal phosphate transport. In: McMillan JA, Feigin RD, DeAngelis CD, Jones MD, eds. *Oski's Pediatrics: Principles and Practice*. 4th ed. Philadelphia, PA: Lippincott Williams & Wilkins; 2006:1898-1901.

Greenbaum LA. Rickets and hypervitaminosis D. In: Kleigman RM, Behrman RE, Jenson HB, Stanton BF, eds. *Nelson Textbook of Pediatrics*. 18th ed. Philadelphia, PA: WB Saunders; 2007:253-263.

Hill LL, Chiang ML. Renal tubular acidosis. In: McMillan JA, Feigin RD, DeAngelis CD, Jones MD, eds. *Oski's Pediatrics: Principles and Practice*. 4th ed. Philadelphia, PA: Lippincott Williams & Wilkins; 2006:1886-1892.

Kohaut EC. Chronic renal failure. In: McMillan JA, Feigin RD, DeAngelis CD, Jones MD, eds. *Oski's Pediatrics: Principles and Practice*. 4th ed. Philadelphia, PA: Lippincott Williams & Wilkins; 2006:1841-1844.

Orenstein DM. Cystic fibrosis. In: Rudolph CD, Rudolph AM, Hostetter MK, Lister G, Siegel NJ, eds. *Rudolph's Pediatrics*. 21st ed. New York, NY: McGraw-Hill; 2003: 1967-1980.

Root AW. Rickets and osteomalacia. In: Rudolph CD, Rudolph AM, Hostetter MK, Lister G, Siegel NJ, eds. *Rudolph's Pediatrics*. 21st ed. New York, NY: McGraw-Hill; 2003:2156-2160.

Rosenstein BJ. Cystic fibrosis. In: McMillan JA, Feigin RD, DeAngelis CD, Jones MD, eds. *Oski's Pediatrics: Principles and Practice*. 4th ed. Philadelphia, PA: Lippincott Williams & Wilkins; 2006:1425-1438.

Vogt BA, Avner ED. Toxic nephropathies-renal failure. In: Kleigman RM, Behrman RE, Jenson HB, Stanton BF, eds. *Nelson Textbook of Pediatrics*. 18th ed. Philadelphia, PA: WB Saunders; 2007:2204-2205.

Watkins SL. Chronic renal insufficiency. In: Rudolph CD, Rudolph AM, Hostetter MK, Lister G, Siegel NJ, eds. *Rudolph's Pediatrics*. 21st ed. New York, NY: McGraw-Hill; 2003:1718-1724.

# Case 8

A family reports that their 5-year-old son has been increasingly confused over the last several hours. His emergency department vital signs show a heart rate of 180 beats/min, a blood pressure of 80/50 mm Hg, a temperature of 36.1°C (97°F), and slow, deep respirations. His capillary refill is 5 seconds, and he has skin tenting as well as altered mental status. His mother reports that he has had a several pounds of weight loss over the last few weeks, has been increasingly tired for several days, and that she has been concerned about his 2- or 3-day history of thirst, frequent daytime urination, and new onset of nocturnal enuresis.

➤ What is the most likely diagnosis?

➤ What is the best therapy?

# ANSWERS TO CASE 8: Diabetic Ketoacidosis

*Summary:* A 5-year-old with weight loss, polydipsia, and polyuria who presents with dehydration and Kussmaul breathing.

- **Most likely diagnosis:** Diabetic ketoacidosis (DKA).
- **Best therapy:** Fluid rehydration, insulin, and close monitoring of serum glucose level and acidemia.

## ANALYSIS

### Objectives

1. Understand the presentation of patients in DKA.
2. Appreciate the initial treatment strategies in the management of DKA.
3. Become familiar with pitfalls in the treatment of DKA.

### Considerations

This patient is **in extremis**. He is tachycardic, hypotensive, hypothermic, and has delayed capillary refill with tenting of the skin. The **ABCs** of medicine apply. He is confused but not obtunded; he probably requires neither his **air**way controlled nor his **b**reathing regulated. His examination suggests at least 10% dehydration; his **c**irculatory status is marginal and requires rapid volume restoration. His history and physical examination suggest diabetes; a fingerstick glucose test confirms the diagnosis. The therapy for DKA rests on (1) aggressive volume repletion, (2) glucose control with insulin, and (3) correction of metabolic abnormalities.

# APPROACH TO Diabetic Ketoacidosis

## DEFINITIONS

**KETOACIDOSIS:** A condition resulting from deficient insulin availability, leading to lipid oxidation and metabolism rather than glucose metabolism. The insulin absence results in free fatty acid (FFA) released from adipose tissue and in unregulated hepatic FFA oxidation and ketogenesis.

**TYPE I DIABETES:** Known by a variety of names, it is caused by a severe endogenous insulin deficiency and a requirement for exogenous insulin to prevent ketoacidosis.

**TYPE II DIABETES:** Known by a variety of names, it usually consists of tissue-level insulin resistance (although exogenous insulin is often required) and rarely leads to ketoacidosis.

**KUSSMAUL BREATHING:** Deep, rapid respirations associated with acidosis.

## CLINICAL APPROACH

**Patients with DKA represent a medical emergency.** Such patients may require intubation, but usually this is seen later in the disease course. Children more commonly present with signs and symptoms of severe dehydration and acidosis. **The history often is positive for polyuria, nausea, vomiting, and abdominal complaints. Hypothermia, hypotension, Kussmaul respirations, and acetone on the breath are common.** As these signs and symptoms may be nonspecific, especially in younger children, a high index of suspicion is required to make the diagnosis.

Laboratory data demonstrate an **elevated glucose level** (often 400-800 mg/dL), **metabolic acidosis** (with anion gap, ie, excess endogenous anion production such as from lactic acid), and **hyperketonemia**. Serum electrolyte levels usually show hyponatremia and normal or slightly elevated potassium (despite intracellular potassium depletion). Elevated blood urea nitrogen and creatinine levels are commonly seen, reflecting the dehydration. White blood cell counts (WCBs) often are elevated, especially if a bacterial infection is exacerbating the condition.

**Treating DKA includes initial vascular volume expansion (often with normal saline) and then correction of the hyperglycemia and hyperketonemia.** Intravenous (IV) fluid boluses sufficient to stabilize the heart rate and blood pressure are sometimes required, and then a slower IV rate (usually a saline solution with or without some glucose) to replace fluid losses and to ensure adequate urine flow is initiated. **Potassium is added to IV fluids after urine output** is established to counteract the patient's total body potassium depletion (treatment of the hyperglycemia and acidosis drives potassium intracellularly; hypokalemia is an avoidable complication). A continuous insulin infusion at a rate of approximately 0.1 U/kg/h is also started (a bolus of 0.1 U/kg is often given initially), with the IV rate adjusted based on the results of hourly glucose measurements. Glucose is added to IV fluids when the serum glucose level drops to approximately 250 or 300 mg/dL, and additional insulin rates adjustments are made based on serum glucose levels. The **low plasma pH and elevated serum ketone levels will correct significantly in the first 8 to 10 hours**; the serum bicarbonate level may remain low for approximately 24 hours or more. Improvement is characterized by a decrease in IV insulin rates and resolution of the ketonuria; then, the patient can take oral feedings, and insulin is converted from the IV to subcutaneous route.

Several pitfalls should be avoided during the treatment of DKA. IV fluids with insulin and **improvement in acidosis levels often are associated with a fall in serum potassium levels**; addition of potassium to the IV fluids usually is indicated to prevent serious hypokalemia. Bicarbonate infusion usually is avoided except in extreme situations, because it may (1) precipitate hypokalemia, (2) shift the oxygen dissociation curve to the left, worsening organ oxygen delivery, (3) overcorrect the acidosis, and (4) result in worsening cerebral acidosis while the plasma pH is being corrected (transfer into the cerebrum of $CO_2$ formed when the bicarbonate is infused in an acid serum). Cerebral edema (etiology unknown) sometimes occurs, manifesting as headache, personality changes, vomiting, and decreased reflexes. Treatment of cerebral edema consists of reduction in IV fluid, administration of IV mannitol, and hyperventilation. **Episodes of DKA (especially in the known diabetic) can be precipitated by bacterial infection.** An **evaluation for infection sources** with institution of antibiotics (if appropriate) is required.

## Comprehension Questions

8.1 A 14-year-old adolescent female from another state was followed for 7 years for a history of insulin-dependent diabetes mellitus. At your clinic her hemoglobin $A_{1C}$ is 14.9%. This laboratory test indicates which of the following?

A. Her glucose control is poor.
B. She does not have insulin-dependent diabetes.
C. She has entered the "honeymoon phase" of her diabetes.
D. She has an underlying infection.
E. She is demonstrating the Somogyi phenomenon.

8.2 Six months after being diagnosed with what appears to be insulin-dependent diabetes, the 5-year-old in the case presentation has a significant decrease in his insulin requirement. Which of the following is the most likely explanation?

A. His diagnosis of insulin-dependent diabetes was incorrect.
B. He had a chronic infection that is now under control.
C. He has followed his diabetes diet so well that he requires less insulin.
D. He is demonstrating the Somogyi phenomenon.
E. He has entered the "honeymoon phase" of his diabetes.

8.3 A 15-year-old adolescent female has experienced abdominal pain, vomiting, and lethargy for 3 days. Her chest and throat examinations are clear, but her abdominal examination is significant for right lower quadrant pain. Rectal examination is equivocal for pain, and her pelvic examination is remarkable for pain upon movement of her cervix. Laboratory data include a white blood cell count of 18,000/$mm^3$, serum glucose level of 145 mg/dL, and serum bicarbonate level of 21 mEq/dL. Her urinalysis is remarkable for 1+ white blood cells, 1+ glucose, and 1+ ketones. Which of the following is the most likely diagnosis?

A. Appendicitis
B. Diabetic ketoacidosis (DKA)
C. Gastroenteritis
D. Pelvic inflammatory disease (PID)
E. Right lower lobe pneumonia

8.4 A 16-year-old obese adolescent female has enuresis, frequent urination, a white vaginal discharge, and a dark rash around her neck. Her serum glucose level is 250 mg/dL, and her urinalysis is positive for 2+ glucose but is otherwise negative. Which of the following is the most likely diagnosis?

A. Chemical vaginitis
B. Chlamydia cervicitis
C. Psoriasis
D. Type II diabetes
E. Urinary tract infection (UTI)

## ANSWERS

8.1 **A.** The patient likely has poor diabetes control. The hemoglobin $A_{1C}$, commonly used to follow glucose control, measures the average glucose levels over the previous 2 or 3 months. The hemoglobin $A_{1C}$ goal for most diabetics is 6% to 9%. Levels greater than 12% suggest poor control, and levels 9% to 12% represent fair control. In the Somogyi phenomenon, a patient has nocturnal hypoglycemic episodes manifested as night terrors, headaches, or early morning sweating and then presents a few hours later with hyperglycemia, ketonuria, and glucosuria. Counter-regulatory hormones, in response to the hypoglycemia, cause the hyperglycemia.

8.2 **E.** Up to 75% of newly diagnosed diabetics have a progressive decrease in the daily insulin requirement in the months after their diabetes diagnosis; a few patients temporarily require no insulin. This "honeymoon" period usually lasts a few months, and then an insulin requirement returns. Patients are told that the "honeymoon" period is not a cure and that they should expect a return to insulin requirement.

8.3 **D.** The patient likely has PID; glucosuria is a stress response to the infection and does not represent glucose metabolism problems. All of the options in the question can cause abdominal pain. Although diabetes mellitus is in the differential, DKA more likely presents with ketoacidosis (significantly decreased serum bicarbonate levels) and high serum glucose levels.

8.4 **D.** The description is of an obese adolescent female with candida vaginitis (the vaginal discharge) and acanthosis nigricans (the nuchal dark rash) consistent with type II diabetes. This condition is far more common in overweight children, especially those with a family history of the condition.

## Clinical Pearls

- Diabetic ketoacidosis (DKA) is a medical emergency that can present with nonspecific signs of dehydration, polyuria, nausea, vomiting, and abdominal complaints. Hypothermia, hypotension, Kussmaul respirations, and acetone on the breath are also seen. A high index of suspicion is required to make the diagnosis, especially in the younger child.
- Cerebral edema is a potentially life-threatening complication in diabetic ketoacidosis treatment presenting as headache, personality changes, vomiting, and decreased reflexes.
- Electrolyte disturbances are common in diabetic ketoacidosis. Hypokalemia can occur during treatment if adequate sources are not provided. Bicarbonate administration usually is avoided except in extreme situations for a variety of physiologic reasons.

## REFERENCES

Alemzadeh R, Wyatt DT. Diabetes mellitus. In: Kleigman RM, Behrman RE, Jenson HB, Stanton BF, eds. *Nelson Textbook of Pediatrics*. 18th ed. Philadelphia, PA: WB Saunders; 2007:2404-2432.

Cooke DW. Type 2 diabetes mellitus. In: McMillan JA, Feigin RD, DeAngelis CD, Jones MD, eds. *Oski's Pediatrics: Principles and Practice*. 4th ed. Philadelphia, PA: Lippincott Williams & Wilkins; 2006:2115-2122.

Gitelman SE. Diabetes mellitus. In: Rudolph CD, Rudolph AM, Hostetter MK, Lister G, Siegel NJ, eds. *Rudolph's Pediatrics*. 21st ed. New York, NY: McGraw-Hill; 2003: 2111-2136.

Plotnick LP. Type 1 (insulin-dependent) diabetes mellitus. In: McMillan JA, Feigin RD, DeAngelis CD, Jones MD, eds. *Oski's Pediatrics: Principles and Practice*. 4th ed. Philadelphia, PA: Lippincott Williams & Wilkins; 2006:2103-2115.

# Case 9

A 2-month-old child you have followed since birth arrives for his routine "baby shots." His mother's pregnancy was uncomplicated, and he has been healthy without significant problems.

➤ What is the next step in the care of this patient?

# ANSWER TO CASE 9:
# Routine Well-Child Care

*Summary:* A healthy 2-month-old infant due for a routine well-child visit.

➤ **Next step:** Gather interval history (feeding, sleep), obtain appropriate measurements (length, weight, and head circumference), review sensory and developmental or behavioral screenings (ensure that he can see and hear, and that he is developing normally), perform a physical examination, perform general and specialized procedures (ensure that his neonatal state screen is normal and provide immunizations), and offer anticipatory guidance.

## ANALYSIS

### Objectives

1. Become familiar with the goals of the routine well-child (or health supervision) session.
2. Become familiar with the American Academy of Pediatrics (AAP) Recommended Childhood and Adolescent Immunization Schedule.
3. Learn the side effects and contraindications of common childhood immunizations.

### Considerations

Well-child care for this healthy infant is uncomplicated. For children with special needs, such as Down syndrome or sickle cell disease, guidelines outline their specific considerations. For children with multiple handicaps, such as those resulting from extreme prematurity, no specific guidelines exist; the providers adapt national "well-child care" guidelines as appropriate.

# APPROACH TO
# Childhood Well-Child Care

## CLINICAL APPROACH

**Goals of a health supervision visit** include evaluating a child's physical, developmental, psychosocial, and educational status to identify problems early; prompt intervention then can be instituted. Anticipatory guidance aims to foster good health habits, prevent illness, and assist in family communication.

Most pediatric providers follow commonly available preventive health-care guidelines. The AAP periodically updates its Recommendations for Preventive Pediatric Health Care, which outlines questions, medical procedures, and counseling areas for children's birth through 21 years. Other sources include guidelines from the Agency for Healthcare Research and Quality and "Bright Futures" (National Center for Education in Maternal and Child Healthcare). Regardless of the source, guidelines are modified to fit local practice and to best serve the patients' needs.

## IMMUNIZATIONS

Immunizations are part of the well-child visit. They are cost-effective and efficacious in improving children's general health and well-being. Vaccination programs have eliminated smallpox and reduced the incidence of other diseases (*Haemophilus influenzae* type b [Hib], polio, measles, tetanus, rubella, and diphtheria) such that medical students and residents are unlikely to see a single case. The Recommended Childhood and Adolescent Immunization Schedule (Figure 9–1), updated annually and available on the Internet, is supported by a variety of organizations, including the AAP, the American Academy of Family Practice, and the Centers for Disease Control and Prevention.

Pediatric immunizations are extraordinarily safe. The side effects risk is extremely low, especially when compared to the benefit of preventing morbidity and mortality from communicable diseases. However, vaccine safety sometimes is scrutinized by the news media and by parents. The health-care provider must have access to scientifically sound and updated side effect data to allay these fears (Table 9–1).

Many American children are incompletely immunized because of a lack of access to immunizations, poor family understanding of the need for immunizations, cost, or fear of side effects. True contraindications to giving immunizations are rare. **Mild upper respiratory infections, gastroenteritis, and low-grade fever are not contraindications.**

**True contraindications** to a particular vaccine include **immediate hypersensitivity** reactions to the given vaccine, the vaccine component, or the preservative in the agent. **True egg hypersensitivity is a contraindication to influenza and yellow fever vaccination** (both grown in chick embryo tissue cultures) but not for measles-mumps-rubella (MMR) vaccination (contains only minute amounts of egg products). Patients having encephalopathy or encephalitis after receiving the diphtheria, tetanus, and pertussis vaccine do not receive subsequent doses. **In general, live virus vaccines are not given to pregnant and severely immunocompromised patients**, but they are given to a child living in the home with a pregnant woman. Giving MMR or varicella to an asymptomatic patient with human immunodeficiency virus (HIV) is permitted. Expert consultation in some cases is warranted.

| Vaccine ▼ Age ► | Birth | 1 month | 2 months | 4 months | 6 months | 12 months | 15 months | 18 months | 19–23 months | 2–3 years | 4–6 years |
|---|---|---|---|---|---|---|---|---|---|---|---|
| Hepatitis B[1] | HepB | HepB | | *see footnote 1* | HepB | | | | | | |
| Rotavirus[2] | | | RV | RV | *RV*[2] | | | | | | |
| Diphtheria, Tetanus, Pertussis[3] | | | DTaP | DTaP | DTaP | *see footnote 3* | DTaP | | | | DTaP |
| *Haemophilus influenzae* type b[4] | | | Hib | Hib | *Hib*[4] | Hib | | | | | |
| Pneumococcal[5] | | | PCV | PCV | PCV | PCV | | | | PPSV | |
| Inactivated Poliovirus | | | IPV | IPV | IPV | | | | | | IPV |
| Influenza[6] | | | | | Influenza (Yearly) | | | | | | |
| Measles, Mumps, Rubella[7] | | | | | | MMR | | | *see footnote 7* | | MMR |
| Varicella[8] | | | | | | Varicella | | | *see footnote 8* | | Varicella |
| Hepatitis A[9] | | | | | | HepA (2 doses) | | | | HepA Series | |
| Meningococcal[10] | | | | | | | | | | MCV | |

Range of recommended ages / Certain high-risk groups

This schedule indicates the recommended ages for routine administration of currently licensed vaccines, as of December 1, 2008, for children aged 0 through 6 years. Any dose not administered at the recommended age should be administered at a subsequent visit, when indicated and feasible. Licensed combination vaccines may be used whenever any component of the combination is indicated and other components are not contraindicated and if approved by the Food and Drug Administration for that dose of the series. Providers should consult the relevant Advisory Committee on Immunization Practices statement for detailed recommendations, including high-risk conditions: http://www.cdc.gov/vaccines/pubs/acip-list.htm. Clinically significant adverse events that follow immunization should be reported to the Vaccine Adverse Event Reporting System (VAERS). Guidance about how to obtain and complete a VAERS form is available at http://www.vaers.hhs.gov or by telephone, 800-822-7967.

**Figure 9–1.** Recommended childhood adolescent immunization schedule: 2009. (*Reproduced from the Centers for Disease Control and Prevention, www.cdc.gov.*)

**Table 9–1 VACCINE ADVERSE EVENTS, CONTRAINDICATIONS, AND PRECAUTIONS**

| AGENT | ADVERSE EVENT | CONTRAINDICATIONS OR PRECAUTIONS |
| --- | --- | --- |
| *H influenzae* type b vaccine | Pain, redness, and/or swelling at the injection site in 25% of recipients. | Anaphylactic reaction to vaccine. |
| DPT/DTaP* vaccine (In general, only the acellular (DTaP) pertussis vaccine is available; all of the adverse events listed are far more common with the cellular (DTP) form.) | Local and febrile reaction.<br>Redness, edema, induration, and tenderness at the injection site.<br>Drowsiness, fretfulness, anorexia, vomiting, crying.<br>Slight to moderate fever.<br>Bacterial or sterile abscesses at the site of injection (6-10 cases per million injections).<br>Allergic reactions (2 cases per 100,000 injections), transient urticarial rash.<br>Seizures (incidence occurring within 48 h is 1 case per 1750 doses).<br>Hypotonic-hyporesponsive (also called "collapse" or "shocklike state") episodes (1 case per 1750 doses).<br>Fever ≥40.5°C (105°F) (0.3% of recipients).<br>Persistent, severe, inconsolable screaming or crying (1 case per 100 doses). | Contraindications<br>• Anaphylactic reaction to vaccine or vaccine constituent.<br>• Moderate or severe illness with or without a fever.<br>• Encephalopathy within 7 d of administration of previous dose of DTP/DTaP.<br>Precautions<br>• Fever ≥40.5°C (105°F) within 48 h of vaccination with a prior dose of DTP/DTaP.<br>• Collapse or shocklike state (hypotonic-hyporesponsive episode) within 48 h of receiving a prior dose of DTP/DTaP.<br>• Seizures within 3 d of receiving a prior dose of DTP/DTaP (acetaminophen given prior to administering DTaP or DTP and every 4 h thereafter for 24 h should be considered for children with a personal or family history of convulsions in siblings or parents).<br>• Persistent, inconsolable crying lasting >3 h within 48 h of receiving a prior dose of DTP/DTaP.<br>• Guillain-Barré syndrome within 6 wk after a dose of DTP/DTaP. |

(*Continued*)

**Table 9–1** VACCINE ADVERSE EVENTS, CONTRAINDICATIONS, AND PRECAUTIONS (CONTINUED)

| AGENT | ADVERSE EVENT | CONTRAINDICATIONS OR PRECAUTIONS |
|---|---|---|
| Hepatitis B vaccine | Pain at injection site and temperature >37.7°C (99.86°F) (1%-6% of recipients).<br>Anaphylaxis reported to be 1 in 600,000 doses. | Contraindications<br>• Anaphylactic reaction to vaccine or vaccine constituent.<br>• Anaphylactic reaction to baker's yeast.<br>Precautions<br>• Moderate or severe illness with or without a fever. |
| MMR vaccine | Fever up to 39.4°C (103°F) occurs in 5%-15% of vaccines 7-12 d after injection, lasting 1-2 d.<br>Rash in about 5% of vaccines.<br>Transient thrombocytopenia.<br>Encephalitis and encephalopathy occurs in 1 per million doses, less often with revaccination.<br>Allergic reaction: reactions to the MMR vaccine are rare even in children with documented egg allergy.<br>Clinically apparent thrombocytopenia within 2 mo of the vaccine occurs in <1 per 25,000-40,000 vaccinated children, clustered about 2-3 wk after the vaccine, and is generally transient and benign in nature.<br>Subacute sclerosing panencephalitis is possibly a rare complication. | Contraindications<br>• Anaphylactic reaction to neomycin or gelatin.<br>• Pregnancy.<br>• Known altered immunodeficiency (hematologic and solid tumors, severe HIV infection, congenital immunodeficiency, and long-term immunosuppressive therapy).<br>Precautions<br>• Recent immunoglobulin administration (within 3-11 mo depending on product).<br>• Thrombocytopenia or history of thrombocytopenic purpura. |
| Inactivated poliovirus vaccine (IPV) | None. | Contraindications<br>• Anaphylactic reaction to streptomycin, polymyxin B, and neomycin.<br>Precautions<br>• Pregnancy. |

**Table 9–1 VACCINE ADVERSE EVENTS, CONTRAINDICATIONS, AND PRECAUTIONS (CONTINUED)**

| AGENT | ADVERSE EVENT | CONTRAINDICATIONS OR PRECAUTIONS |
|---|---|---|
| Varicella vaccine | Rash within 1 mo of immunization, a mild maculopapular or varicelliform rash (median of about 2-5 lesions) at the injection site or elsewhere, develops in about 7% of children and about 8% of susceptible adolescents/adults.<br>Pain, redness, and/or swelling at the injection site in 20% of children and 25%-35% of adolescents.<br>Transmission of the vaccine virus from healthy vaccines to other persons is rare (<1%) and appears to occur only if vaccine develops rash. Transmission of this vaccine virus appears to cause mild or no disease.<br>Zoster-like illness (rash and minimal or absent system symptoms) has been reported in vaccines (about 18 cases per 100,000 person years); no cases have been severe. | Contraindications<br>• Anaphylactic reaction to neomycin and gelatin.<br>• Infection with HIV.<br>• Known altered immunodeficiency (hematologic and solid tumors, congenital immunodeficiency, and long-term immunosuppressive therapy).<br>Precautions<br>• Recent immunoglobulin administration (within 5 mo).<br>• Family history of immunodeficiency. |
| Pneumococcal vaccine | Up to about 1 of 4 infants had redness, tenderness, or swelling where the shot was given.<br>About 1 of 3 infants had a fever >38°C (>100.4°F), and up to about 1 in 50 had a higher fever >39°C (>102.2°F).<br>Some children also became fussy or drowsy, or had a loss of appetite. | Known anaphylactic reaction. |

(*Continued*)

**Table 9–1 VACCINE ADVERSE EVENTS, CONTRAINDICATIONS, AND PRECAUTIONS (CONTINUED)**

| AGENT | ADVERSE EVENT | CONTRAINDICATIONS OR PRECAUTIONS |
| --- | --- | --- |
| Hepatitis A vaccine | Soreness where the shot was given (about 1 of 2 adults and up to 1 of 5 children).<br>Headache (about 1 of 6 adults and 1 of 20 children).<br>Loss of appetite (about 1 of 12 children).<br>Fatigue (about 1 of 14 adults).<br>If these problems occur, they usually come 3-5 d after vaccination and last for 1 or 2 d. | Known anaphylactic reaction. |

Abbreviations: DTaP, diphtheria and tetanus toxoids and acellular pertussis [vaccine]; DTP, diphtheria and tetanus toxoids and pertussis [vaccine]; HIV, human immunodeficiency virus; MMR, measles-mumps-rubella.

*In general, only the acellular (DTaP) pertussis vaccine is available; all of the adverse events listed are far more common with the cellular (DTP) form.

*(Data from Pickering LK, ed.* 2006 Red Book: Report of the Committee on Infectious Diseases. *27th ed. Elk Grove Village, IL: American Academy of Pediatrics, 2006 and Centers for Disease Control and Prevention available at www.cdc.gov).*

## Comprehension Questions

9.1 A healthy, well-developed 6-year-old child arrives as a new patient to your clinic. His immunization card reveals that he received an immunization at birth and some when he was 2 months old, but none since. Which of the following statements about him is correct?

A. He should receive the live oral poliovirus vaccine rather than the inactivated (injectable) poliovirus vaccine (IPV).
B. The pertussis vaccine is contraindicated at his age and is replaced with the tetanus-diphtheria vaccine.
C. He is too old to receive the *H influenzae* type b vaccine.
D. His vaccinations at birth and 2 months are repeated because too much time has elapsed for them to be effective.
E. He is too young for the varicella vaccine.

9.2 Appropriate advice for a mother of a 2-week-old child here for a "well-child" visit includes which of the following?

A. By age 1 month the child should be sleeping through the night.
B. Children should be able to roll over by age 2 months and to sit by age 4 months.
C. Half-strength fruit juices can be initiated at age 2 months.
D. Potty training should begin at age 1 year.
E. Sleep in the supine position is recommended.

9.3 During a "well-child" visit, the parents of a healthy 5-month-old offer a great amount of information. Which of the following bits of information is of most concern?

A. A diet that includes baby cereal, five different baby vegetables, and one baby fruit
B. Consuming 32 oz of infant formula per day
C. Intermittent tugging on the ears
D. Limited eye contact with parents
E. Rolling from front to back but not back to front

9.4 Which of the following statements about "routine" screening tests is accurate?

A. All children undergo tuberculosis skin testing at age 12 months.
B. Lead testing is obtained on all 12- and 14-month-old infants.
C. Pelvic examinations are part of the examination of a sexually active adolescent.
D. Screening hematocrit levels are obtained on all infants at age 2 months.
E. Universal cholesterol screening begins at age 11 months.

## ANSWERS

9.1 **C.** The Hib vaccine generally is not recommended for children 5 years of age or older.

9.2 **E.** Juices (undiluted) are avoided until approximately 6 months of age (in a cup and not in the bottle). At 1 month of age an infant should be able to fix and follow, but not be expected to sleep through the night by age 2 to 3 months. Realistic targets for development include rolling over at 4 months and sitting by 6 months. Potty training starts when the child shows interest, usually no earlier than age 2 years. Parents are told to place healthy children on their backs (or side) for sleep to reduce the incidence of sudden infant death syndrome.

9.3 **D.** Children fix and follow on the human face from birth. A 5-month-old child who does not engage in eye contact is abnormal.

9.4 **C.** Tuberculosis and lead testing are performed on at-risk children. Pelvic examinations are performed when girls become sexually active or by age 18 to 21 years. Screening hematocrits are done at age 9 to 12 months, and cholesterol tests are done for children with familial risk factors.

### Clinical Pearls

- True contraindications for vaccinations are rare but include immediate hypersensitivity reactions to the vaccine, the vaccine component, or the preservative in the agent.
- Conditions that are *not* contraindications for vaccinations include mild upper respiratory infections, gastroenteritis, and low-grade fever.
- In general, pregnant and severely immunocompromised patients should not receive live virus vaccinations, but the vaccines are given to children living in the home with a pregnant woman. Measles-mumps-rubella (MMR) and varicella vaccinations can be given to asymptomatic patients with HIV.

## REFERENCES

Agency for Healthcare Research and Quality. Guide to clinical preventive services. Available at: http://www.ahrq.gov/clinic/cpsix.htm.

American Academy of Pediatrics. Recommendations for preventive pediatric health care. Available at: http://www.aap.org.

Bright Futures. Guidelines for health supervision of infants, children, and adolescents. Available at: http://www.brightfutures.org.

Centers for Disease Control and Prevention. Vaccine side effects. Available at: http://www.cdc.gov/vaccines/vac-gen/side-effects.htm#dtap.

Halsey NA. Immunization. In: McMillan JA, Feigin RD, DeAngelis CD, Jones MD, eds. *Oski's Pediatrics: Principles and Practice*. 4th ed. Philadelphia, PA: Lippincott Williams & Wilkins; 2006:118-134.

Orenstein WA, Pickering LK. Immunization practices. In: Kleigman RM, Behrman RE, Jenson HB, Stanton BF, eds. *Nelson Textbook of Pediatrics*. 18th ed. Philadelphia, PA: WB Saunders; 2007:1058-1070.

Overby KJ. Pediatric health supervision. In: Rudolph CD, Rudolph AM, Hostetter MK, Lister G, Siegel NJ, eds. *Rudolph's Pediatrics*. 21st ed. New York, NY: McGraw-Hill; 2003:2-4, 19-30, 37-53.

# Case 10

A 4-year-old boy has a 2-day history of runny nose, productive cough, and wheezing. Subjective fever and decreased appetite also were noted today. He has no known cardiorespiratory disease, and his immunizations are current. His two younger siblings are recovering from "colds." On examination, he is febrile to 103.2°F (39.6°C), with a respiratory rate of 22 breaths/min. His examination is remarkable for congested nares, clear rhinorrhea, coarse breaths sounds in all lung fields, and bibasilar end-expiratory wheezes.

- What is the most likely diagnosis?
- What is the next step in evaluation?

# ANSWERS TO CASE 10:
## Pneumonia

*Summary:* A toddler presents with cough, fever, and an abnormal chest examination.

- **Most likely diagnosis:** Pneumonia.
- **Next step in evaluation:** A chest x-ray (CXR) often is indicated to ascertain if radiographic changes support clinical findings. In addition to chest radiography, pulse oximetry and selected laboratory tests (complete blood count [CBC], blood culture, and nasal wash for selected viral antigens) may help elucidate the etiology and extent of infection, as well as direct possible antimicrobial therapy.

## ANALYSIS

### Objectives

1. Describe the etiologies of pneumonia and their age predilections.
2. Describe various clinical and radiographic findings in pneumonia.
3. Describe the evaluation and treatment of pneumonia.

### Considerations

The most important initial goal in managing this patient is to ensure adequacy of the **ABC**s (maintaining the **A**irway, controlling the **B**reathing, and ensuring adequate **C**irculation). A patient with pneumonia may present with varying degrees of respiratory compromise. Oxygen may be required, and in severe cases respiratory failure may be imminent, necessitating intubation and mechanical ventilation. The patient with pneumonia and sepsis also may have evidence of circulatory failure (septic shock) and require vigorous fluid resuscitation. After the basics of resuscitation have been achieved, further evaluation and management can be initiated.

# APPROACH TO
## The Child with Pneumonia

## DEFINITIONS

**RALES:** Wet or "crackly" inspiratory breath sounds due to alveolar fluid or debris; usually heard in pneumonia or congestive heart failure (CHF).

**PLEURAL RUB:** Inspiratory and expiratory "rubbing" or scratching breath sounds heard when inflamed visceral and parietal pleurae come together.

**STACCATO COUGH:** Coughing spells with quiet intervals, often heard in croup and chlamydial pneumonia.

**PLEURAL EFFUSION:** Fluid accumulation in the pleural space; may be associated with chest pain or dyspnea; can be transudate or exudate depending on results of fluid analysis for protein and lactate dehydrogenase; origins include cardiovascular (congestive heart failure), infectious (mycobacterial pneumonia), and malignant (lymphoma).

**EMPYEMA:** Purulent infection in the pleural space; may be associated with chest pain, dyspnea, or fever; usually seen in conjunction with bacterial pneumonia or pulmonary abscess.

**PULSE OXIMETRY:** Noninvasive estimation of arterial oxyhemoglobin concentration ($SaO_2$) using select wavelengths of light.

## CLINICAL APPROACH

Pneumonia or lower respiratory tract infection (LRTI) is a diagnosis made clinically and radiographically. The typical pediatric patient with pneumonia may have traditional findings (fever, cough, tachypnea, and toxicity) or very few signs, depending on the organism involved and the patient's age and health status.

### Pathophysiology

LRTI typically begins with organism acquisition via inhalation of infected droplets or contact with a contaminated surface. Depending on the organism, spread to distal airways occurs over varying intervals. Bacterial infection typically progresses rapidly over a few days; viral pneumonia may develop more gradually. With infection progression, an inflammatory cascade ensues with airways affected by humoral and cellular mediators. The resulting milieu adversely affects ventilation–perfusion, and respiratory symptoms develop.

### Clinical and Radiologic Findings

The pneumonia process may produce few findings or may present with increased work of breathing manifested as nasal flaring, accessory muscle use, or tachypnea, the latter being a relatively sensitive indicator of pneumonia. Associated symptoms may include malaise, headache, abdominal pain, nausea, or emesis. Toxicity can develop, especially in bacterial pneumonia. Fever is not a constant finding. Subtle temperature instability may be noted in neonatal pneumonia. Clinically, pneumonia can be associated with decreased or abnormal breathing (rales or wheezing). Chest examination may be equivocal, especially in the neonate. Hypoxia can be seen. Pneumonia complications (pleural effusion) may be identified by finding localized decreased breath sounds or rubs.

Radiographic findings in LRTI may be limited, nonexistent, or lag the clinical symptoms, especially in the dehydrated patient. Findings may include single or multilobar consolidation (pneumococcal or staphylococcal pneumonia), air trapping with flattened diaphragm (viral pneumonia with bronchospasm), or perihilar lymphadenopathy (mycobacterial pneumonia). Alternatively, an interstitial pattern may predominate (mycoplasmal pneumonia). Finally, pleural effusion and abscess formation are more consistent with bacterial infection.

## Causative Organisms

LRTI occurs more frequently in the fall and winter and with greater frequency in younger patients, especially those in group environments (large households, day care facilities, and elementary schools). When all age groups are considered, approximately 60% of pediatric pneumonias are bacterial in origin, with pneumococcus topping the list. Viruses (respiratory syncytial virus [RSV], adenovirus, influenza, parainfluenza, enteric cytopathic human orphan [ECHO] virus, and coxsackie virus) run a close second.

Identifying an organism in pediatric pneumonia may prove difficult; causative organisms are identified in only 40% to 80% of cases. Routine culturing of the nasopharynx (poor sensitivity/specificity) or sputum (difficulty obtaining specimens in young patients) usually is not performed. Thus, diagnosis and treatment usually are directed by a patient's symptoms, physical and radiographic findings, and age.

**In the first few days of life, *Enterobacteriaceae* and group B *Streptococcus* (GBS) are the primary bacterial etiologies; other possibilities include *Staphylococcus aureus, Streptococcus pneumoniae* (pneumococcus), and *Listeria monocytogenes*.** In the newborn with pneumonia, broad-spectrum antimicrobials (ampicillin with either gentamicin or cefotaxime) are customarily prescribed. **During the first few months of life, *Chlamydia trachomatis* is a possibility, particularly in the infant with staccato cough and tachypnea, with or without conjunctivitis or known maternal chlamydia history.** These infants also have **eosinophilia, and bilateral infiltrates with hyperinflation on chest radiograph;** treatment is erythromycin. **Viral etiologies include herpes simplex virus (HSV), enterovirus, influenza, and RSV;** of these, HSV is the most concerning and prevalent viral pneumonia in the first few days of life. Acyclovir is an important consideration if HSV is suspected.

Beyond the newborn period and **through approximately 5 years of age, viral pneumonia is common; adenovirus, rhinovirus, RSV, influenza, and parainfluenza are possibilities. Bacterial etiologies include pneumococcus and nontypeable *Haemophilus influenzae*.** Patients with nasal and chest congestion with increased work of breathing, wheezing, and hypoxemia regularly present to the emergency room during the winter months and are admitted for observation, oxygen, and bronchodilator therapies. The diagnosis of a viral process may be made clinically or with CXR findings (perihilar interstitial infiltrates). Nucleic acid (PCR) amplification of secretions from a nasal swab or wash often is performed to confirm a viral etiology. A mixed viral and bacterial pneumonia can be present in approximately 20% of patients. Antibacterial coverage should be considered if the clinical scenario, examination, or x-ray findings suggest bacterial infection.

**The pediatric patient older than approximately 5 years of age with LRTI typically has mycoplasma. However, most of the viral and bacterial etiologies previously listed are possible, except GBS and *Listeria*.** Antibiotics in this age group are directed toward mycoplasma and typical bacteria (pneumococcus). Treatment options include macrolides (azithromycin) or cephalosporins (ceftriaxone or cefuroxime).

**Pneumonia in the intubated intensive care patient with central lines may be related to *Pseudomonas aeruginosa* or fungal species (*Candida*).** *Pseudomonas* and *Aspergillus* are possibilities in the patient with chronic lung disease (cystic fibrosis). Varicella-zoster virus should be considered in the patient with typical skin findings and pneumonia; cytomegalovirus (CMV) if concomitant retinitis is present; *Legionella pneumophila* if the patient has been exposed to stagnant water; and *Aspergillus* if a patient has refractory asthma or a classic "fungal ball" on chest radiograph. Travel to the southwestern United States exposes patients to *Coccidioides immitis*, infected sheep or cattle expose patients to *Coxiella brunetti*, and spelunking or working on a farm east of the Rocky Mountains exposes patients to *Histoplasma capsulatum*.

**One important subset of LRTI is tuberculosis.** *Mycobacterium tuberculosis* has become more problematic over the past decade; multidrug resistance is increasingly seen. Patients may present with symptoms ranging from a traditional cough, bloody sputum, fever, and weight loss to subtle or nonspecific symptoms. A positive purified protein derivative (PPD) is defined by induration diameter in the context of a patient's exposure history, radiographic findings, and immune status. For instance, 5-mm induration may be considered a "positive" PPD at 48 to 72 hours in a patient with confirmed exposure, abnormal chest radiograph, or immunodeficiency. This same measurement in an otherwise healthy child without exposures would not be considered positive. Possible sources for acid-fast bacilli for stain and culture (depending on the age of the patient) include first-morning sputum samples, gastric aspirates, bronchial washes or biopsy obtained via bronchoscopy, and empyema fluid analysis or pleural biopsy if surgical intervention is required. Standard antituberculous therapy while awaiting culture and sensitivities includes isoniazid, rifampin, and pyrazinamide. For possible drug-resistant organisms, ethambutol can be added temporarily as long as visual acuity can be followed. The typical antibiotic course consists of an initial phase of approximately 2 months' duration on three or four medications, followed by a continuation phase of 4 to 7 months on isoniazid and rifampin. Total therapy duration is dependent upon the extent of CXR abnormalities, resistance patterns, and results of follow-up sputum samples. Directly observed therapy should be routinely advised.

## Comprehension Questions

10.1 A 6-week-old boy, born by vaginal delivery after an uncomplicated term gestation, has experienced cough and "fast breathing" for 2 days. His mother relates that he has a 1-week history of nasal congestion and watery eye discharge, but no fever or change in appetite. He has a temperature of 99.4°F (37.4°C) and a respiratory rate of 44 breaths/min. He has nasal congestion, clear rhinorrhea, erythematous conjunctivae bilaterally, and watery, right eye discharge. His lungs demonstrate scattered crackles without wheezes. Which of the following is the most likely pathogen?

A. *C trachomatis*
B. *L monocytogenes*
C. Respiratory syncytial virus
D. Rhinovirus
E. *S pneumoniae*

10.2 A 2-year-old girl has increased work of breathing. Her father notes she has had cough and subjective fever over the past 3 days. She has been complaining that her "belly hurts" and has experienced one episode of posttussive emesis but no diarrhea. Her immunizations are current, and she is otherwise healthy. Her temperature is 102°F (38.9°C). She is somnolent but easily aroused. Respirations are 28 breaths/min, and her examination is remarkable for decreased breath sounds at the left base posteriorly with prominent crackles. Which of the following acute interventions is the next best step in your evaluation?

A. Blood culture
B. Chest radiography
C. Pulse oximetry
D. Sputum culture
E. Viral nasal swab

10.3 You are evaluating a previously healthy 8-year-old boy with subjective fever, sore throat, and cough over the past week. There has been no rhinorrhea, emesis or diarrhea, and his appetite is unchanged. According to your clinic records, his immunizations are current and his weight was at the 25th percentile on his examination 6 months ago. Today he is noted at the 10th percentile for weight. He is afebrile, with clear nares and posterior oropharynx, and a normal respiratory effort. He has bilateral cervical and right supraclavicular lymphadenopathy. Chest auscultation is notable for diminished breath sounds at the left base. Beyond obtaining a chest radiograph, which of the following is the best next step in your evaluation?

A. Rapid strep throat swab
B. Viral nasal swab
C. PPD placement
D. Lymph node biopsy
E. *Bordetella pertussis* direct fluorescent antibody testing

10.4 A 13-year-old adolescent female complains of dry cough, slight fever, and fatigue over the past 2 weeks. She noted increased chest congestion and coughing yesterday when walking outside in the cold air. She denies nasal congestion, rhinorrhea, emesis, or diarrhea. Her mother declares her daughter is generally healthy with a history of only summertime allergies. Her vital signs, respiratory effort, and chest examination are normal. Which of the following is the most likely pathogen?

A. *H influenzae*
B. *M pneumoniae*
C. Respiratory syncytial virus
D. *S aureus*
E. *S pneumoniae*

## ANSWERS

10.1 **A.** Cough and increased respiratory effort in an afebrile infant with eye discharge are consistent with *Chlamydia*. Transmission typically occurs during vaginal delivery. Approximately 25% of infants born to mothers with *Chlamydia* develop conjunctivitis; about half of these develop pneumonia. Most infants present with respiratory infection in the second month of life, but symptoms can be seen as early as the second week. Inner eyelid swabs are sent for PCR, and oral erythromycin or sulfisoxazole (latter only in infants older than 2 months of age) is given for 2 weeks for either conjunctivitis or pneumonia.

10.2 **C.** Tachypnea and lethargy are prominent in this patient with clinical pneumonia. Pulse oximetry should urgently be performed to ascertain whether oxygen is required. Sputum culturing is reasonable, but an adequate and diagnostically useful specimen can only be obtained from a 2-year-old by endotracheal aspirate or bronchoscopy. In this otherwise healthy toddler for whom concerns for atypical pneumonia are high, invasive maneuvers are not indicated. Viruses (RSV and adenovirus) are prominent at this age; one might consider performing a nasal swab for viral antigens. Abdominal pain, as noted in this question, can be seen as a presenting symptom in pneumonia, probably as a result of irritation of the diaphragm by pulmonary infection.

10.3 **C.** The scenario is typical for pediatric tuberculosis. Neck and perihilar or mediastinal lymphadenopathy and pulmonary or extrapulmonary manifestations can occur, with miliary disease and meningitis more common in infants and younger children. Fever, weight loss, and lower respiratory tract signs and symptoms (possible left pleural effusion in this patient) are archetypal tuberculosis (TB) findings. A PPD should be placed, and consideration given to hospitalizing this patient in negative pressure isolation for further evaluation beyond PPD placement (pleurocentesis, bronchoalveolar lavage, gastric aspirates) and possible antituberculous treatment.

10.4 **B.** All of these findings are consistent with mycoplasmal infection ("walking pneumonia"). The incubation period for mycoplasma is 5 to 7 days, and most symptoms are noted during the second to third week of infection. Hemolysis occurs as antibodies attach to red blood cells, prompting reticulocyte production. If necessary, nasopharyngeal aspirate for PCR or measurement of cold agglutinins may help aid in the diagnosis. Auscultatory and radiographic findings vary in this infection; a normal CXR or one with an interstitial pattern, effusion, or atelectasis could be seen.

## Clinical Pearls

- The etiology of pneumonia varies according to the patient's age. Neonates have the greatest risk of group B *Streptococcus*, toddlers are more likely to have respiratory syncytial virus, and adolescents usually contract mycoplasma.
- Efforts in tuberculosis management should be directed toward isolating an organism and obtaining sensitivities, thus allowing selection of the optimal antituberculous regimen.

## REFERENCES

Kennedy WA. Disorders of the lungs and pleura. In: Osborn LM, DeWitt TG, First LR, Zenel JA, eds. *Pediatrics*. 1st ed. Philadelphia, PA: Elsevier-Mosby; 2005:803-818.

Moscona A, Murrell MT, Horga M, Burroughs M. Respiratory infections. In: Katz SL, Hotez PJ, Gerson AA, eds. *Krugman's Infectious Diseases of Children*. 11th ed. Philadelphia, PA: Mosby; 2005:493-524.

Roosevelt GE. Acute inflammatory upper airway obstruction. In: Kliegman RM, Behrman RE, Jenson HB, Stanton BF, eds. *Nelson Textbook of Pediatrics*. 18th ed. Philadelphia, PA: WB Saunders; 2007:1762-1766.

Sectish TC, Prober CG. Pneumonia. In: Kliegman RM, Behrman RE, Jenson HB, Stanton BF, eds. *Nelson Textbook of Pediatrics*. 18th ed. Philadelphia, PA: WB Saunders; 2007:1795-1799.

# Case 11

You are moonlighting in a rural emergency room when a father rushes his 3-year-old daughter into the waiting area. You quickly determine that he and the child have been at a relative's farm where they were spraying for bugs in an old barn. The child had been fine, but while at the farm developed abdominal cramping, cough, drooling, and tearing. While in route the child seems to be having increased respiratory difficulty, and the dad notes she soiled and urinated upon herself.

- What is the most likely diagnosis?
- How is the diagnosis made?
- What is the best therapy?

# ANSWERS TO CASE 11: Organophosphate Poisoning

*Summary:* A 3-year-old, previously healthy child who, while helping her father spray for bugs, develops salivation, lacrimation, respiratory distress, and gastrointestinal (GI) symptoms.

- **Most likely diagnosis:** Organophosphate poisoning.
- **Making the diagnosis:** High index of suspicion so therapy is not delayed; confirmation via decreased serum pseudocholinesterase and erythrocyte cholinesterase levels.
- **Best therapy:** Decontamination of the child, supportive care, administration of atropine or pralidoxime.

## ANALYSIS

### Objectives

1. Understand the signs, symptoms, and treatment of organophosphate poisoning.
2. Be familiar with the treatment options of various commonly ingested agents.

### Considerations

This child is demonstrating evidence of organophosphate poisoning, the leading cause of nonpharmaceutical ingestion fatality in children. She was exposed during the spraying for insects in the barn, and is at risk for ongoing absorption of toxin until decontamination of her clothing is achieved.

*Note:* For some children exposed to a toxic substance, parents are able to provide a container of the toxic agent. For others either the container is not available or the symptoms are not obviously related to a toxic exposure. In all cases a thorough history and physical examination, along with a high index of suspicion in younger children, is required to ensure the diagnosis of accidental toxic exposure is made.

# APPROACH TO
## Organophosphate Poisoning

## DEFINITIONS

**NICOTINIC SYMPTOMS:** Cardiac (hypertension, tachycardia, arrhythmia); muscle (fasciculations, weakness, tremors); respiratory failure due to diaphragm paralysis; hypertension.

**MUSCARINIC SYMPTOMS:** Gastrointestinal (emesis, urinary and fecal incontinence); respiratory (bronchorrhea, bronchospasm); cardiac (hypotension, bradycardia); tearing and drooling; miosis.

## CLINICAL APPROACH

Millions of children are poisoned each year with about 90% of exposures occurring in the home. About half of all accidental poisonings occur in children younger than 5 years of age. Children aged from about 6 to 12 years are much less likely to be exposed, and those with toxic exposures beyond 12 years of age often do so intentionally. Death due to accidental poisonings has become unusual since a variety of measures have been implemented, including poison prevention as part of all well-child visits, development of regional poison control centers, child-resistant packaging, and improved medical management.

Organophosphate poisoning can occur across skin or mucous membranes, by inhalation, or by ingestion. Commonly found in such pesticides as parathion, malathion, and diazinon, organophosphates bind irreversibly to cholinesterase of neurons and erythrocytes, as well as to liver pseudocholinesterase. The common finding is failure to terminate the effects of acetylcholine at the receptor sites.

Signs and symptoms of cholinergic excess are often remembered with the mnemonic "dumb bells" which includes

D diarrhea/defecation
U urination
M miosis
B brachycardia
B bronchorrhea
E emesis/excitation of muscles
L lacrimation
S salivation

In addition to these muscarinic and nicotinic effects, central effects including obtundation, seizures, and apnea are seen.

Confirmation of the exposure can be confirmed by finding decreased serum pseudocholinesterase and erythrocyte cholinesterase levels, but the correlation to these levels to the magnitude of exposure or the symptoms observed is poor. Thus, a high index of suspicion must be maintained to quickly and accurately diagnose organophosphate exposure.

Treatment of the patient exposed to organophosphate consists of rapid decontamination by removing all clothing and washing of all skin surfaces. For ingestions, gastric lavage or activated charcoal may be attempted, but the compounds are rapidly absorbed and the benefits somewhat limited. The **ABC**s of medicine apply: preserve the **A**irway (intubation may be required); maintain **B**reathing (excessive secretions may require frequent suctioning); and ensure appropriate **C**irculation.

Two specific therapies to counter the effects of organophosphate poisonings include atropine and pralidoxime. Atropine works by antagonizing the muscarinic receptor; large, repeated, and sometimes continuous doses may be required. Often the amount and number of atropine doses required correlates to the degree of exposure and may assist in the prediction of course duration. Pralidoxime is a cholinesterase-reactivating oxime, often used for patients with significant muscle weakness, especially if mechanical ventilation is required owing to muscle failure.

Careful attention to a child's environment can help prevent countless instances of toxic ingestion. Counseling parents to "poison proof" their home is a first step toward prevention. Written and video materials are readily available through the American Academy of Pediatrics, local and state health departments, and poison control centers. All families are taught to become familiar with the national network of poison control centers, reached toll-free at 1-800-222-1222.

## Comprehension Questions

11.1 Students attending a school built in 1951 are at risk for which of the following?

A. Arsenic
B. Asbestos
C. Dichlorodiphenyltrichloroethane (DDT)
D. Mercury
E. Polychlorinated biphenyls (PCBs)

11.2 An 8-year-old, mentally delayed child ingests the contents of a mercury thermometer. Which of the following symptoms are most likely to be seen?

A. Ataxia, dysarthria, and paresthesias
B. Chest pain and dyspnea
C. Gingivostomatitis, tremor, and neuropsychiatric disturbances
D. No symptoms
E. Pulmonary fibrosis

11.3 A 4-year-old child is found with a bottle of insecticide that contains arsenic. Which of the following symptoms is most likely to occur?
A. Bradycardia with third-degree heart block
B. Constipation
C. Hemorrhagic gastroenteritis with third spacing of fluids
D. Hyperreflexia
E. Hypothermia

11.4 Exposure to environmental toxins can occur in a number of ways. Which of the following is the most likely mechanism of exposure?
A. Asbestos exposure from hazardous arts and crafts materials
B. Exposure of a child to beryllium from the child's parents' clothing
C. Iron intoxication from vehicular emissions
D. Lead toxicity from ingesting pieces of a pencil
E. Transplacental exposure to benzene

## ANSWERS

11.1 **B.** Between 1947 and 1973 asbestos was commonly sprayed on school ceilings as a fire retardant. Deterioration results in release of microscopic fibers into the air. Drop ceilings or placement of barriers usually is sufficient protection against this carcinogen.

11.2 **D.** The child in the question is unlikely to develop symptoms (the quantity of mercury is small); a larger acute elemental ingestion might result in a variety of gastrointestinal (GI) complaints. If the elemental mercury were in vapor form, GI complaints would be seen, along with fever, chills, headaches, visual changes, cough, chest pain, and possibly pneumonitis and pulmonary edema. Exposure to inorganic mercury salts (pesticides, disinfectants, explosives, dry batteries) can cause gastroesophageal burns, nausea, vomiting, abdominal pain, hematemesis, hematochezia, cardiovascular collapse, or death. Ataxia, dysarthria, and paresthesias are seen in methyl mercury intoxication (contaminated fish exposure). Gingivostomatitis, tremor, and neuropsychiatric disturbances are seen with chronic inorganic mercury intoxication; indeed, the term "mad as a hatter" originates from the occupational hazard of workers' exposure in the early industrial period to mercury-containing vapors during the process of felt hat making.

11.3 **C.** Acute arsenic ingestions can cause nausea, vomiting, abdominal pain, and diarrhea. The third spacing and hemorrhage in the gut can lead to hypovolemic shock. Cardiac symptoms include ventricular tachycardia (QT prolongation) and congestive heart failure (CHF). These patients can develop seizures, cerebral edema, encephalopathy, and coma. Early on, patients develop loss of deep tendon reflexes, paralysis, painful dysesthesias, and respiratory failure similar to Guillain-Barré syndrome. Fever, anemia, alopecia, hepatitis, and renal failure also can be seen.

11.4 **B.** Fat-soluble compounds can be transmitted transplacentally (but benzene would be unusual). Parents' work clothes can transmit potentially hazardous compounds. Arts and crafts supplies likely do not contain asbestos. Vehicular emissions are responsible for a number of pollutants, many of which are carcinogens, but iron intoxication would be unusual. Pencil "lead" is actually graphite (carbon) and not elemental lead.

## Clinical Pearls

- Organophosphate poisoning is the leading cause of nonpharmacologic ingestion fatality in the United States.
- The mnemonic "dumb bells" outlines the signs and symptoms of cholinergic excess.
- Therapy for organophosphate toxicity includes supportive care and use of either atropine or pralidoxime.

## REFERENCES

Fortenberry JD, Mariscalco MM. General principles of poisoning management. In: McMillan JA, Feigin RD, DeAngelis CD, Jones MD, eds. *Oski's Pediatrics: Principles and Practice*. 4th ed. Philadelphia, PA: Lippincott Williams & Wilkins; 2006:747-754.

Rodgers GC, Condurache T, Reed MD, Bestic M, Gal P. Poisonings. In: Kleigman RM, Behrman RE, Jenson HB, Stanton BF, eds. *Nelson Textbook of Pediatrics*. 18th ed. Philadelphia, PA: WB Saunders; 2007:339-357.

Tenenbein M. Toxic ingestions and exposures. In: Rudolph CD, Rudolph AM, Hostetter MK, Lister G, Siegel NJ, eds. *Rudolph's Pediatrics*. 21st ed. New York, NY: McGraw-Hill; 2003:354–379.

# Case 12

A mother brings her 8-year-old daughter to your office because she has noticed a "yellowish" stain on her daughter's panties. The mother reports the girl recently started using many sexually explicit words, her grades have dropped significantly, and she has become quiet and reluctant to interact. When interviewed alone, the child begins crying and states that her mother's boyfriend touches her "private with his private part." The child's physical examination is normal, except for a yellowish vaginal discharge and erythema of the perihymenal tissue. A wet mount microscopic examination is negative for trichomonads, bacterial vaginosis, and yeast. A nucleic acid amplification test (NAAT) from the vagina is negative for *Chlamydia trachomatis* but is positive for *Neisseria gonorrhoeae*.

- ➤ What is the best management for this condition?
- ➤ What is your next step in the evaluation?

# ANSWERS TO CASE 12:
# Sexual Abuse

*Summary:* An 8-year-old girl has a positive NAAT for *N gonorrhoeae*. She disclosed that her mother's boyfriend sexually abused her.

- **Best management:** Confirm the test result by performing a second test (either a true culture for *N gonorrhoeae* or a second NAAT that targets a different portion of the organism's genome) and then administer treatment in the form of a single dose of ceftriaxone 125 mg intramuscularly.
- **Next step:** A blood test for human immunodeficiency virus (HIV) antibody and rapid plasma reagin (RPR) for syphilis should be obtained. Children's Protective Services and/or law enforcement *must* be notified.

## ANALYSIS

### Objectives

1. Know how to approach the medical evaluation of a child who complains that she has been sexually abused.
2. Know that most children who are sexually abused have no physical findings of abuse.
3. Be familiar with the different diagnostic testing methods for chlamydia and gonorrhea.

### Considerations

Nucleic acid amplification tests (NAATs) are highly sensitive and specific tests commonly used to detect infections caused by *C trachomatis* and *N gonorrhoeae*. The gravity of these diagnoses in children dictates confirmation of a positive test with either a true culture or a second NAAT that targets a different portion of the organism's genome. Consultation with a child abuse pediatrician or pediatric infectious disease specialist is also recommended in these cases.

Transmission of *N gonorrhoeae* occurs only via sexual contact. Therefore, a confirmed diagnosis indicates that this child was sexually abused. An attempt to identify when the last sexual contact is thought to have occurred is important because periodic testing for HIV and syphilis is indicated for at least 6 months. It is important to determine if this child's home environment is safe. Children's Protective Services and law enforcement officials generally work in tandem to ensure the safety of the child and to perform criminal investigations of child sexual abuse. Child abuse specialists can help coordinate this child's care and provide assistance in medical management.

# APPROACH TO
## Sexual Abuse in the Child

## DEFINITIONS

**SEXUAL ABUSE:** Sexual activity in which a child engages but which the child cannot comprehend, cannot give consent to, or is not developmentally prepared for; or sexual activity that is a violation of the law or societal taboos. Coercion, power imbalance, or a significant age gap may be present.

**NUCLEIC ACID AMPLIFICATION TEST (NAAT):** A nonculture method that may be used on swab or urine specimens to test for C *trachomatis* and N *gonorrhoeae*.

## CLINICAL APPROACH

It is estimated that by age 18 years, one in four women and one in six men in the United States are victims of sexual abuse. Abuse can be noncontact (exhibitionism, voyeurism, pornography) or contact (fondling, anogenital contact). **Most victims of sexual abuse know their abusers; they may be family members, friends, or acquaintances.**

Supportive and sensitive history taking, detailed documentation of the child's disclosure, and careful examination are imperative. **More than three quarters of sexually abused children** have **no sign of physical trauma on examination** (in part because anogenital area tissues heal rapidly and often without scarring), and even fewer have a sexually transmitted disease (STD). When injury does occur, it may be **nonspecific** (erythema); occasionally there are signs of penetrating trauma, such as a tear of the posterior hymen (ie, between the 3 and 9 o'clock positions) or a deep tear into the anal muscle. If the suspected abuse occurred near the time of medical evaluation (eg, within approximately 72 hours), forensic evidence may be available from the child's body or the clothing worn at the time of the assault. An "evidence collection kit" is used for such specimen collection; contents are kept in police laboratories and are analyzed if legal proceedings require.

Pediatric sexual assault victims are tested for sexually transmissible diseases (chlamydia, gonorrhea, trichomonas, HIV, and syphilis) whenever anal-genital, genital-genital, or oral-genital contact has occurred. Historically, true cultures for chlamydia and gonorrhea have been preferred in prepubertal children and nonsexually active teens because of their high specificities. However, it may be desirable to perform a more sensitive NAAT. Because of its potential implications, a positive NAAT result for a prepubertal child or nonsexually active teen must be confirmed with either a culture or a second NAAT that amplifies a different gene sequence. In the acute setting, prophylactic STD and pregnancy medications may be indicated. All sexual abuse victims require psychological support. Social workers can be helpful in identifying and mitigating stressors in the child's environment.

## Comprehension Questions

12.1 A developmentally delayed 18-year-old adolescent female tells her mother that someone at her day care facility has been "messing with her." The mother brings her to you for evaluation for sexual abuse. Which of the following statements about this child's possible sexual abuse is more likely to be accurate?

A. This developmentally delayed girl is at a lower risk for abuse than a developmentally appropriate child.
B. This girl was most likely sexually abused by a stranger.
C. If this child is a victim of chronic sexual abuse, physical evidence is unlikely.
D. Most children, like this girl, immediately disclose their sexual abuse.
E. If this nonsexually active adolescent develops a culture positive for chlamydia or gonorrhea, a nonsexual mode of transmission must be sought.

12.2 An 18-month-old boy is brought to clinic by his father because the child has perianal "skin tags." The child lives with his mother and father, and the father reports no history of potential sexual abuse. The mother has a 15-year history of venereal warts. Examination reveals cauliflower-like warts in the perianal area. Which of the following is the most likely cause of this finding?

A. Condyloma acuminata (human papillomavirus [HPV]) acquired at sexual abuse
B. Condyloma acuminata (HPV) acquired from birth
C. Herpes type I
D. Herpes type II
E. *Molluscum contagiosum*

12.3 A 7-year-old girl has itching for 1 week in her "front and back private parts." She has no history of skin disorders. She has not changed her soap, clothes washing detergents, or clothing. She states that no one has touched her inappropriately in her private places. The mother reports that her daughter's appetite has decreased over the past month, and she occasionally complains of abdominal pain. Examination is normal except for some mild perianal erythema. Which of the following is the most likely cause of her problem?

A. Eczema
B. Gonorrhea
C. Lichen sclerosus
D. Pinworms
E. Psoriasis

12.4 A 9-year-old boy has bright red rectal bleeding off and on for a few months. He has a history of constipation and intermittent encopresis. He denies inappropriate touching in the area. Upon examination, the child's anus has lost its stellate pattern and its tone. He has three deep fissures in the anus and a scar at 8 o'clock. Which of the following is a likely cause of the boy's findings?

A. Constipation
B. Eczema
C. Hemorrhoids
D. Hirschsprung disease
E. Penetrating anal trauma

## ANSWERS

12.1 **C.** Many girls abused over time neither report the abuse nor show physical evidence of penetrating vaginal trauma. Physical complaints that *sometimes* are associated with sexual abuse include dysuria, enuresis, frequent urinary tract infections (UTIs), genital irritation and itching, vaginal or penile discharge, vaginal bleeding, genital or anal pain, abdominal pain, and encopresis. Nonspecific behavioral findings *may* include nightmares, sleep disorders, developmentally inappropriate sexual behaviors, regressive behaviors, eating disorders, acting out aggressively, poor school performance, and poor peer relationships. The list of alternative diagnoses includes dermatologic conditions, nonsexual trauma, constipation, vaginal foreign bodies, psychosocial stressors, and psychiatric illness. In most cases, the perpetrator of sexual abuse is known to the victim. Developmentally delayed children are at higher risk. Except in cases of vertical transmission, Chlamydia and gonorrhea are diagnostic of sexual contact.

12.2 **B.** Anal condylomata in children younger than age 3 years are often acquired at birth through direct contact with genital condylomata in the birth canal. A full history is important to determine the risk of abuse versus the risk of acquiring the infection at birth.

12.3 **D.** Pinworms cause intense itching, loss of appetite, and episodic abdominal pain; humans are the only natural host (see also Case 38). Viewing under a microscope adhesive tape placed over the anus can identify the worm's eggs (and, less likely, a tiny, threadlike worm). Treatment usually consists of a single dose of mebendazole, which is repeated in 2 weeks. Family members who sleep in the child's bed also are treated. Bed clothes are washed at the time of treatment because ova can remain viable for 2 to 3 weeks in moist environments. Eczema could involve more than just the perianal region.

12.4 **E.** Repeated penetrating anal trauma causes loss of stellate pattern of the anus, loss of tone, and deep fissures. Constipation would be less likely to cause such dramatic findings. Sexual abuse must be suspected, and further history is indicated.

## Clinical Pearls

- It is estimated that by age 18 years, one in four women and one in six men in the United States are victims of sexual abuse.
- Most victims of sexual abuse know their abusers; they may be family members, friends, or acquaintances.
- Most sexually abused children have no physical signs of abuse.
- Careful attention must be paid to the method of testing for chlamydia and gonorrhea in children; serologies for human immunodeficiency virus and syphilis should be periodically checked until at least 6 months have elapsed following the assault.

## REFERENCES

Centers for Disease Control and Prevention. Sexually transmitted diseases treatment guidelines, 2006. *MMWR Morb Mortal Wkly Rep*. 2006;55(RR11):1-94.

Heger A, Ticson L, Velasquez O, Bernier R. Children referred for possible sexual abuse: medical findings in 2384 children. *Child Abuse Negl*. 2002;26:645-659.

Kellogg N and the Committee on Child Abuse and Neglect. The evaluation of sexual abuse in children. *Pediatrics*. 2005;116:506-512.

# Case 13

A 4-year-old child complains of ear pain. He has a temperature of 102.1°F (38.9°C) and has had a cold for several days, but he has been eating well and his activity has been essentially normal.

- ➤ What is the most likely diagnosis?
- ➤ What is the best therapy?

# ANSWERS TO CASE 13: Acute Otitis Media

*Summary:* A toddler presents with ear pain and fever.

- **Most likely diagnosis:** Acute otitis media (AOM)
- **Best therapy:** Oral antibiotics

## ANALYSIS

### Objectives

1. Be familiar with the epidemiology of otitis media (OM) in children.
2. Understand the treatment option for this condition.
3. Learn the consequences of severe infection.

### Considerations

Otitis media is high on the differential diagnosis for this child with upper respiratory infection (URI) and ear pain. The diagnosis can be confirmed by pneumatic otoscopy and treatment started. A "telephone diagnosis" should be avoided. Figure 13–1 illustrates the anatomy of the middle ear.

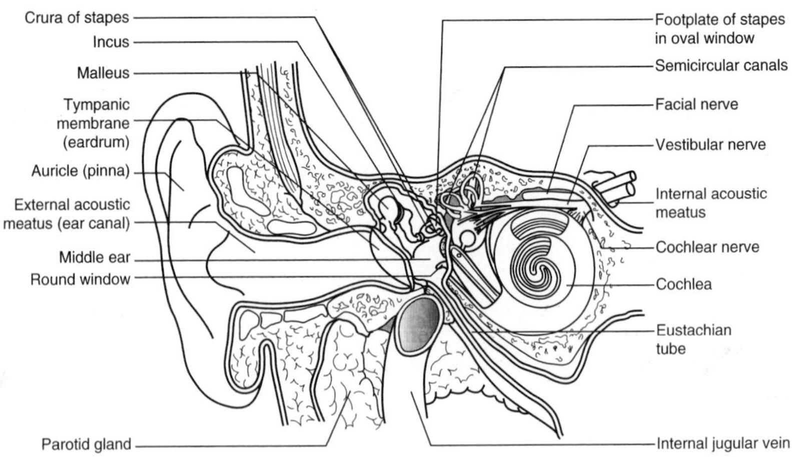


**Figure 13–1.** Anatomy of the middle ear. (*Redrawn, with permission, from Rudolph CD, Rudolph AM, Hostetter MK, Lister G, Siegel NJ, eds.* Rudolph's Pediatrics. *21st ed. New York, NY: McGraw-Hill; 2003:1240.*)

# APPROACH TO
## Acute Otitis Media

## DEFINITIONS

**ACUTE OTITIS MEDIA (AOM):** A condition of otalgia (ear pain), fever, and other symptoms along with findings of a red, opaque, poorly moving, bulging tympanic membrane (TM).

**MYRINGOTOMY AND PLACEMENT OF PRESSURE EQUALIZATION TUBES:** A surgical procedure involving TM incision and placement of pressure equalization (PE) tubes (tiny plastic or metal tubes anchored into the TM) to ventilate the middle ear and help prevent reaccumulation of middle ear fluid.

**OTITIS MEDIA WITH EFFUSION:** A condition in which fluid collects behind the TM but without signs and symptoms of AOM. Sometimes called serous OM.

**PNEUMATIC OTOSCOPY:** The process of obtaining a tight ear canal seal with a speculum and then applying slight positive and negative pressure with a rubber bulb to verify TM mobility.

**TYMPANOCENTESIS:** A minor surgical procedure in which a small incision is made into the TM to drain pus and fluid from the middle ear space. This procedure is rarely done in the primary care office, but rather is done by the specialist.

## CLINICAL APPROACH

Otitis media is a common childhood diagnosis. **Common bacterial pathogens include *Streptococcus pneumoniae*, nontypeable *Haemophilus influenzae*, and *Moraxella catarrhalis*.** Other organisms, *Staphylococcus aureus*, *Escherichia coli*, *Klebsiella pneumoniae*, and *Pseudomonas aeruginosa*, are seen in neonates and patients with immune deficiencies. Viruses can cause AOM, and in many cases the etiology is unknown. Acute OM is diagnosed in a child with fever (usually <104°F [40°C]), ear pain (often nocturnal awakening child from sleep), and generalized malaise. Systemic symptoms include anorexia, nausea, vomiting, diarrhea, and headache. Examination findings include a **red, bulging TM that does not move well with pneumatic otoscopy.** The TM may be opaque with pus behind it, the middle ear landmarks may be obscured, and, if the TM has ruptured, pus may be seen in the ear canal. Normal landmarks are shown in Figure 13–2.

Depending on a community's bacterial resistance patterns, amoxicillin at doses up to 80 to 90 mg/kg/d for 7 to 10 days is often the initial treatment. If clinical failure is noted after 3 treatment days, a change to amoxicillin-clavulanate,

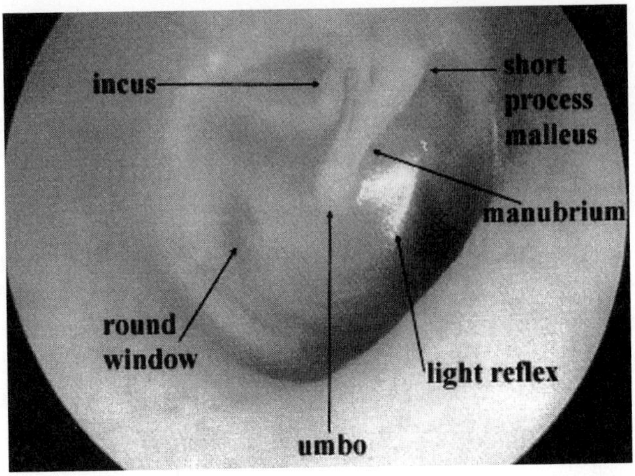


**Figure 13–2.** The tympanic membrane. (*Reproduced, with permission, from Rudolph CD, Rudolph AM, Hostetter MK, Lister G, Siegel NJ, eds.* Rudolph's Pediatrics. *21st ed. New York, NY: McGraw-Hill; 2003:1240.)*

cefuroxime axetil, azithromycin, cefixime, ceftriaxone, or tympanocentesis is considered. Adjuvant therapies (analgesics or antipyretics) are often indicated, but other measures (antihistamines, decongestants, and corticosteroids) are ineffective.

**After an AOM episode, middle ear fluid can persist for up to several months.** If hearing is normal, middle ear effusion often is treated with observation; some practitioners treat with antibiotics. **When the fluid does not resolve or recurrent episodes of suppurative OM occur, especially if hearing loss is noted, myringotomy with PE tubes is often used.**

Rare but serious OM **complications** include **mastoiditis, temporal bone osteomyelitis, facial nerve paralysis**, epidural and subdural abscess formation, meningitis, lateral sinus thrombosis, and otitic hydrocephalus (evidence of increased intracranial pressure with OM). An AOM patient whose clinical course is unusual or prolonged is evaluated for one of these conditions.

## Comprehension Questions

13.1 An 8-year-old boy has severe pain with ear movement. He has no fever, nausea, vomiting, or other symptoms. He has been in good health, having just returned from summer camp where he swam, rode horses, and water-skied. Ear examination reveals a somewhat red pinna that is extremely tender with movement, a very red and swollen ear canal, but an essentially normal TM. Which of the following is the most appropriate next course of therapy?

A. Administration of topical mixture of polymyxin and corticosteroids
B. High-dose oral amoxicillin
C. Intramuscular ceftriaxone
D. Intravenous vancomycin
E. Tympanocentesis and culture

13.2 Three days after beginning oral amoxicillin therapy for OM, a 4-year-old boy has continued fever, ear pain, and swelling with redness behind his ear. His ear lobe is pushed superiorly and laterally. He seems to be doing well otherwise. Which of the following is the most appropriate course of action?

A. Change to oral amoxicillin-clavulanate
B. Myringotomy and parenteral antibiotics
C. Nuclear scan of the head
D. Topical steroids
E. Tympanocentesis

13.3 A 5-year-old girl developed high fever, ear pain, and vomiting 1 week ago. She was diagnosed with OM and started on amoxicillin-clavulanate. On the third day of this medication she continued with findings of OM, fever, and pain. She received ceftriaxone intramuscularly and switched to oral cefuroxime. Now, 48 hours later, she has fever, pain, and no improvement in her OM; otherwise she is doing well. Which of the following is the most logical next step in her management?

A. Addition of intranasal topical steroids to the oral cefuroxime
B. Adenoidectomy
C. High-dose oral amoxicillin
D. Oral trimethoprim-sulfamethoxazole
E. Tympanocentesis and culture of middle ear fluid

13.4 A 1-month-old boy has a fever to 102.7°F (39.3°C), is irritable, has diarrhea, and has not been eating well. On examination he has an immobile red TM that has pus behind it. Which of the following is the most appropriate course of action?

A. Admission to the hospital with complete sepsis evaluation
B. Intramuscular ceftriaxone and close outpatient follow-up
C. Oral amoxicillin-clavulanate
D. Oral cefuroxime
E. High-dose oral amoxicillin

## ANSWERS

13.1 **A.** The patient likely has an otitis externa that was caused by his swimming (also known as swimmer's ear). Treatment is the application of a topical agent as described. Insertion of a wick may assist in excess fluid absorption in the macerated ear canal. Causative organisms include *Pseudomonas* species (or other gram-negative organisms), *S aureus*, and occasionally fungus (*Candida* or *Aspergillus* species).

13.2 **B.** The child has mastoiditis, a clinical diagnosis that can require CT scan confirmation. Treatment includes myringotomy, fluid culture, and parenteral antibiotics. Surgical drainage of the mastoid air cells may be needed if improvement is not seen in 24 to 48 hours.

13.3 **E.** After failing several antibiotic regimens, tympanocentesis and culture of the middle ear fluid are indicated.

13.4 **A.** Very young children with OM (especially if irritable or lethargic) are at higher risk for bacteremia or other serious infection. Hospitalization and parenteral antibiotics often are needed.

## Clinical Pearls

- The most common bacterial pathogens causing otitis media (OM) are *S pneumoniae*, nontypeable *H influenzae*, and *M catarrhalis*.
- Examination findings of otitis media include a red, bulging tympanic membrane that does not move well with pneumatic otoscopy, an opaque tympanic membrane with pus behind it, obscured middle-ear landmarks, and, if the tympanic membrane has ruptured, pus in the ear canal.
- Initial treatment of otitis media often includes amoxicillin (depending on local rate of resistant *S pneumonia*). If a clinical failure is seen on day 3, a change to amoxicillin-clavulanate, cefuroxime axetil, ceftriaxone, or a tympanocentesis is indicated.
- Complications are rare but include mastoiditis, temporal bone osteomyelitis, facial nerve palsy, epidural and subdural abscess formation, meningitis, lateral sinus thrombosis, and otitic hydrocephalus.

## REFERENCES

Haddad J. External otitis (otitis externa). In: Kleigman RM, Behrman RE, Jenson HB, Stanton BF, eds. *Nelson Textbook of Pediatrics*. 18th ed. Philadelphia, PA: WB Saunders; 2007:2629-2632.

Kerschner JE. Otitis media. In: Kleigman RM, Behrman RE, Jenson HB, Stanton BF, eds. *Nelson Textbook of Pediatrics*. 18th ed. Philadelphia, PA: WB Saunders; 2007:2632-2646.

Kline MW. Otitis externa. In: McMillan JA, Feigin RD, DeAngelis CD, Jones MD, eds. *Oski's Pediatrics: Principles and Practice*. 4th ed. Philadelphia, PA: Lippincott Williams & Wilkins; 2006:1496-1497.

Kline MW. Mastoiditis. In: McMillan JA, Feigin RD, DeAngelis CD, Jones MD, eds. *Oski's Pediatrics: Principles and Practice*. 4th ed. Philadelphia, PA: Lippincott Williams & Wilkins; 2006:1501-1502.

Rutter MJ, Choo D. Otitis media. In: Rudolph CD, Rudolph AM, Hostetter MK, Lister G, Siegel NJ, eds. *Rudolph's Pediatrics*. 21st ed. New York, NY: McGraw-Hill, 2003:1249-1256.

Schwarzwald H, Kline MW. Otitis media. In: McMillan JA, Feigin RD, DeAngelis CD, Jones MD, eds. *Oski's Pediatrics: Principles and Practice*. 4th ed. Philadelphia, PA: Lippincott Williams & Wilkins; 2006:1497-1500.

# Case 14

You are called stat to the delivery room because a now 2-minute-old infant was born floppy and blue and has not responded well to stimulation and blow-by oxygen. The obstetrician who is resuscitating the infant informs you that the child was born by a spontaneous vaginal delivery to a 24-year-old gravida 1 woman. Her pregnancy was uncomplicated. Fetal heart tones were stable throughout the labor. Spinal anesthesia was partially effective and was supplemented with intravenous (IV) meperidine (Demerol) and promethazine (Phenergan). The amniotic fluid was not bile-stained, and the mother had no evidence of intraamniotic infection.

➤ What is the next step?

# ANSWER TO CASE 14:
# Neonatal Resuscitation

*Summary:* A newborn is born floppy, blue, and has responded poorly to initial resuscitation efforts.

- **Next step:** Evaluate for heart rate (HR) and respirations. If no respirations are found or if HR is less than100 bpm (beats/min), initiate positive-pressure ventilation (PPV) by bag and mask. Because this mother received meperidine during the labor process, naloxone (Narcan) administration is an important step in resuscitation.

## ANALYSIS

### Objectives

1. Understand the steps of newborn delivery room resuscitation.
2. Become familiar with use of the Apgar score.
3. Become familiar with conditions causing newborn transition problems.

### Considerations

This depressed infant was born to a healthy mother without prenatal or delivery complications other than failed epidural anesthesia. PPV was initiated and naloxone administered. The provider must appreciate the timing of maternal meperidine administration and its continued neonatal effects.

# APPROACH TO
# Neonatal Resuscitation

## DEFINITIONS

**NARCOSIS:** The condition of deep stupor or unconsciousness produced by a chemical substance such as a drug or anesthesia.

**PERINATAL HYPOXIA:** Inadequate oxygenation of a neonate that, if severe, can lead to brainstem depression and secondary apnea unresponsive to stimulation.

**POSITIVE-PRESSURE VENTILATION (PPV):** Mechanically breathing using a bag and mask.

## CLINICAL APPROACH

Delivery room resuscitation follows the **ABC** rules of resuscitation for patients of all ages: establish and maintain the **airway,** control the **breathing,** and maintain the **circulation** with medications and chest compressions (if necessary).

In this case, the meperidine given during labor probably is responsible for the infant's apnea and poor respiratory effort. Neonates with narcosis usually have a good HR response but poor respiratory effort in response to bag-and-mask ventilation. The **therapy for narcotic-related depression** is intravenous (IV), intramuscular (IM), subcutaneous (SQ), or endotracheal administration of **naloxone** (Narcan); repeated doses may be required should respiratory depression recur.

The **Apgar score** (Table 14–1) is widely used to evaluate a neonate's transition from the intra- to extrauterine environment. Scores of 0, 1, or 2 are given at 1 and 5 minutes of life for the listed signs. The 1-minute score helps to determine an infant's well-being, and scores less than 3 historically have been used to indicate the need for immediate resuscitation. In current practice HR, color, and respiratory rate (RR) rather than the 1-minute Apgar score are used to determine this need. The 5-minute score is one indicator of how successful the resuscitation efforts were. Some continue to measure Apgar scores beyond the 5-minute period to determine the continued effects of resuscitation efforts. The Apgar score alone cannot determine neonatal morbidity or mortality.

**Table 14–1** APGAR EVALUATION OF A NEWBORN

| SIGN | 0 | 1 | 2 |
|---|---|---|---|
| Heart rate | Absent | <100 bpm | >100 bpm |
| Respiratory effort | Absent | Slow, irregular | Good, crying |
| Muscle tone | Limp | Some flexion of extremities | Flexed, active motion |
| Reflex irritability (response to catheter in nose) | No response | Grimace | Cough or sneeze |
| Color | Blue, pale | Body pink, acrocyanosis (extremities blue) | Completely pink |

## Comprehension Questions

14.1 A girl is born via stat cesarean section to a 34-year-old mother whose pregnancy was complicated by hypertension and abnormal fetal heart monitoring. At delivery she is covered in thick, green meconium and is limp, apneic, and bradycardic. Which of the following is the best first step in her resuscitation?

A. Administer IV bicarbonate.
B. Administer IV naloxone.
C. Initiate bag-and-mask ventilation.
D. Initiate chest compressions immediately.
E. Intubate with an endotracheal tube and suction meconium from the trachea.

14.2 A term male is delivered vaginally to a 22-year-old mother. Immediately after birth he is noted to have a scaphoid abdomen, cyanosis, and respiratory distress. Heart sounds are heard on the right side of the chest, and the breath sounds seem to be diminished on the left side. Which of the following is the most appropriate next step in his resuscitation?

A. Administer IV bicarbonate.
B. Administer IV naloxone.
C. Initiate bag-and-mask intubation.
D. Initiate chest compressions immediately.
E. Intubate with an endotracheal tube.

14.3 A 37-week-gestation boy is born after an uncomplicated pregnancy to a 33-year-old mother. At birth he was lethargic and had a slow HR. Oxygen was administered via bag and mask, and he was intubated; his HR remained at 40 bpm. Which of the following is the most appropriate next step?

A. Administer IV bicarbonate.
B. Administer IV atropine.
C. Administer IV epinephrine.
D. Administer IV calcium chloride.
E. Begin chest compressions.

14.4 A term infant is born vaginally after an uncomplicated pregnancy. She appears normal but has respiratory distress when she stops crying. When crying she is pink; when not she makes vigorous respiratory efforts but becomes dusky. Which of the following is the likely explanation for her symptoms?

A. Choanal atresia
B. Diaphragmatic hernia
C. Meconium aspiration
D. Neonatal narcosis
E. Pneumothorax

## ANSWERS

14.1 **E.** An attempt is made to remove the meconium from the oropharynx and the airway prior to initiation of respirations. Ideally, the obstetrician will begin suctioning the meconium upon delivery of the head, and the pediatrician will further remove meconium with an aspirator or through endotracheal intubation with suction. Ventilation is initiated after meconium is removed. The goal is to remove airway meconium and to prevent its aspiration into the small airways where ventilation-perfusion mismatch may occur with deleterious effects.

14.2 **E.** The case describes diaphragmatic hernia. As a result of herniated bowel contents into the chest, these children often have pulmonary hypoplasia. Bag-and-mask ventilation will cause accumulation of bowel gas (which is located in the chest) and further respiratory compromise. Therefore, endotracheal intubation is the best course of action.

14.3 **E.** If the HR is still less than 60 bpm despite PPV with 100% oxygen, then chest compressions are given for 30 seconds. If the HR is still less than 60 bpm, then drug therapy (usually epinephrine) is indicated.

14.4 **A.** Infants are obligate nose breathers. When crying they can breathe through their mouth, but they must have a patent nose when quiet. Choanal atresia is identified by passing a feeding tube through each nostril or by identification of mist on cold metal held under the infant's nose. Should choanal atresia be diagnosed, endotracheal intubation bypasses the airway obstruction until surgical repair can be completed.

### Clinical Pearls

- An infant with slow heart rate, poor color, and inadequate respiratory effort requires immediate resuscitation.
- The therapy for narcosis (newborn respiratory depression due to maternal pain control) is intravenous, intramuscular, subcutaneous, or endotracheal administration of naloxone (Narcan).
- A child with diaphragmatic hernia often presents with immediate respiratory distress, scaphoid abdomen, cyanosis, and heart sounds displaced to the right side of the chest.
- Choanal atresia results in respiratory distress when a child stops crying; immediate treatment is intubation until surgical correction can be completed.

## REFERENCES

Ekrenkranz RA. Newborn resuscitation. In: McMillan JA, Feigin RD, DeAngelis CD, Jones MD, eds. *Oski's Pediatrics: Principles and Practice*. 4th ed. Philadelphia, PA: Lippincott Williams & Wilkins; 2006:207-213.

Sola A, Gregory GA. Delivery room emergencies and newborn resuscitation. In: Rudolph CD, Rudolph AM, Hostetter MK, Lister G, Siegel NJ, eds. *Rudolph's Pediatrics*. 21st ed. New York, NY: McGraw-Hill; 2003:97-103.

Stoll BJ, Adams-Chapman I. Delivery room emergencies. In: Kleigman RM, Behrman RE, Jenson HB, Stanton BF, eds. *Nelson Textbook of Pediatrics*. 18th ed. Philadelphia, PA: WB Saunders; 2007:723-728.

Stoll BJ. Routine delivery room care. In: Kleigman RM, Behrman RE, Jenson HB, Stanton BF, eds. *Nelson Textbook of Pediatrics*. 18th ed. Philadelphia, PA: WB Saunders; 2007:679-681.

Wilkinson AR, Charlton VE, Phibbs RH, Amiel-Tison C. Nose. In: Rudolph CD, Rudolph AM, Hostetter MK, Lister G, Siegel NJ, eds. *Rudolph's Pediatrics*. 21st ed. New York, NY: McGraw-Hill; 2003:88.

# Case 15

A 12-month-old boy whom you have followed since birth arrives for a well-child visit. The mother is concerned that the baby's manner of crawling, where he drags his legs rather than using a four-limbed movement, is abnormal. She says that the child only recently began crawling and he does not pull to a stand. You noted at his 6-month visit that he was not yet rolling over nor sitting; previous visits were unremarkable as was the mother's pregnancy and vaginal delivery. On examination today, you note that he positions his legs in a "scissoring" posture when held by the axillae.

- What is the initial step in the evaluation of this child?
- What is the most likely diagnosis?
- What is the next step in the evaluation?

# ANSWERS TO CASE 15: Cerebral Palsy

*Summary:* A 12-month-old boy crawls using primarily his upper extremities, and holds his legs in a "scissoring" posture when suspended.

- **Initial step:** Gather detailed history, focusing on developmental questions; obtain a thorough pregnancy, birth, social, and family histories; and perform a detailed neurologic examination.
- **Most likely diagnosis:** Cerebral palsy (CP).
- **Next step:** Vision and hearing testing, consider a brain magnetic resonance imaging (MRI) scan, and arrange for therapy with a developmental specialist.

## ANALYSIS

### Objectives

1. Know the definition of CP.
2. Recognize the classifications of CP.
3. Know the basic therapeutic approach to CP.

### Considerations

The spasticity of the baby's lower extremities described is abnormal and is **suggestive of CP**. He has gross motor delay. A complete developmental and neurologic assessment is crucial for initiating therapies that will help him achieve maximal functional outcome. Although often of low yield, an attempt should be made to identify the etiology of the child's CP. Knowing the etiology can aid in developing a treatment plan, in family planning (especially if the etiology is inherited), and in assuaging parental guilt for this child's condition.

# APPROACH TO Cerebral Palsy

## DEFINITIONS

**CEREBRAL PALSY (CP):** A disorder of movement and posture that results from an insult to or anomaly of the immature central nervous system (CNS). This definition recognizes the central origin of the dysfunction, thus distinguishing it from neuropathies and myopathies.

**DEVELOPMENTAL DELAY:** Failure of a child to reach developmental milestones of gross motor, fine motor, language, and social-adaptive skills at anticipated ages.

**NEUROLOGIC DEFICIT:** Abnormal functioning or lack of function of a part of the nervous system.

## CLINICAL APPROACH

With a prevalence of at least 1 to 2 cases per 1000 live births, **CP is the most common childhood movement disorder. Approximately one-third of CP patients also have seizures, and approximately 60% are mentally retarded.** Deafness, visual impairments, swallowing difficulty with concomitant aspiration, limb sensory impairments, and behavioral disturbances are common comorbidities. The effect of aggressive neonatal medical therapies on CP prevalence is unclear; improved premature infant outcomes may mitigate the impact of increased survival of very low-birth-weight infants.

Most children with CP have no identifiable risk factors. **Current research indicates that CP most likely is the result of antenatal insults.** Difficulties during the **pregnancy, delivery**, and the **perinatal period** are thought to reflect these insults and are **probably not the primary cause of CP**.

Cerebral palsy, or "static" encephalopathy, is the result of a one-time CNS insult. In contrast, progressive encephalopathies destroy brain function with time. The term *static* is misleading, however, because the manifestations of CP change with age. Contractures and postural deformities may become more severe with time or may improve with therapy. Also, a child's changing developmental stages early in life can alter the expression of his or her neurologic deficits.

Immaturity of the CNS at birth makes diagnosis of CP nearly impossible in a neonate. If a CNS insult is suspected, head imaging (by ultrasound or MRI) can be helpful in recognizing CP early. Possible imaging findings include periventricular leukomalacia, atrophy, or focal infarctions. Beyond infancy, CP is suspected when a child fails to meet anticipated developmental milestones.

Examples of concerning findings are

- A stepping response after age 3 months
- A Moro reflex beyond 6 months
- An asymmetrical tonic neck reflex beyond 6 months

Cerebral palsy can be classified in terms of physiologic, topographic, or functional categories. Physiologic descriptors identify the major motor abnormality and are divided into pyramidal (spastic) and extrapyramidal (nonspastic) categories. Extrapyramidal types can be subdivided further into choreoathetoid, ataxic, dystonic, or rigid types.

The topographic classification categorizes CP types according to limb involvement. **Hemiplegia** refers to involvement of a single lateral side of the body, with greater impairment of the upper extremities than the lower extremities. **Diplegia** describes four-limb involvement, with greater impairment of the lower extremities. **Spastic quadriplegia** is four-limb involvement with significant impairment of all extremities, although the upper limbs may be less impaired than lower limbs. (The term *paraplegia* is reserved for spinal and lower motor neuron disorders.)

The functional classification of CP relies on the "motor quotient" to place patients into minimal, mild, moderate, and severe (profound) categories. The motor quotient is derived by dividing the child's "motor age" (ie, motor skills developmental age) with the chronologic age. A motor quotient of 75 to 100 represents minimal impairment, 55 to 70 mild impairment, 40 to 55 moderate impairment, and lesser quotients severe impairment. These categories help clinicians identify children with less obvious impairments so that early treatment can be provided.

The evaluation of CP is based on the history and physical examination. The yield of diagnostic findings with brain imaging and metabolic or genetic testing is low but can be helpful in managing the patient, in future family planning, and in reassuring the parents. Identification of comorbid conditions includes cognitive testing for mental retardation and electroencephalography (EEG) for seizures.

Treatment goals include maximizing motor function and preventing secondary handicaps. During the preschool years, the child's communication ability is important. School performance and peer acceptance become important issues for older children. Physical therapy for motor deficits may be supplemented with pharmacologic and surgical interventions. Occupational therapy improves positioning and allows for better interaction with the environment and eases care as the child grows. The family's psychological and social needs should not be overlooked; children may require extensive physical and emotional support.

## Comprehension Questions

15.1 A term infant requires resuscitation after a spontaneous vaginal delivery. The Apgar scores at 1, 5, and 10 minutes were 2, 7, and 9, respectively. The mother's medical records show that she received routine prenatal care with normal prenatal ultrasonogram, triple screen, and glucose tolerance tests. The nurse tells you that the father seemed very agitated and mentioned "suing the obstetrician if the baby does not turn out normal." Your examination of the baby reveals no abnormalities. In counseling the family, which of the following is most appropriate?

A. Tell them that your examination findings indicate that everything is fine.
B. Tell them that the low Apgar scores at 1 and 5 minutes indicate that the baby suffered perinatal asphyxia.
C. Tell them that because the pregnancy was uncomplicated, any neurologic deficit that the baby may develop likely can be attributed to events occurring at delivery.
D. Tell them that your examination findings are reassuring, and that you will perform a careful developmental assessment at every well-child visit.
E. Avoid speaking to the parents until you have had a chance to speak with the obstetrician and to see the cord blood gas results.

15.2 A 4-year-old child with CP comes to your clinic for the first time for a routine visit. He walks with the help of leg braces and a walker, and his speech is slurred and limited to short phrases. He has never been hospitalized and he does not have swallowing problems. He began walking at age 2.5 years, and he is unable to take off his clothes and use the toilet without help. On examination you find that the boy has only minimally increased tone in the upper extremities but good fine motor coordination; he has significantly increased tone and deep tendon reflexes in the lower extremities. How would you categorize this child's CP?

A. Mild, diplegic
B. Mild, hemiplegic
C. Moderate, diplegic
D. Moderate, quadriplegic
E. Severe, diplegic

15.3 An infant girl is born via spontaneous vaginal delivery at 28-week gestation because of an incompetent cervix. Which of the following features of her clinical course in the neonatal intensive care unit (ICU) is most likely to correlate with her clinical outcome 5 years from now?

A. Administration of surfactant
B. Apnea of prematurity
C. Grade IV intraventricular hemorrhage
D. Retinopathy of prematurity stage 1 on initial ophthalmologic examination
E. Umbilical artery catheterization

15.4 The parents of a 2-year-old girl, recent immigrants from Guatemala, bring their child to you for the first time. The child was born at term after an uncomplicated pregnancy and delivery, and her neonatal course was uneventful. She sat without support at 6 months of age, pulled to a stand at 10 months, and walked at 14 months. She has a 10-word vocabulary, is able to drink from a cup, and feeds herself with a spoon. A previous child in the family died at age 5 years from "heart trouble." On physical examination, you note lower extremity contractures, hand stiffness, somewhat coarse facial features, and hepatosplenomegaly. The child's growth is within normal limits, and her examination is otherwise normal. Which of the following is the most appropriate next step to diagnose this child's condition?

A. Abdominal computerized tomography (CT)
B. Brain magnetic resonance imaging (MRI)
C. Chromosomal analysis
D. Tests for a storage disorder
E. Thyroid function studies

## ANSWERS

15.1 **D.** The Apgar score at 1 minute reflects the neonatal environment immediately prior to birth; the 5-minute score correlates the infant's response to resuscitation. The Apgar scores are not an accurate reflection of morbidity. An examination is a better indicator of the child's outcome, but CP cannot be ruled out on the basis of a normal neonatal physical examination. A discussion of the events of delivery is best left to the obstetrician; the majority of difficult deliveries are the result of a previously unidentified antenatal insult. However, avoidance of the parents will likely only further their anxiety and may impede your efforts to provide care for the child.

15.2 **C.** In diplegia all four extremities are affected, with greater impairment of the lower extremities. As most children walk by age 14 months, this child's motor quotient is 14 months/30 months = 0.47, which classifies him as moderately impaired.

15.3 **C.** Intraventricular hemorrhage is a complication in preterm infants. It is associated with seizures, hydrocephalus, and periventricular leukomalacia. A grade IV bleed involves the brain parenchyma, putting this child at higher risk for neurodevelopmental handicap.

15.4 **D.** The enlarged liver and spleen, the coarse facies, and the history of death in a previous child from "heart trouble" point to a storage disorder. Her joint contractures and hand stiffness may be explained by an abnormal metabolism rather than a CNS deficit as in CP.

## Clinical Pearls

- Cerebral palsy is a disorder of movement or posture resulting from an insult to, or an anomaly of, the central nervous system.
- Most children with cerebral palsy have no identifiable risk factors for the disorder.
- Optimal treatment plans for cerebral palsy use a multidisciplinary approach.

## REFERENCES

American Academy of Pediatrics. Use and abuse of the Apgar score. Available at: http://www.aap.org.

Johnson MV. Cerebral palsy. In: Kliegman RM, Behrman RE, Jenson HB, Stanton BF, eds. *Nelson Textbook of Pediatrics*. 18th ed. Philadelphia, PA: WB Saunders; 2007:2494-2495.

Shapiro BK, Capute AJ. Cerebral palsy. In: McMillan JA, Feigin RD, DeAngelis CD, Jones MD, eds. *Oski's Pediatrics: Principles and Practice*. 4th ed. Philadelphia, PA: Lippincott Williams & Wilkins; 2006:2251-2258.

Wollack JB, Nichter CA. Cerebral palsy. In: Rudolph CD, Rudolph AM, Hostetter MK, Lister G, Siegel NJ, eds. *Rudolph's Pediatrics*. 21st ed. New York, NY: McGraw-Hill; 2003:2197-2202.

# Case 16

A 5-year-old girl comes to your clinic for the first time with complaints of fever, malaise, and a cough for 2 days. She has a history of asthma for which she uses a steroid inhaler daily and an albuterol inhaler as needed. She has been tried on various over-the-counter cold and allergy remedies, but her respiratory symptoms have been worsening over the past several months. Her past medical history is notable for an episode of rectal prolapse and "sinusitis" during each of the past two winter seasons. Her mother also reports that her daughter has "always been small for her age." Your examination reveals a moderately ill-appearing child whose height and weight are at the fifth percentile for age. Her temperature is 101°F (38.3°C) and respiratory rate 32 breaths/min. She has scant purulent rhinorrhea bilaterally, wheezy breath sounds in all lung fields, and diminished breath sounds on the right side. Heart sounds and capillary refill are normal, yet she has digital clubbing.

- What is the diagnostic approach in the evaluation of this child?
- What is the most likely diagnosis?
- What is the next step in evaluation?

# ANSWERS TO CASE 16:
# Cystic Fibrosis

*Summary:* A small-appearing, 5-year-old girl previously diagnosed with asthma, rectal prolapse, and sinusitis presents with fever, scant purulent rhinorrhea, abnormal breath sounds, and digital clubbing.

- **Diagnostic approach:** Gather perinatal, past medical, family, and dietary histories, and a thorough systems review. Plot the child's height and weight on a standard growth curve.
- **Most likely diagnosis:** Cystic fibrosis (CF).
- **Next step in evaluation:** Obtain a chest radiograph and perform a sweat chloride test.

## ANALYSIS

### Objectives

1. Know the historical clues and physical signs to distinguish CF from more common conditions.
2. Know how to accurately diagnose CF.
3. Have a basic understanding of the implications and limitations of genetic testing for CF.

### Considerations

A careful review of this child's frequency and severity of respiratory symptoms, response to medications, and general health is warranted. Her small size and digital clubbing (unusual findings for asthma) suggest alternative diagnoses for her respiratory problems. Recurrent sinusitis is uncommon in young children because their nasal passages are not fully pneumatized; this girl likely was incorrectly diagnosed or has an underlying, predisposing condition for this problem.

# APPROACH TO
# Cystic Fibrosis

## DEFINITIONS

**CLUBBING:** Increase in the angle between the nail and nail base of 180° or greater, and softening of the nail base to palpation. Although the condition can be familial, clubbing is uncommon in children, usually indicating chronic pulmonary, hepatic, cardiac, or gastrointestinal disease.

**CYSTIC FIBROSIS (CF):** The major cause of chronic debilitating pulmonary disease and pancreatic exocrine deficiency in the first three decades of life. It is characterized by the triad of chronic obstructive pulmonary disease, pancreatic exocrine deficiency, and abnormally high sweat electrolyte concentrations. Characteristic pancreatic changes give the disease its name.

## CLINICAL APPROACH

Cystic fibrosis (CF) afflicts 1 of 3300 whites, 1 of 16,300 African Americans, and 1 of 32,100 Asian Americans. It almost always involves the **respiratory tract**; most patients develop **bronchiectasis** by age 18 months, although some may not experience respiratory difficulty for several years. Children are commonly misdiagnosed as asthmatic, but a careful history and physical examination ultimately demonstrates clues of CF. **Persistent bronchial obstruction from impaired mucus secretion** predisposes patients to secondary bacterial infection, which leads to a cycle of inflammation, tissue damage, further obstruction, and chronic infection. **Bacterial pneumonia** is initially caused by *Staphylococcus aureus*, and then by *Pseudomonas aeruginosa*. Most patients with advanced disease harbor **heavy, slime-producing mucoid** variants of *P aeruginosa*, rarely found in other conditions. Once established, these bacteria are virtually impossible to eradicate. Colonization with *Burkholderia cepacia* may be associated with rapid clinical deterioration.

Airway reactivity is present in 50% of patients, but bronchodilator response is unpredictable and varies. Pneumothorax, hemoptysis, and *cor pulmonale* are frequent complications with advanced disease; pulmonary problems ultimately cause respiratory and cardiac failure. Chronic nasal congestion and sinus opacification is common, but acute sinusitis occurs infrequently. Children with CF may develop nasal polyps, with resultant nasal obstruction, headaches, and mouth breathing.

**Children with CF grow poorly** due to **maldigestion from exocrine pancreatic insufficiency**. They may have abdominal distention, rectal prolapse, subcutaneous fat and muscle tissue deficiency, and frequent passage of oily, malodorous stools; these stools predispose to obstruction, volvulus, or intussusception.

**Fatty liver infiltration** or focal biliary cirrhosis occurs in many CF patients. Hepatomegaly, esophageal varices, and hypersplenism caused by portal hypertension develop in a small proportion of teens; neonates may have prolonged jaundice. Gallbladder disease is common in adults. Abdominal pain is relatively common. Other symptoms are **azoospermia**, enlarged submaxillary glands, **osteoarthropathy**, and a "salty taste" on the skin (due to eccrine sweat gland dysfunction). Patients and their families require extensive psychosocial support.

The diagnosis of CF is usually based on a positive sweat test in conjunction with one of the following: typical chronic obstructive pulmonary disease, documented exocrine pancreatic insufficiency, and/or a positive family history. Persons with CF have **elevated sweat electrolyte concentrations** because of **abnormalities in the CF transmembrane conductance regulator (CFTR) protein.** Appropriate technique is important when attempting to measure sweat chloride in infants, in whom the collection of an adequate sweat quantity may be difficult. Elevated sweat electrolyte levels (false positives) have been reported in conditions such as anorexia nervosa, hypothyroidism, and nephrogenic diabetes insipidus. False-negative results can occur in CF patients with edema and hypoproteinemia. Because the implications of false test results are great, sweat testing is most appropriately obtained when a reasonable clinical suspicion of CF exists (see Table 16–1 for indications) and repeated when the initial test results are in doubt.

**Genetic CF testing** may be used when CF is suspected but the results of sweat testing are negative or equivocal. Disease is caused by **long arm of chromosome 7 mutations**, the most common being a single phenylalanine deletion at **amino acid 508 (Δ508).** Available tests detect more than 90% of individuals who carry two CF gene mutations; some children have only one or no detectable mutations by this methodology.

Because research demonstrates that newborn screening improves nutritional status, growth, and reduces hospitalizations, routine testing for CF is now performed for all newborns in most states in the United States. The blood spot screening test detects the pancreatic enzyme immunoreactive trypsinogen (IRT), which is elevated in infants with CF. Second-tier testing for samples with high IRT levels relies on a second IRT test or DNA testing. Infants with positive results on the newborn screen undergo sweat chloride testing for definitive confirmation. False-negative results are possible with the IRT newborn screen, so infants with symptoms suggestive of CF (such as meconium ileus) should undergo further testing even if newborn screen results are negative.

**Long-term management of CF patients** is best coordinated by experienced pediatric **pulmonary specialists** and includes minimizing airway reactivity and infections, optimizing nutritional status, and providing ongoing psychosocial support. The prognosis varies depending on disease severity. Infants with severe lung disease can die in early childhood, but most patients reach

**Table 16–1 INDICATIONS FOR SWEAT TESTING**

**GASTROINTESTINAL**

Chronic diarrhea
Steatorrhea
Meconium ileus or plug syndrome
Rectal prolapse
Cirrhosis/portal hypertension
Prolonged neonatal jaundice
Pancreatitis
Deficiency of fat-soluble vitamins (especially A, E, K)

**RESPIRATORY TRACT**

Upper
- Nasal polyps
- Pansinusitis on radiographs

Lower
- Chronic cough
- Recurrent "wheezing" bronchiolitis
- Recurrent or intractable asthma
- Obstructive pulmonary disease
- Staphylococcal pneumonia
- *Pseudomonas aeruginosa* (especially mucoid) from throat, sputum, or bronchoscopy cultures

**OTHER**

Digital clubbing
Family history of cystic fibrosis
Failure to thrive
Hyponatremic, hypochloremic alkalosis
Severe dehydration or heat prostration incompatible with history
"Tastes salty"
Male infertility

*(Reproduced, with permission, from Rudolph CD, Rudolph AM, Hostetter MK, Lister G, Siegel NJ, eds.* Rudolph's Pediatrics. *21st ed. New York, NY: McGraw-Hill; 2003:1973.)*

adolescence or adulthood. Mean survival for persons with CF now exceeds 35 years. Male survival is slightly longer than female, for reasons that are poorly understood; children from socioeconomically disadvantaged homes have a poorer prognosis.

## Comprehension Questions

16.1 A term infant delivered vaginally develops vomiting and abdominal distention at age 10 hours. No stool passage has been noted. An abdominal radiograph shows distended bowel loops and a "bubbly" pattern in a portion of intestine; the colon is narrow. Which of the following should you tell the parents?

A. You would like to consult a pediatric surgeon because you suspect that their child has Hirschsprung disease.
B. The child most likely has necrotizing enterocolitis, a condition more commonly seen in premature infants. Therefore you question the child's supposed gestational age.
C. You are concerned about the possibility of meconium ileus and would like to obtain some family history.
D. You believe that the child simply is constipated and would like to change to a soy-based formula to see whether the baby tolerates this better.
E. The child's symptoms and radiograph findings most likely are normal.

16.2 Appropriate clinical management of the patient in Question 16.1 includes which of the following?

A. Change from enteral to intravenous feeds; obtain genetics consultation for the next morning.
B. Change from enteral to intravenous feeds, obtain a blood culture, and initiate antibiotics.
C. Change from enteral to intravenous feeds and obtain a **STAT** pediatric surgery consultation.
D. Change from cow's milk to soy-based infant formula and continue to observe the infant.
E. Do not change your current management.

16.3 A 10-year-old boy has a history of recurrent sinusitis and multiple episodes of pneumonia. A sweat electrolyte test result is within the normal range. Your differential diagnosis now includes atopy, primary ciliary dyskinesia, and which of the following?

A. Tuberculosis
B. Chronic granulomatous disease
C. Coccidioidomycosis
D. Cystic fibrosis
E. Severe combined immunodeficiency

16.4 A 2-month-old infant arrives with bulging of his anterior fontanelle. He is fussy, refuses to nurse or to take a bottle, and has vomited once en route to the hospital. He has had no fever. Computerized tomographic (CT) scan of the head is negative for trauma or tumor. In addition to meningitis, your differential diagnosis should include which of the following?

A. Colic
B. Intussusception
C. Sinusitis
D. Pneumonia
E. Vitamin A excess

## ANSWERS

16.1 **C.** Meconium ileus, inspissated meconium obstructing the distal ileum, is thought to be caused by deficiency of proteolytic enzymes. Obstruction begins *in utero*, resulting in underdevelopment of distal lumina. It almost always is associated with CF. Intestinal atresia and Hirschsprung disease (congenital aganglionic megacolon) cause similar clinical pictures, but the radiographic findings for this child are most consistent with meconium ileus. Necrotizing enterocolitis also causes emesis and abdominal distension but occurs primarily in extremely low-birth-weight infants (ie, $<1000$ g); the colon would be expected to be of normal size. Constipation is not consistent with this baby's clinical picture or the described radiographic picture.

16.2 **C.** Meconium ileus is a surgical emergency, as volvulus and perforation peritonitis are not uncommon complications.

16.3 **D.** CF cannot be ruled out (false-negative test results); the sweat chloride test should be repeated and/or other CF diagnostic modalities considered. Bronchiectasis and chronic sinusitis are characteristic of ciliary dyskinesia syndromes. If associated with visceral situs inversus, the diagnosis of Kartagener disease is given. Sinusitis is not a common complaint among patients with tuberculosis, chronic granulomatous disease, or coccidioidomycosis. In addition to severe pulmonary infections, chronic diarrhea and wasting dominate the clinical picture in children with severe combined immunodeficiency.

16.4 **E.** Malabsorption of fats and protein are major causes of morbidity for patients with CF. In addition to carefully planned diets, most children with CF take supplements of the fat-soluble vitamins D, E, K, and A. Disorders of vitamin A metabolism can result in pseudotumor cerebri (increased intracranial pressure), which cause headache, vomiting, and neurologic abnormalities. Thus, a bulging fontanelle may be the presenting sign of CF in an infant.

## Clinical Pearls

- Cystic fibrosis (CF) involves a defect in mucus secretion and eccrine sweat gland function, resulting in various visceral lumina obstructions and excessive electrolyte secretion.
- Extrapulmonary signs and symptoms, such as digital clubbing, recurrent sinusitis, growth retardation, and fat malabsorption, are clues to the diagnosis of cystic fibrosis.
- A negative sweat chloride test result does not preclude cystic fibrosis.
- Meconium ileus in the newborn period is nearly pathognomonic for cystic fibrosis.

## REFERENCES


Boat TF, Acton JD. Cystic fibrosis. In: Kliegman RM, Behrman RE, Jenson HB, Stanton BF, eds. *Nelson Textbook of Pediatrics*. 18th ed. Philadelphia, PA: WB Saunders; 2007:1803-1817.

Comeau AM, Accurso FJ, White TB, et al. Guidelines for implementation of cystic fibrosis newborn screening programs: cystic fibrosis foundation workshop report. *Pediatrics*. 2007;119:e495-e518.

Hazinski TA. Dysmotile cilia syndrome. In: Rudolph CD, Rudolph AM, Hostetter MK, Lister G, Siegel NJ, eds. *Rudolph's Pediatrics*. 21st ed. New York, NY: McGraw-Hill; 2003:1949.

*National Newborn Screening Status Report*, updated 12/08/2008. National Newborn Screening and Genetics Resource Center. Available at http://genes-r-us.uthscsa.edu/nbsdisorders.pdf. Accessed 1/5/2008.

Orenstein DM. Cystic fibrosis. In: Rudolph CD, Rudolph AM, Hostetter MK, Lister G, Siegel NJ, eds. *Rudolph's Pediatrics*. 21st ed. New York, NY: McGraw-Hill; 2003:1967-1980.

Rosenstein BJ. Cystic fibrosis. In: McMillan JA, Feigin RD, DeAngelis CD, Jones MD, eds. *Oski's Pediatrics: Principles and Practice*. 4th ed. Philadelphia, PA: Lippincott Williams & Wilkins; 2006:1425-1438.

# Case 17

A mother brings her previously healthy 6-year-old son to your clinic because he has been limping and complaining of left leg and knee pain for 1 week. He has experienced no recent trauma, and his past medical history is unremarkable. His physical examination reveals a temperature of 100°F (37.8°C) orally with no lower extremity swelling, misalignment, or weakness. He has tenderness over the right knee, hepatosplenomegaly, and petechiae on his cheeks and chest.

- What is the most likely diagnosis?
- What is the next step in the evaluation?

# ANSWERS TO CASE 17:
# Acute Lymphoblastic Leukemia

*Summary:* A 6-year-old boy with a 1-week history of leg pain and limping. He has a low-grade fever, hepatosplenomegaly, and petechiae on his face and chest.

- **Most likely diagnosis:** Acute lymphoblastic leukemia (ALL).
- **Next step in the evaluation:** Complete blood count with platelets and differential.

## ANALYSIS

### Objectives

1. Describe the clinical manifestations of ALL.
2. Describe the laboratory and radiologic tests used in diagnosing ALL.
3. Know the treatment plan for a child with newly diagnosed ALL.
4. Understand the long-term survival and follow-up issues for children with ALL.

### Considerations

This patient has several manifestations of ALL, including leg and joint pain, fever, petechiae, and hepatosplenomegaly. Most of the signs and symptoms of ALL result from either replacement of normal bone marrow components with clonal proliferation of a single lymphoblast that has undergone malignant transformation, or from infiltrates of extramedullary sites by these malignant lymphoid cells. Rapid diagnosis and referral to a pediatric cancer center can increase survival.

# APPROACH TO
# Acute Lymphoblastic Leukemia

## DEFINITIONS

**EXTRAMEDULLARY:** Areas of the body outside of the bone marrow.

**GRANULOCYTOPENIA:** A reduction in total circulating leukocytes.

**LYMPHOBLAST:** A large, primitive, undifferentiated precursor cell not normally seen in the peripheral circulation.

**PANCYTOPENIA:** A reduction in circulating erythrocytes, leukocytes, and platelets.

**THROMBOCYTOPENIA:** A reduction in circulating platelets.

## CLINICAL APPROACH

**Leukemia is the most common childhood cancer**, accounting for **approximately 40% of all pediatric malignancies. Acute lymphoblastic leukemia** affects the **lymphoid cell line** and comprises approximately **75% of leukemia cases in children**. Acute myeloblastic leukemia (AML) affects the myeloid cell line (granulocytes, monocytes, and can affect erythrocytes or megakaryocytes) and comprises approximately 20% of childhood leukemia. The clinical manifestations of AML and ALL are similar. In the United States, childhood **ALL has a peak incidence at age 4 years** and occurs more frequently in **boys.**

ALL is often called the "great imitator" because of its nonspecific symptoms, including anorexia, irritability, lethargy, pallor, bleeding, petechiae, leg and joint pain, and fever. A physical examination includes the child's general appearance and energy level, vital signs (note if antipyretics taken), bleeding, bruising, petechiae, pallor, pain upon palpating bones or joints, and hepatosplenomegaly. Differential diagnoses include idiopathic thrombocytopenic purpura (ITP), aplastic anemia, mononucleosis, juvenile rheumatoid arthritis, and leukemoid reaction:

- Idiopathic thrombocytopenic purpura is a common cause of bruising and petechiae due to low platelet levels; however, anemia, leukocyte disturbances, and hepatosplenomegaly are absent.
- Aplastic anemia causes pancytopenia and fever; lymphadenopathy, arthralgias, bone pain, and hepatosplenomegaly are unusual findings.
- Children with infectious mononucleosis (ie, Epstein-Barr virus) or other acute viral illnesses may present with fever, malaise, adenopathy, splenomegaly, and lymphocytosis. Atypical lymphocytes resembling leukemic lymphoblasts are characteristic of these viral illnesses.
- Leukemoid reactions may be observed in bacterial sepsis, pertussis, acute hemolysis, granulomatous disease, and vasculitis. The leukemoid reaction resolves as the underlying disease is treated.

Children with ALL who present with fever, arthralgias, arthritis, or a limp frequently are diagnosed initially with juvenile rheumatoid arthritis (JRA). Anemia, leukocytosis, and mild splenomegaly may also be seen in JRA, causing even more confusion. **A bone marrow examination may be required to differentiate ALL from other diagnoses.**

Infiltration of the marrow by other types of malignant cells (neuroblastoma, rhabdomyosarcoma, Ewing sarcoma, and retinoblastoma) occasionally produces pancytopenia. These tumor cells usually are found in clumps in the normal marrow but occasionally replace the marrow completely.

**Almost half of the children with newly diagnosed leukemia have total leukocyte counts less than 10,000/mm$^3$.** Leukemic blasts may not be seen in the peripheral blood smear. Therefore, the diagnosis of leukemia is established by **examination of bone marrow,** most commonly aspirated from the posterior iliac crest. **A normal marrow contains less than 5% blasts; a minimum of 25% blasts confirms the diagnosis.** Approximately two-thirds of children with ALL have leukemic cell karyotypic abnormalities, including changes in chromosome number (ie, hypodiploidy or hyperdiploidy) or chromosome structure (translocation, deletions, inversions).

A variety of markers can help gauge prognosis. In general, **girls have a better prognosis. African-American and Hispanic populations** have **lower remission and higher relapse rates**. Children with ALL **younger than 1 year and those older than 10 years** have a **worse prognosis. Higher leukocyte counts,** especially if higher than 50,000/mm$^3$, have an unfavorable prognosis. Patients with **mature B-cell or T-cell immunophenotypes** typically have a worse outcome than those with B-precursor ALL. The karyotypes of leukemic cells have diagnostic, prognostic, and therapeutic significance. Patients with hyperdiploidy generally have a more favorable prognosis; those with hypoploidy and pseudodiploidy do less well. Translocations with a poor outcome include t(9;22) (Philadelphia chromosome) in patients with pre-B ALL, and t(4;11) seen in infants with AML.

Workup includes a **lumbar puncture** to examine the central nervous system (CNS) for early leukemic involvement; a **higher number of blasts in the cerebrospinal fluid is associated with a worse prognosis.** A **chest radiograph** is performed to detect a **mediastinal mass.** Bone radiographs may show altered medullary trabeculation, cortical defects, or transverse radiolucent lines; these radiologic findings lack prognostic significance and usually are unnecessary.

**Combination chemotherapy is the principal therapy**. The therapy involves remission induction and consolidation, prophylactic CNS therapy, and maintenance. Induction therapy, a combination of prednisone, vincristine, and asparaginase, produces remission within 4 weeks in approximately 98% of children with non–high-risk ALL. Consolidation treatment, aimed at further reducing residual leukemia, delivers multiple chemotherapies in a relatively short period of time. Prophylactic therapy with intrathecal cytarabine and/or methotrexate (± craniospinal irradiation) has decreased the incidence of CNS leukemia as a primary site of relapse from 50% to approximately 3% to 6%. Maintenance therapy with methotrexate and 6-mercaptopurine, vincristine, and prednisone is given for 2 to 3 years to prevent relapse; therapy is discontinued for children who remain in complete remission for 2 to 3 years.

**The 5-year survival rate for childhood ALL has steadily improved over the last 40 years and now is greater than 80%.** Late effects to be considered include neuropsychological deficits, seizures, and endocrine disturbances (ie, growth hormone deficiency) related to CNS prophylaxis; spermatogenesis dysfunction related to cyclophosphamide; delayed sexual maturation in boys who received irradiation of gonadal tissue due to leukemic invasion of the testes; leukoencephalopathy and neurodevelopmental problems (especially in post–CNS radiation patients); and secondary malignancies.

## Comprehension Questions

17.1 A mother brings her 3-year-old son with Down syndrome to the clinic because his gums have been bleeding for 1 week. She reports he has been less energetic than usual. Examination reveals that the child has a temperature of 100°F (37.8°C) orally, pallor, splenomegaly, gingival bleeding, and bruises on the lower extremities. Which of the following is most likely?

A. Aplastic anemia
B. Idiopathic thrombocytopenic purpura
C. Leukemia
D. Leukemoid reaction
E. Megaloblastic anemia

17.2 A father brings to the clinic his 6-year-old son who currently is undergoing induction chemotherapy for ALL. The school will not allow the child to register until his immunizations are up-to-date. Which of the following is the best course of action?

A. Call the school nurse or principal to inform him or her that this child should not receive immunizations while he is taking chemotherapy.
B. Update all immunizations except for measles-mumps-rubella (MMR) and varicella.
C. Update all immunizations except for oral polio vaccine.
D. Update all immunizations.
E. Call the school nurse or principal to inform him or her that this child will never receive immunizations because of the alteration in his immune system.

17.3 A mother brings to the clinic her 4-year-old son who began complaining of right knee pain 2 weeks ago, is limping slightly, is fatigued, and has had a fever to 100.4°F (38°C). Which of the following laboratory tests is most important?

A. Antinuclear antibodies
B. Complete blood count (CBC) with differential and platelets
C. Epstein-Barr virus titer
D. Rheumatoid factor
E. Sedimentation rate

17.4 Two weeks after a viral syndrome, a 2-year-old develops bruising and generalized petechiae that is more prominent over the legs. He has neither hepatosplenomegaly nor lymph node enlargement. Laboratory testing reveals a normal hemoglobin, hematocrit, and white blood cell count and differential. The platelet count is 15,000/mm³. Which of the following is the most likely diagnosis?

A. Acute lymphoblastic leukemia
B. Aplastic anemia
C. Immune thrombocytopenic purpura
D. Thrombotic thrombocytopenic purpura
E. von Willebrand disease

## ANSWERS

17.1 **C.** A high susceptibility to leukemia is associated with certain heritable diseases (Klinefelter syndrome, Bloom syndrome, Fanconi syndrome, ataxia telangiectasia, neurofibromatosis) and chromosomal disorders such as Down syndrome. Children with Down syndrome have a 10- to 15-fold increased risk for developing leukemia. Siblings of an ALL patient have a two- to fourfold increased risk for ALL. A few cases of ALL are associated with p53 gene aberrations. Overall, these genetic links account for a small number of total ALL cases.

17.2 **A.** Live virus vaccines are contraindicated for the child with ALL (and all members of the household) during chemotherapy and for at least 6 months after completion of treatment. Although the viruses in the vaccine are attenuated, immunosuppression from treatment can be profound and viral disease can result. Immunizations without live virus (diphtheria, tetanus, inactivated poliovirus vaccine, hepatitis A and B) are not absolutely contraindicated in this case, but the immunosuppression with chemotherapy often inhibits antibody responses.

17.3 **B.** This child has symptoms of JRA and leukemia. The CBC with differential and platelets is the best initial screening test. The leukocyte and platelet counts are normal to increased in JRA, and no blast cells are present. Frequently, blast cells are found on the peripheral smear with ALL. The child in the question ultimately may require a bone marrow aspiration.

17.4 **C.** Immune (or idiopathic) thrombocytopenic purpura (ITP) is common in children. In most cases, a preceding viral infection can be documented. The platelet count frequently is less than 20,000/mm³, but other laboratory test results are normal, including the bone marrow aspiration (which may show an increase in megakaryocytes). Treatment consists of observation or possibly intravenous immunoglobulin (IVIG), anti-RhD, immunosuppressives, or steroids. The history is explored for other possible causes of thrombocytopenia, including recent MMR vaccination, drug ingestion, and human immunodeficiency virus.

## Clinical Pearls

- Leukemias are the most common childhood cancers, and acute lymphoblastic leukemia (ALL) represents approximately 75% of all leukemia cases in children.
- Acute lymphoblastic leukemia has a peak incidence at age 4 years, and boys are affected more frequently.
- Acute lymphoblastic leukemia is often called the "great imitator" because of its nonspecific symptoms of anorexia, irritability, lethargy, pallor, bleeding, petechiae, leg and joint pain, and fever.
- Combination chemotherapy is the principal therapy for childhood acute lymphoblastic leukemia. Induction therapy (prednisone, vincristine, and asparaginase) produces remission within 4 weeks in approximately 98% of children with average-risk acute lymphoblastic leukemia.

## REFERENCES

Campana D, Pui CH. Childhood leukemia. In: Abeloff MD, Armitage JD, Niederhuber JE, Kastan MB, McKenna WG, eds. *Abeloff's Clinical Oncology*. 4th ed. Philadelphia, PA: Churchill Livingston Elsevier; 2008:2139-2160.

Freeman MH. Idiopathic (immune) thrombocytopenic purpura (ITP). In: Rudolph CD, Rudolph AM, Hostetter MK, Lister G, Siegel NJ, eds. *Rudolph's Pediatrics*. 21st ed. New York, NY: McGraw-Hill; 2003:1556-1557.

Mahoney DH. Acute lymphoblastic leukemia. In: McMillan JA, Feigin RD, DeAngelis CD, Jones MD, eds. *Oski's Pediatrics: Principles and Practice*. 4th ed. Philadelphia, PA: Lippincott Williams & Wilkins; 2006:1750-1758.

Steuber CP, Poplack DG. Acute lymphoblastic leukemia. In: Rudolph CD, Rudolph AM, Hostetter MK, Lister G, Siegel NJ, eds. *Rudolph's Pediatrics*. 21st ed. New York, NY: McGraw-Hill; 2003:1594-1600.

Tubergen DT, Bleyer A. The leukemias. In: Kliegman RM, Behrman RE, Jenson HB, Stanton BF, eds. *Nelson Textbook of Pediatrics*. 18th ed. Philadelphia, PA: Saunders Elsevier; 2007:2116-2122.

Wallace CA, Sherry DD. Juvenile rheumatoid arthritis. In: Rudolph CD, Rudolph AM, Hostetter MK, Lister G, Siegel NJ, eds. *Rudolph's Pediatrics*. 21st ed. New York, NY: McGraw-Hill; 2003:836-840.

# Case 18

You are called to the operating room to manage an infant recently born by emergency cesarean delivery. The mother, an 18-year-old with one previous child, received no prenatal care and arrived at the hospital approximately 1 hour prior to delivery. At delivery you find a large (4500 g), grayish-colored infant with poor tone, no spontaneous respirations, and a pulse of 100 beats per minute (bpm).

- What is the first step in the evaluation of this child?
- What is the most likely diagnosis?
- What is the next step in evaluation?

# ANSWERS TO CASE 18:
# Infant of a Diabetic Mother

*Summary:* A very large newborn with respiratory depression.

- **First step:** Resuscitation of the infant focuses on the **ABCs**: **A** (airway), **B** (breathing), and **C** (circulation). Oxygen is provided and the infant is stimulated to breathe on his own. If these simple measures fail, bag-and-mask ventilation and endotracheal intubation may be required. Upon oxygenation, the infant's poor tone, color, and slow heart rate should resolve.
- **Most likely diagnosis:** Respiratory distress in an infant of a diabetic mother (IDM).
- **Next step:** Once the infant's cardiorespiratory status is stabilized, frequent checks for hypoglycemia are indicated.

## ANALYSIS

### Objectives

1. Recognize the clinical features of the IDM.
2. Know the management of the IDM.
3. Know the infant anomalies that are associated with pregestational diabetes.

### Considerations

**Fetal hyperinsulinism** is a response to **poorly controlled maternal hyperglycemia resulting in fetal macrosomia and increased fetal oxygen requirements.** These two factors can make the birth process difficult and result in neonatal distress. High infant insulin levels cause him to become **hypoglycemic** when he is removed from the high-sugar *in utero* environment and must be managed immediately to prevent further complications. A blood glucose level of 25 to 40 mg/dL requires immediate feeding. A level less than 25 mg/dL (or higher levels in symptomatic infants) is treated with intravenous glucose. **Polycythemia, hypocalcemia, and hyperbilirubinemia** are other sequelae of gestational diabetes that may require management.

# APPROACH TO
# Infant of a Diabetic Mother

## DEFINITIONS

**GESTATIONAL DIABETES:** Persistent hyperglycemia during pregnancy, with untreated serum glucose levels greater than 100 mg/dL in the fasting state or greater than 130 mg/dL otherwise.

**HYPOGLYCEMIA:** A blood glucose level less than 40 mg/dL is the usual definition, although other definitions exist. Symptoms include lethargy, listlessness, poor feeding, temperature instability, apnea, cyanosis, jitteriness, tremors, seizure activity, and respiratory distress.

**MACROSOMIA:** Larger than normal baby, exceeding the 90th percentile for gestational age.

**POLYCYTHEMIA:** Elevated hematocrit that can lead to thrombosis if the level is significant and remains untreated. Levels greater than 65% in a newborn are often treated by partial exchange transfusion.

**CAUDAL REGRESSION SYNDROME:** Rare congenital malformation found almost exclusively in the IDM, characterized by hypoplasia of the sacrum and lower extremities.

## CLINICAL APPROACH

**Diabetes affects more than 3% of pregnancies.** For most women, the condition is transient, occurring during pregnancy and disappearing after delivery. **Women are screened for gestational diabetes between 24 and 28 weeks of pregnancy.** It is classified according to maternal age when the condition is first diagnosed (onset during gestation, or pregestational), the duration of symptoms, and the presence of vasculopathy (the "White Classification"). Women who require insulin therapy are at higher risk for a poor perinatal outcome than those whose carbohydrate intolerance can be managed by diet alone. Women with preexisting diabetes are followed closely; **many of the congenital malformations associated with gestational diabetes are thought to result from hyperglycemia early in the pregnancy.**

The fetal pancreas begins producing insulin during the fourth month of gestation and becomes functionally significant after week 26, when macrosomia due to maternal hyperglycemia may first be noted. Increased infant weight and length occur because of increased adipose tissue deposition and the growth hormone effects of insulin. Increased glycogen is stored in the infant liver, kidney, skeletal muscle, and heart. Head circumference is less significantly affected because insulin does not affect brain growth. Thus, the weight of an IDM typically is in its shoulders and abdomen.

Macrosomia, increased oxygen requirements, and placental insufficiency can lead to perinatal asphyxia and increased production of erythropoietin. The resultant **polycythemia** contributes to elevated bilirubin levels and can cause renal vein thrombosis. **Hypocalcemia** is common and results in irritability or decreased myocardial contractility.

**IDMs are at increased risk for congenital malformations,** including **congenital heart disease, neural tube defects,** and the **caudal regression syndrome.** Their large size at birth can complicate vaginal delivery; shoulder dystocia is a common problem in the vaginal delivery of a large IDM. Conversely, an IDM may be small for gestational age if the mother's diabetes is associated with severe vascular disease and resultant placental insufficiency. IDMs may be small in childhood but are often overweight in adolescence. They may be at risk for problems of obesity later in life.

## Comprehension Questions

18.1 A 35-week-gestation infant is delivered via cesarean section because of macrosomia and fetal distress. The mother has class D pregestational diabetes (insulin-dependent, with vascular disease); her hemoglobin $A_1C$ is 20% (normal 8%). This infant is at risk for birth asphyxia, cardiac septal hypertrophy, polycythemia, and which of the following?

A. Congenital dislocated hip
B. Dacryostenosis
C. Hyaline membrane disease
D. Hyperglycemia
E. Pneumothorax

18.2 A term infant weighing 4530 g is born without complication to a mother with class A pregestational diabetes (non-insulin requiring). His initial glucose level is 30 mg/dL, but the level after he consumes 30 cc of infant formula is 50 mg/dL, and another level obtained 30 minutes later is 55 mg/dL. His physical examination is unremarkable except for his large size. Approximately 48 hours later he appears mildly jaundiced. Vital signs are stable, and he is eating well. Which of the following serum laboratory tests are most likely to help you evaluate this infant's jaundice?

A. Total protein, serum albumin, and liver transaminases
B. Total and direct bilirubin, liver transaminases, and a hepatitis panel
C. Total bilirubin and a hematocrit
D. Total bilirubin and a complete blood count
E. Total and direct bilirubin and a complete blood count with differential and platelets

18.3 A premature infant of a class B pregestational (insulin-requiring, but without vascular disease) diabetic mother is delivered via cesarean section due to fetal distress. The mother's axillary temperature at delivery is 98.6°F (37°C). The child has poor color and tone, no spontaneous cry, minimal respiratory effort, and a weak pulse of 80 bpm. After endotracheal intubation, the color and tone improve a bit, but she still has perioral cyanosis and her heart rate is 90 bpm. Which of the following is the most likely cause of her persistent distress?

A. Hypocalcemia
B. Hypoglycemia
C. Impaired cardiac function
D. Renal failure
E. Sepsis

18.4 A term infant born to a mother with class C pregestational diabetes (insulin-dependent, but without vascular disease) requires endotracheal intubation at delivery for poor respiratory effort, tone, and color. His initial serum glucose level is 10 mg/dL, and the level stabilizes over 36 hours with intravenous administration of glucose. On the third day of life, his physical examination is remarkable for macrosomia and a new abdominal mass. Which of the following is the most likely cause of the abdominal mass?

A. Hydronephrosis
B. Infarction of the spleen
C. Intraintestinal air
D. Liver engorgement
E. Volvulus

## ANSWERS

18.1 **C.** Infants born to mothers with poorly controlled diabetes are at risk for respiratory distress syndrome (surfactant deficiency) at later gestational ages than seen in infants born to mothers who do not have diabetes.

18.2 **C.** This baby most likely has hyperbilirubinemia secondary to liver immaturity, possibly complicated by polycythemia. He should have a high level of unconjugated bilirubin and, in the absence of intrahepatic disease, a normal conjugated (or direct) portion. While choices D and E include the correct answer, additional tests are unnecessary for this otherwise healthy-appearing infant who continues to feed well. Therefore, C is the best answer to the question.

18.3 **C.** Infants born to mothers with poorly controlled gestational diabetes are at risk for congenital heart anomalies, cardiomyopathy, septal hypertrophy, and subaortic stenosis. This child's symptoms and the maternal diabetes history indicate a risk for cardiac problems. Sepsis can cause similar symptoms, but no risk factors for infectious disease are noted. This child is at risk for hypoglycemia, but hypoglycemia alone would less likely explain all of his symptoms.

18.4 **A.** Renal vein thrombosis can present as an abdominal mass (hydronephrosis), as a complication of polycythemia in IDMs. Such infants may have gross hematuria, but microscopic hematuria is more common. Hypertension is uncommon following an acute thrombosis but may occur as a late complication. The affected kidney may recover normal function or it may atrophy. Bilateral thrombosis can lead to chronic renal failure. If this child has delayed passage of meconium, small left colon syndrome (also seen in IDM) should be considered as a cause of the abdominal mass.

## Clinical Pearls

- Infants of diabetic mothers are at risk for perinatal complications, including hypoglycemia, hyperbilirubinemia, birth trauma, and congenital malformations.
- Infants of diabetic mothers usually are heavier and longer than expected, but head circumference usually is normal. Infants of diabetic mothers can be small for gestational age if placental insufficiency is present.
- Routine prenatal care includes screening for gestational diabetes.

## REFERENCES

Ogata ES. Infant of the diabetic mother. In: Rudolph CD, Rudolph AM, Hostetter MK, Lister G, Siegel NJ, eds. *Rudolph's Pediatrics*. 21st ed. New York, NY: McGraw-Hill; 2003:124-127.

Stoll BJ. Infants of diabetic mothers. In: Kliegman RM, Behrman RE, Jenson HB, Stanton BF, eds. *Nelson Textbook of Pediatrics*. 18th ed. Philadelphia, PA: WB Saunders; 2007:783-785.

Warshaw JB, Hay WW. Infant of the diabetic mother. In: McMillan JA, Feigin RD, DeAngelis CD, Jones MD, eds. *Oski's Pediatrics: Principles and Practice*. 4th ed. Philadelphia, PA: Lippincott Williams & Wilkins; 2006:423-427.

# Case 19

A mother is concerned that her 4-day-old son's face and chest are turning yellow. This Asian infant was delivered vaginally after an uncomplicated term pregnancy. The family history is unremarkable. With the exception of a large cephalohematoma, his physical examination is normal. He is breast-feeding well and shows no signs of illness.

- ➤ What is the most likely diagnosis?
- ➤ What is the next step in evaluating this patient?

# ANSWERS TO CASE 19:
## Neonatal Hyperbilirubinemia

*Summary*: A healthy, 4-day-old jaundiced, breast-feeding Asian male has a cephalohematoma.

➤ **Most likely diagnosis:** Neonatal hyperbilirubinemia.

➤ **Next step:** Serum or transcutaneous bilirubin level.

## ANALYSIS

### Objectives

1. Understand the etiology of physiologic neonatal jaundice.
2. Identify the causes of pathologic jaundice in a newborn.
3. Know the treatment for neonatal jaundice.

### Considerations

Neonatal hyperbilirubinemia results from higher rates of bilirubin production and a limited ability to excrete it. It includes physiologic jaundice and nonphysiologic jaundice. **This infant has several risk factors for neonatal physiologic jaundice: male gender, cephalohematoma, Asian origin, and breast-feeding.** Other possible risk factors are maternal diabetes, prematurity, polycythemia, trisomy 21, cutaneous bruising, delayed bowel movement, upper gastrointestinal obstruction, hypothyroidism, swallowed maternal blood, and a sibling with physiologic jaundice. A variety of pathologic conditions can cause nonphysiologic jaundice when excessive unconjugated bilirubin accumulates:

- Red blood cells (RBCs) are lysed at too rapid a rate.
- Transmission of unconjugated bilirubin to the liver is interrupted.
- Liver enzyme deficiencies preclude appropriate metabolism of the unconjugated material.

Neonatal jaundice may present at birth or appear at any time during the neonatal period. Untreated severe unconjugated hyperbilirubinemia is potentially neurotoxic. Conjugated hyperbilirubinemia, although not neurotoxic, often signifies a serious underlying illness (Table 19–1).

**Table 19–1 DIFFERENTIAL DIAGNOSIS OF NEONATAL JAUNDICE**

| |
|---|
| Hemolytic disease (isoimmune)—ABO, Rh, or minor group incompatibility |
| • Structural or metabolic red cell abnormalities (Hereditary spherocytosis, Glucose-6-phosphate dehydrogenase deficiency) |
| • Hereditary defects in bilirubin conjugation (Crigler-Najjar syndrome, Gilbert disease) |
| Bacterial sepsis |
| Breast-milk jaundice |
| Physiologic jaundice |
| Congenital biliary atresia |
| Extrahepatic biliary obstruction |
| Neonatal hepatitis—bacterial, viral, nonspecific |
| Inspissated bile syndrome |
| Postasphyxia |
| Neonatal hemosiderosis |

*(Adapted, with permission, from Cashore WJ. Neonatal hyperbilirubinemia. In: McMillan JA, Fegin RD, DeAngelis CD, Jones MD, eds.* Oski's Pediatrics: Principles and Practice. *4th ed. Philadelphia, PA: Lippincott Williams & Wilkins; 2006:237.)*

# APPROACH TO Neonatal Jaundice

## DEFINITIONS

**CONJUGATED (DIRECT) BILIRUBIN:** Bilirubin chemically attached to a glucuronide by an enzymatic process in the liver.

**ERYTHROBLASTOSIS FETALIS:** Increased RBC destruction due to transplacental maternal antibody passage active against the infant's RBC antigens.

**HEMOLYSIS:** Rapid breakdown of RBCs. Clinical and laboratory findings might include a rapid rise of serum bilirubin level (>0.5 mg/dL/h), anemia, pallor, reticulocytosis, and hepatosplenomegaly.

**KERNICTERUS:** A neurologic syndrome resulting from unconjugated bilirubin deposition in brain cells, especially the basal ganglia, globus pallidus, putamen, and caudate nuclei. Less mature or sick infants have greater susceptibility. Lethargy, poor feeding, and loss of Moro reflex are common initial signs.

**POLYCYTHEMIA:** A central hematocrit of 65% or higher, which can lead to blood hyperviscosity.

**UNCONJUGATED (INDIRECT) BILIRUBIN:** Bilirubin yet to be enzymatically attached to a glucuronide in the liver.

## CLINICAL APPROACH

**Physiologic jaundice comprises primarily unconjugated hyperbilirubinemia observed during the first week of life in approximately 60% of full-term infants and 80% of preterm infants.** Physiologic jaundice is established by precluding known jaundice causes via history and clinical and laboratory findings. Newborn infants have a limited ability to conjugate bilirubin and cannot readily excrete unconjugated bilirubin. Jaundice usually begins on the face and then progresses to the chest, abdomen, and feet. **Full-term newborns usually have peak bilirubin concentrations of 5 to 6 mg/dL between the second and fourth days of life.**

**Findings suggestive of nonphysiologic jaundice** include (1) appearance in the first 24 to 36 hours of life; (2) bilirubin rate of rise greater than 5 mg/dL/24 h; (3) bilirubin greater than 12 mg/dL in a full-term infant without other physiologic jaundice risk factors listed; and (4) jaundice that persists after 10 to 14 days of life. Nonphysiologic etiologies are commonly diagnosed in a jaundiced infant who has a family history of hemolytic disease or in an infant with concomitant pallor, hepatomegaly, splenomegaly, failure of phototherapy to lower bilirubin, vomiting, lethargy, poor feeding, excessive weight loss, apnea, or bradycardia. **Causes of nonphysiologic jaundice** include **septicemia, biliary atresia, hepatitis, galactosemia, hypothyroidism, cystic fibrosis, congenital hemolytic anemia** (eg, spherocytosis, maternal Rh or blood type sensitization), or **drug-induced hemolytic anemia.**

**Jaundice presenting within the first 24 hours of life requires immediate attention**; causes include **erythroblastosis fetalis, hemorrhage, sepsis, cytomegalic inclusion disease, rubella, and congenital toxoplasmosis.** Unconjugated hyperbilirubinemia can cause **kernicterus**, the signs of which mimic sepsis, asphyxia, hypoglycemia, and intracranial hemorrhage. Lethargy and poor feeding are common initial signs, followed by a gravely ill appearance with respiratory distress and diminished tendon reflexes.

**Approximately 2% of breast-fed full-term infants develop significant unconjugated bilirubin elevations (breast-milk jaundice) after the seventh day of life; concentrations up to 30 mg/dL** during the second to third week can be seen. If breast-feeding is continued, the levels gradually decrease. Formula substitution for breast milk for 12 to 24 hours results in a rapid bilirubin level decrease; breast-feeding can be resumed without return of hyperbilirubinemia.

Full-term, asymptomatic, low-risk but jaundiced infants are monitored with serum bilirubin levels. Significant hyperbilirubinemia requires a diagnostic evaluation, including measurement of indirect and direct bilirubin concentrations, hemoglobin level, reticulocyte count, blood type, Coombs test (indirect Coombs measures antibodies to RBCs in the blood; direct Coombs test identifies antibodies on surface of the infant's RBCs), and peripheral blood smear examination. Estimates of serum bilirubin concentrations that are based solely on clinical examination are not reliable. **Noninvasive, transcutaneous measurement** using multiwavelength spectral reflectance is an alternative to serum measurement.

**Phototherapy** is often used to treat unconjugated hyperbilirubinemia, with the unclothed infant placed under a bank of lights, the eyes shielded, and hydration maintained. The light changes the skin's bilirubin isomerization into an extractible form. For full-term infants without hemolysis, **phototherapy** is initiated at the following bilirubin levels: 16-18 mg/dL at an age of 24 to 48 hours; 16-18 mg/dL at 49 to 72 hours; and more than or equal to 20 mg/dL at 72 hours or more.

**Exchange transfusion** is needed in a small number of jaundiced infants who do not respond to conservative measures. Small aliquots of the infant's blood are removed via a blood vessel catheter and replaced with similar aliquots of donor blood. Risks of this procedure include air embolus, volume imbalance, arrhythmias, acidosis, respiratory distress, electrolyte imbalance, anemia or polycythemia, blood pressure fluctuation, infection, and necrotizing enterocolitis.

## Comprehension Questions

19.1 Which of the following decreases the risk of neurologic damage in a jaundiced newborn?

A. Acidosis
B. Displacement of bilirubin from binding sites by drugs such as sulfisoxazole
C. Hypoalbuminemia
D. Sepsis
E. Maternal ingestion of phenobarbital during pregnancy

19.2 You are about to return a telephone call to the mother of an 8-day-old infant who continues to have jaundice which was first noted on the second day of life; you are about to report to her that his latest total and direct bilirubin levels are 12.5 and 0.9 mg/dL, respectively. You look over your chart and see that he and his mother have O type blood, the direct and indirect Coombs test is negative, his reticulocyte count is 15%, and a smear of his blood reveals no abnormal cell shapes. He is bottle-feeding well, produces normal stools and urine, and has gained weight well. Which of the following diagnoses remains in your differential diagnosis?

A. Gilbert syndrome.
B. Disseminated intravascular coagulation (DIC)
C. Spherocytosis
D. Polycythemia
E. An undiagnosed blood group isoimmunization

19.3 The hyperbilirubinemia associated with Crigler-Najjar syndrome type I is caused by which of the following?

A. Increased production of bilirubin
B. Impaired conjugation of bilirubin
C. Deficient hepatic uptake of bilirubin
D. Severe deficiency of uridine diphosphate glucuronosyltransferase
E. Glucose-6-phosphate dehydrogenase deficiency

19.4 A 30-hour-old full-term infant has face and chest jaundice. He is breast-feeding well and has an otherwise normal examination. His bilirubin level is 15.5 mg/dL. Which of the following is the most appropriate course of action?

A. Recommend cessation of breast-feeding for 48 hours and supplement with formula.
B. Start phototherapy.
C. Wait 6 hours and retest the serum bilirubin level.
D. Start an exchange transfusion.
E. No action is needed.

## ANSWERS

19.1 **E.** Administration of phenobarbital induces glucuronyl transferase, thus reducing neonatal jaundice. Sepsis and acidosis increases the risk of neurologic damage by increasing the blood-brain barrier's permeability to bilirubin. Hypoalbuminemia reduces the infant's ability to transport unconjugated bilirubin to the liver, and similarly drugs that displace bilirubin from albumin elevate free levels of unconjugated bilirubin in the serum.

19.2 **A.** Gilbert syndrome would present with a negative Coombs test, a normal (or low) hemoglobin, a normal (or slightly elevated) reticulocyte count, and prolonged hyperbilirubinemia. Red cell morphology would be abnormal in DIC and spherocytosis, polycythemia would present with an elevated hemoglobin level (that listed above is normal for a newborn), and blood group isoimmunization would present with a positive Coombs test.

19.3 **D.** Although all infants are relatively deficient in uridine diphosphate glucuronosyltransferase, those with Crigler-Najjar syndrome type I have a severe deficiency, causing high bilirubin levels and encephalopathy. Treatment is phototherapy. Encephalopathy is rare with Crigler-Najjar syndrome type II, in which bilirubin levels rarely exceed 20 mg/dL.

19.4 **B.** Although the etiology of the hyperbilirubinemia must be investigated, phototherapy should be started.

## Clinical Pearls

- Physiologic jaundice, observed during the first week of life in the majority of infants, results from higher bilirubin production rates and a limited ability of excretion. The diagnosis is established by precluding known causes of jaundice based on history and clinical and laboratory findings.
- Nonphysiologic jaundice is caused by septicemia, biliary atresia, hepatitis, galactosemia, hypothyroidism, cystic fibrosis, congenital hemolytic anemia, drug-induced hemolytic anemia, or antibodies directed at the fetal RBC.
- High levels of unconjugated bilirubin may lead to kernicterus, an irreversible neurologic syndrome resulting from brain cell bilirubin deposition, especially in the basal ganglia, globus pallidus, putamen, and caudate nuclei. Less mature or sick infants are at greater risk. The signs and symptoms of kernicterus may be subtle and similar to those of sepsis, asphyxia, hypoglycemia, and intracranial hemorrhage.

## REFERENCES

American Academy of Pediatrics. Management of hyperbilirubinemia in the newborn infant 35 or more weeks of gestation. *Pediatrics*. 2004;114:297-316.

Cashore WJ. Neonatal hyperbilirubinemia. In: McMillan JA, DeAngelis CD, Feigin RD, Jones MD, eds. *Oski's Pediatrics: Principles and Practice*. 4th ed. Philadelphia, PA: Lippincott Williams & Wilkins; 2006:235-245.

Piazza AJ, Stoll BJ, Kliegman RM. Jaundice and hyperbilirubinemia in the newborn. In: Kliegman RM, Behrman RE, Jenson HB, Stanton BF, eds. *Nelson Textbook of Pediatrics*. 18th ed. Philadelphia, PA: WB Saunders; 2007:756-766.

Stevenson DK, Madan A. Jaundice in the newborn. In: Rudolph CD, Rudolph AM, Hostetter MK, Lister G, Siegel NJ, eds. *Rudolph's Pediatrics*. 21st ed. New York, NY: McGraw-Hill; 2003:164-169.

# Case 20

A 10-year-old boy in respiratory distress arrives late in the evening to the emergency department (ED); he has a 2-hour history of rapid breathing and a complaint that his chest hurts. His mother gave him two nebulizer treatments without improvement. She tells you that this is the fourth time in 3 months that he has required ED visits for similar symptoms. Your initial examination reveals an afebrile male with a respiratory rate of 60 breaths per minute and a heart rate of 120 beats/min (bpm). You note that his pulse varies in amplitude with respiration. His blood pressure is normal, but his capillary refill is somewhat sluggish at 1 to 2 seconds. He is pale, appears drowsy, has mild perioral cyanosis, and is using accessory chest muscles to breathe. You hear only faint wheezing on chest auscultation.

- ➤ What are the initial steps in evaluating this patient?
- ➤ What is the most likely diagnosis?
- ➤ What is the next step in evaluation?

# ANSWERS TO CASE 20: Asthma Exacerbation

*Summary:* A 10-year-old boy with a multiple episodes of respiratory difficulty presents with tachypnea, perioral cyanosis, likely pulsus paradoxus, use of accessory muscles of breathing, slight wheezing, delayed capillary refill, and drowsiness.

- **Initial steps:** Treating this patient's respiratory distress is of immediate concern. The airway is evaluated first, followed by an evaluation of breathing, and finally assessment of the circulatory status (the "ABCs"). Initial management includes administration of oxygen, an inhaled β-agonist, and a systemic dose of prednisone. Intravenous administration of fluids and medications is indicated for a patient with this degree of distress. A stat blood gas determination and monitoring oxygen saturation levels will aid further management.
- **Most likely diagnosis:** Asthma exacerbation.
- **Next step in evaluation:** After initial stabilization, past medical and family histories (medications, triggers, frequency and severity of previous episodes, previous hospitalization or ICU admissions), and a review of systems are obtained. The physical examination, blood gas report, and response to initial treatments will determine subsequent management.

## ANALYSIS

### Objectives

1. Know the acute management of asthma exacerbation.
2. Know how to classify the severity of an asthma exacerbation.
3. Know the approach to long-term management of asthma and prevention of exacerbations.

### Considerations

This child's history of ED visits for respiratory difficulty and his presenting symptoms point to asthma as the most likely diagnosis; less likely conditions include cystic fibrosis, foreign-body aspiration, and congestive heart failure. The National Institutes of Health, National Heart, Lung, and Blood Institute (NHLBI) asthma guidelines suggest this child's exacerbation is severe and requires immediate, intensive treatment. **His drowsiness is of particular concern, indicating impending respiratory failure**; his respiratory and circulatory status must be assessed frequently. The **paucity of wheezes** results from **severe airway obstruction** and reduced air movement; **wheezing is likely to increase as therapy allows more air movement.**

# APPROACH TO Asthma Exacerbation

## DEFINITIONS

**ASTHMA:** The diagnosis when (1) episodic symptoms of airflow obstruction are present; (2) airflow obstruction is at least partially reversible; and (3) alternative diagnoses are excluded.

**ASTHMA EXACERBATION:** Characterized by the triad of bronchoconstriction, airway inflammation, and mucus plugging.

**PULSUS PARADOXUS:** A blood pressure that varies more widely with respiration than normal. A variance of greater than 10 mm Hg between inspiration and expiration suggests obstructive airway disease, pericardial tamponade, or constrictive pericarditis.

**SPIROMETRY:** A test of pulmonary function. For patients with asthma, this test demonstrates reversibility and can be used to determine an individual's response to treatment.

## CLINICAL APPROACH

Asthma accounts for approximately three million visits to pediatricians per year in the United States. The **median age at onset is 4 years**, but 20% of children develop symptoms within the first year of life. **Atopy and a family history** of asthma are strong risk factors for its development, as is respiratory infections early in life; between 40% and 50% of children with **respiratory syncytial virus (RSV) bronchiolitis** later develop asthma. More than half of children with asthma have symptom resolution by young adulthood, but many have abnormal pulmonary function tests only to become symptomatic in later adulthood. Heavy exposure to pollution, allergens, or cigarette smoke makes resolution less likely. A chronic nighttime cough might be a harbinger of asthma.

**Airway inflammation in asthma is a result of mast cell activation.** An immediate immunoglobulin (Ig) E response to environmental triggers occurs within 15 to 30 minutes and includes vasodilation, increased vascular permeability, smooth-muscle constriction, and mucus secretion. Common triggers include dust mites, animal dander, cigarette smoke, pollution, weather changes, upper respiratory infections, certain drugs (ie, β-adrenergic antagonists, and some nonsteroidal anti-inflammatory agents), and exercise (particularly when performed in a cold environment). Two to four hours after this acute response, a **late-phase reaction (LPR)** begins. The LPR is **characterized by infiltration of inflammatory cells into the airway parenchyma**; it is responsible for the chronic inflammation seen in asthma. Airway hyperresponsiveness may persist for weeks after the LPR.

Asthma management involves identifying and minimizing exposure to triggers. Allergy testing can be helpful in some situations. Pharmacotherapy for the child's asthma symptoms follows NHLBI guidelines (available at http://www.nhlbi.nih.gov/guidelines/asthma/asthsumm.pdf). Adequate long-term management depends on reinforcement with the patient and family goals of therapy. Repeat objective assessment of lung function is achieved with spirometry performed in the clinic and peak expiratory flow measurements obtained at home.

**Pharmacotherapy** for asthma includes **β-adrenergic agonists, anticholinergics, anti-inflammatory agents, and leukotriene modifiers**. The NHLBI guidelines provide a stepwise approach to administration of these medications.

**β-Adrenergic agonists (ie, albuterol) rapidly reverse bronchoconstriction via $\beta_2$-receptors on bronchial smooth muscle cells**; they **do not significantly inhibit the LPR**. These agents also can be used immediately prior to exercise or exposure to allergens to minimize the acute asthmatic response. Toxicity includes tachycardia and muscle tremor. Increased levels of drug are delivered to the lungs and toxicity is decreased when these medications are delivered via inhalation routes (nebulizer or inhaler) as compared to the oral route. When inhalers are used, a reservoir device ("spacer") is used to maximize drug delivered to the lungs. Patients must not over-rely on short-acting inhalers because this practice is associated with death in severe asthma attacks.

**Anticholinergics** may be useful in the **acute management** of asthma exacerbation but are of **little value in chronic therapy**; they work by inhibiting the vagal reflex at smooth muscles.

**Cromolyn and nedocromil**, anti-inflammatory drugs that act by reducing the immune response to allergen exposure, **become effective after 2 to 4 weeks of therapy**; they are successful in only 75% of patients. **Leukotriene modifiers** are safe and effective anti-inflammatory medications for long-term control for some patients. The **most potent available anti-inflammatory drugs are corticosteroids,** which are useful for acute exacerbations (oral or intravenous prednisone, prednisolone) and for chronic therapy (inhaled corticosteroids).

## Comprehension Questions

20.1 A 12-year-old asthmatic girl presents to the ED with tachypnea, intracostal retractions, perioral cyanosis, and minimal wheezing. You administer oxygen, inhaled albuterol, and intravenous prednisone. Upon reassessment, wheezing increases in all fields, and the child's color has improved. Which of the following is the appropriate explanation for these findings?

A. The girl is not having an asthma attack.
B. The girl is not responding to the albuterol, and her symptoms are worsening.
C. The girl is responding to the albuterol, and her symptoms are improving.
D. The girl did not receive enough albuterol.
E. The albuterol was inadvertently left out of the inhalation treatment, and the girl received only saline.

20.2 A previously healthy 2-year-old girl presents with the complaint of acute-onset wheezing. Her mother denies previous wheezing episodes and denies a family history of asthma or atopy. The mother says that she left the child playing in her older brother's room. Approximately 20 minutes later she heard the child coughing and wheezing. Which of the following is the best next step in management?

A. Determining what the girl was playing with and ordering a chest radiograph
B. Referring the child to a pulmonologist
C. Prescribing antibiotics for a likely pneumonia
D. Administering an injection of intramuscular prednisone and sending her home
E. Accusing the mother of poor supervision of her child's health, because this obviously is not the first time the child has experienced these symptoms

20.3 A well-developed 4-month-old boy presents to the ED on a cold winter's night with the complaint of worsening respiratory distress and decreased oral intake. His parents report that he was well until yesterday, when he developed upper respiratory symptoms and a low-grade fever. Upon examination of the child, you note pallor and perioral cyanosis, a respiratory rate of 65 breaths/min, and tight wheezes throughout the chest. An arterial blood gas shows a pH of 7.15, a $PCO_2$ of 65 mm Hg, and a serum bicarbonate of 20 mmol/L. Which of the following is the the most likely explanation regarding the child's condition?

A. The child most likely has bronchiolitis, and is at risk of respiratory failure.
B. The child most likely has bronchiolitis, and his symptoms should resolve in the emergency department with a couple more albuterol treatments.
C. The child should undergo upper endoscopy, as you suspect a tracheoesophageal fistula.
D. The child most likely has gastroesophageal reflux and has aspirated.
E. The child has a metabolic acidosis that is most likely due to bacterial sepsis.

20.4 A 15-year-old adolescent male uses his albuterol inhaler shortly after he mows the lawn because of a mild feeling of chest "tightness." He later returns home early from dinner at a friend's house when he has the sudden onset of wheezing, cough, and chest pain. Which of the following is the most likely explanation for these circumstances?

A. He likely aspirated a piece of grass.
B. His albuterol inhaler must be empty.
C. His albuterol inhaler must be outdated.
D. He is having a late-phase reaction.
E. He has been exposed to a new allergen that is more irritating than grass.

## ANSWERS

20.1 **C.** This child presented in severe respiratory distress. Her improved color indicates reversible symptoms, confirming the diagnosis of asthma. Increased wheezing is auscultated after albuterol treatment because lung areas previously obstructed are now opening, allowing additional airflow. Less-experienced examiners may misinterpret lack of air movement as "clear" breath sounds, further delaying appropriate medical management.

20.2 **A.** Young children, generally between 4 months and 3 years of age, normally put objects in their mouth, and they are prone to developing foreign-body aspirations. A pulmonologist ultimately may be needed to retrieve the object, but this would not be a first step.

20.3 **A.** The differential diagnosis for a wheezing baby is extensive. However, the sudden onset of respiratory symptoms in a previously healthy infant, particularly in association with fever, is most consistent with the diagnosis of bronchiolitis. Initial treatment for this baby includes oxygen and nebulized albuterol or epinephrine. A blood gas measurement should be obtained immediately for any patient who presents in severe respiratory distress. This child's blood gas indices show a marked respiratory acidosis. He will likely require mechanical ventilation and monitoring in an intensive care setting until his symptoms improve. Infants with wheezing caused by bronchiolitis do not always respond to β-agonists. Chest radiographs in infants with bronchiolitis typically show hyperinflated lungs with areas of atelectasis. Respiratory syncytial virus (RSV) and influenza A are common causes of bronchiolitis in infants in the wintertime, but several other viral causes are also possible. A careful history should be obtained to rule out less common causes of wheezing in an infant, such as recurrent aspiration or a congenital anomaly.

20.4 **D.** A late-phase reaction typically occurs 2 to 4 hours after an initial wheezing episode. It is caused by accumulation of inflammatory cells in the airway.

## Clinical Pearls

- The prevalence of asthma in western countries has been increasing steadily, making this the most frequent admission diagnosis for children in many urban hospitals.
- Atopy and a family history of asthma are risk factors for development of asthma; exposure to pollutants including cigarette smoke makes resolution less likely.
- The late-phase reaction begins 2 to 4 hours after allergen exposure and is responsible for the chronic inflammation seen in asthma.
- Acute and long-term management of asthma is guided by recommendations published by the National Heart, Lung, and Blood Institute.

## REFERENCES

Eggleston PA. Asthma. In: McMillan JA, Feigin RD, DeAngelis CD , Jones MD, eds. *Oski's Pediatrics: Principles and Practice*. 4th ed. Philadelphia, PA: Lippincott Williams & Wilkins; 2006:2404-2410.

Lie AH, Covar RA, Spahn JD, Leung DYM. Childhood asthma. In: Kliegman RM, Behrman RE, Jenson HB, Stanton BF, eds. *Nelson Textbook of Pediatrics*. 18th ed. Philadelphia, PA: WB Saunders; 2007:953-970.

National Heart, Lung and Blood Institute. National Asthma Education and Prevention Program, Expert Panel Report 3: guidelines for the diagnosis and management of asthma, 2007. Available at: http://www.nhlbi.nih.gov/guidelines/asthma/asthsumm.pdf.

Ross MH, Mjaanes CM, Lemanske R. Asthma. In: Rudolph CD, Rudolph AM, Hostetter MK, Lister G, Siegel NJ, eds. *Rudolph's Pediatrics*. 21st ed. New York, NY: McGraw-Hill; 2003:1950-1964

Williams SG, Schmidt DK, Redd SC, Storms W. National asthma prevention program. Key clinical activities for quality asthma care. *MMWR Recomm Rep*. 2003; 52(RR-6):1-8.

# Case 21

The parents of a healthy 8-year-old boy are concerned that he is the shortest child in his class. His height and weight growth curves are shown in Figure 21–1 (see next page). He was a full-term infant, has experienced no significant medical problems, and is developmentally appropriate. Other than being small, his examination is normal. His upper and lower body segment measurements demonstrate normal body proportions. His father is 6 ft 4 in tall; he began pubertal development at 13 years of age. His mother is 5 ft 11 in tall; she had her first menstrual cycle at age 14 years.

- ➤ What is the most likely diagnosis?
- ➤ What is the best diagnostic test?
- ➤ What is the best therapy?

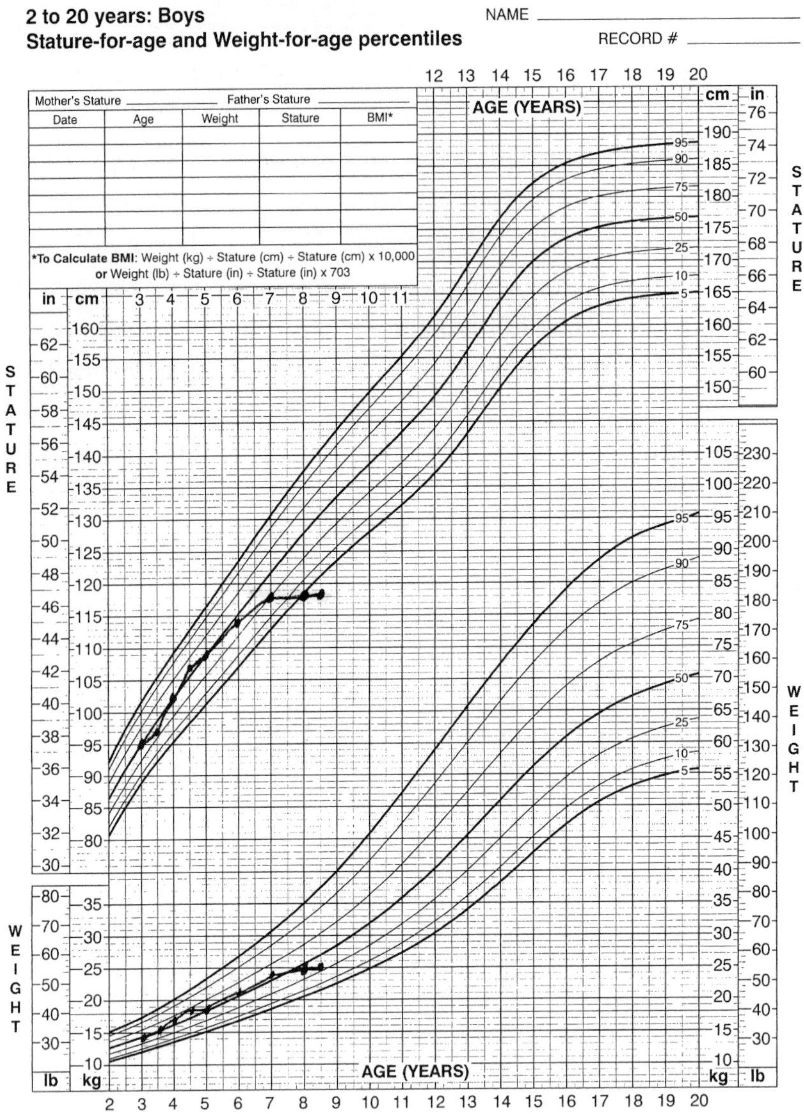


**Figure 21–1.** Childhood growth curve. (*Reproduced from the Center for Disease Control.*)

# ANSWERS TO CASE 21: Growth Hormone Deficiency

*Summary:* An 8-year-old boy with no significant medical history and a normal examination presents with failure to grow.

- **Most likely diagnosis:** Growth hormone (GH) deficiency.
- **Best diagnostic test:** Screening tests might include a complete blood count (CBC) and erythrocyte sedimentation rate (ESR); electrolytes and general health chemistry panel; urinalysis; serum for thyroid function studies, insulinlike growth factor-1 (IGF-1), and insulin like growth factor–binding protein-3 (IGF-BP3); bone age radiograph, and, if this were a girl, possibly chromosomal karyotype.
- **Best therapy:** Replace GH via injection.

## ANALYSIS

### Objectives

1. Understand the common causes of growth delay in children.
2. Appreciate the evaluation strategies for the various forms of growth failure.
3. Learn treatment options for common causes of childhood growth delay.

### Considerations

This patient has essentially stopped growing (or is growing at a rate less than expected). He has no medical problems and a normal examination. His parents are tall, and their pubertal development was not delayed. An evaluation to determine the reason for his growth failure is appropriate.

# APPROACH TO Growth Hormone Deficiency

## DEFINITIONS

**BONE AGE:** Childhood bone development occurs in a predictable sequence. Left wrist radiographs on children older than 2 years (or the knee in those younger) are compared to "normals" to determine how old the bones appear compared to chronologic age, thus providing an estimate of the remaining growth potential of the bones.

**CONSTITUTIONAL GROWTH DELAY:** A condition in which a healthy child's growth is slower than expected but for whom one or more parents demonstrated a pubertal development delay and ultimately normal adult height. In this case, the "bone age" equals the "height age."

**FAMILIAL SHORT STATURE:** A condition in which a short child is born to short parents who had normal timing of their pubertal development.

**HEIGHT AGE:** The age at which a child's measured height is at the 50th percentile.

**IDIOPATHIC SHORT STATURE:** A condition in which a short stature diagnosis cannot be reached.

## CLINICAL APPROACH

Many parents become concerned if their child is noticeably shorter than their child's peers. Many conditions can result in short stature; a growth and social history (to identify psychosocial growth failure), physical examination, and selected screening tests usually help to identify the problem's etiology.

**In the first year of life, children grow at a rate of approximately 23 to 28 cm/y.** This rate **drops to approximately 7.5 to 13 cm per year for children aged 1 to 3 years**. Until puberty, they grow approximately 4.5 to 7 cm per year. At **puberty, growth increases to 8 to 9 cm per year for girls and to 10 to 11 cm per year for boys.** By approximately 24 months of age, most children settle into a percentile growth channel, remaining there for the remainder of their childhood. Significant deviations from these expectations alert the clinician to potential growth problems (ie, "fall off their curve").

**Constitutional growth delay is a common cause of short stature**. These children have no history or examination abnormalities. In contrast to children with GH deficiency, children with constitutional delay have a **growth rate that is normal.** Their family history is positive, however, for one or more parents with pubertal development delays ("late bloomers") who developed normal adult height. A short child in a family with a classic history of "late bloomers" often requires no laboratory or radiographic evaluation. Sometimes a bone age is helpful to reassure the patient and family that much bone growth remains and normal height will be achieved. For some of these children, testosterone injections will hasten pubertal changes (which eventually will begin on its own without treatment); consultation with a pediatric endocrinologist can be helpful.

The child born to short parents often is short (**familial short stature**). The growth curve shows growth parallel to a growth line at or just below the third to fifth percentile. Laboratory and radiographic testing usually are not necessary; a **bone age equals the chronologic age**, indicating no "extra" growth potential. An estimate of a child's ultimate height potential is calculated using the parent's heights. A boy's final height can be predicted as follows: (Father's height in cm + [Mother's height in cm + 13])/2. A girl's final height can be predicted as follows: (Mother's height in cm + [Father's height in cm – 13])/2. Reassurance is indicated for children with familial short stature.

**Growth hormone (GH) deficiency** occurs in approximately 1 in 4000 school-age children. These children demonstrate a **growth rate that is slow, usually falling away from the normal growth curve** (in contrast to constitutional delay where growth parallels the third to fifth percentile curve). On examination these children often appear younger than their stated age and frequently appear chubby (weight age > height age). **Bone ages are delayed,** indicating catch-up growth potential. GH screening tests include serum IGF-1 or somatomedin C and IGF-BP3. Confirmation often requires GH stimulation testing and interpretation by a pediatric endocrinologist. Replacement therapy involves recombinant GH injections several times per week until the child reaches full adult height.

**Clues that growth failure may be caused by an underlying condition** not already mentioned include **poor appetite, weight loss; abdominal pain or diarrhea; unexplained fevers; headaches or vomiting; weight gain out of proportion to height; or dysmorphic features.** Screening tests might include a CBC (anemia), ESR (chronic inflammatory diseases), electrolytes (acidosis or renal abnormalities), general health chemistry panel (hepatitis, liver dysfunction), urinalysis (infection, renal disease), thyroid function tests (hypothyroidism), IGF-1 and IGF-BP3 (GH deficiency), and, for girls, possibly chromosomes (Turner syndrome). Children with growth failure who do not fall into another, more appropriate category are classified as having idiopathic short stature.

## Comprehension Questions

21.1 An 8-year-old boy has short stature. He has begun to gain quite a bit of weight over the last year, has little or no energy, sleeps more than normal, and complains of being cold. His growth curve demonstrates that he has fallen from the 50th percentile to the 5th percentile for height, but his weight has increased to the 90th percentile. On examination, he is obese, has an immature facies, thin hair, and slow reflexes. Which of the following is the most appropriate course of action for this child?

A. Order Epstein-Barr virus titers.
B. Measure thyroid function.
C. Reassure the mother that the child has normal prepubertal development.
D. Determine bone age.
E. Order a somatomedin C level.

21.2 A 16-year-old boy complains that he is the shortest boy in his class. He has a normal past medical history, and although always a bit small for age, he has really noticed that he has fallen behind his peers in the last 2 years. He is Tanner stage 3 and is at the fifth percentile for height. His father began puberty at age 16 and completed his growth at age 19; he is now 6 ft 2 in tall. His mother began her pubertal development at age 10 and had her first menstrual period at age 13; her height is 5 ft 4 in. Which of the following is the single most appropriate intervention?

A. Chromosomal analysis
B. Liver function studies
C. Measurement of bone age
D. Measurement of somatomedin C
E. Pediatric endocrinology referral

21.3 A 17-year-old girl is 4 ft 10 in tall. Her father is 5 ft 10 in tall and her mother is 5 ft 5 in tall. Her past medical history is significant for life-long short stature and cardiac surgery at age 1 year. She has never had a menstrual period. Which of the following is the most appropriate action?

A. Chromosomal analysis
B. Referral to a pediatric endocrinologist
C. Serum testosterone levels
D. Thyroid function studies
E. Ultrasonogram of the abdomen

21.4 You see a 14-year-old boy in the juvenile detention center where he is currently living for arson to an abandoned building. He is tall, slim, underweight, and appears to have especially long legs. His testes are small for age, and his phallus seems somewhat undersized. His mother reports that he had difficulty with reading, spelling, and mathematics early on, but now he has difficulty in all classes. Which of the following diagnostic tests is most likely to identify his problem?

A. Chromosomal analysis
B. Referral to pediatric endocrinology
C. Serum testosterone levels
D. Thyroid function studies
E. Ultrasonogram of the abdomen

## ANSWERS

21.1 **B.** This child has classic symptoms of acquired hypothyroidism. A bone age would be delayed, but thyroid function studies are needed to make the diagnosis. Thyroid hormone replacement therapy should resolve these symptoms, and growth should resume normally.

21.2 **C.** This boy likely has constitutional growth delay, similar to that of his father. Bone age would be delayed, indicating potential growth. He eventually will enter puberty, but the psychosocial ramifications of remaining shorter and appearing more immature than his peers may warrant treatment. Monthly testosterone injections "jump start" the pubertal process without altering final growth potential; a pediatric endocrinologist might be required to assist.

21.3 **A.** Chromosomal analysis is likely to show Turner syndrome (TS) in this child with parents of normal height. The surgery might have been for coarctation of the aorta. Common TS features include female phenotype, short stature, sexual infantilism, streak gonads, broad chest, low hairline, webbed neck, and congenital lymphedema of the hands and feet. Some TS children benefit from GH therapy.

21.4 **A.** Boys with Klinefelter syndrome are tall for their age; the testes are smaller than normal and feel firm and fibrotic. Examination can reveal eunuchoid body habitus and reduced upper body-lower body segment ratio (a long lower segment). Diagnosis is established by karyotyping.

## Clinical Pearls

- Constitutional growth delay is a condition in which a healthy child's growth is slower than expected and for whom at least one parent demonstrated a pubertal development delay but normal adult height ("late bloomers"). Growth parallels the third or fifth percentile growth curve; bone age is delayed.
- Familial short stature is a condition in which a short child is born to short parents who had normal timing of their pubertal development. Growth parallels the third or fifth percentile growth curve; bone age is normal.
- Idiopathic short stature includes children with short stature for whom a more appropriate diagnosis cannot be found.
- Growth hormone (GH) deficiency is a condition in which inadequate GH secretion results in growth failure, delayed bone age, and catch-up growth upon GH replacement.

## REFERENCES

Moshang T, Grimberg A. Neuroendocrine disorders. In: McMillan JA, Feigin RD, DeAngelis CD, Jones MD, eds. *Oski's Pediatrics: Principles and Practice*. 4th ed. Philadelphia, PA: Lippincott Williams & Wilkins; 2006:2097-2103.

Parks JS, Felner EI. Hypopituitarism. In: Kleigman RM, Behrman RE, Jenson HB, Stanton BF, eds. *Nelson Textbook of Pediatrics*. 18th ed. Philadelphia, PA: WB Saunders; 2007:2293-2299.

Plotnick LP, Miller RS. Growth, growth hormone, and pituitary disorders. In: McMillan JA, Feigin RD, DeAngelis CD, Jones MD, eds. *Oski's Pediatrics: Principles and Practice*. 4th ed. Philadelphia, PA: Lippincott Williams & Wilkins; 2006:2084-2092.

Rapaport R. Hypergonadotropic hypogonadism in the male (primary hypogonadism). In: Kleigman RM, Behrman RE, Jenson HB, Stanton BF, eds. *Nelson Textbook of Pediatrics*. 18th ed. Philadelphia, PA: WB Saunders; 2007:2379-2382.

Reiter EO, D'Ercole AJ. Disorders of the anterior pituitary gland, hypothalamus, and growth. In: Rudolph CD, Rudolph AM, Hostetter MK, Lister G, Siegel NJ, eds. *Rudolph's Pediatrics*. 21st ed. New York, NY: McGraw-Hill; 2003:2011-2025.

# Case 22

A 2800-g male is born at 36-weeks' gestation to a 19-year-old mother via vaginal delivery. Delivery occurred 19 hours after membrane rupture. The mother's pregnancy was uncomplicated, but her prenatal records are not available at delivery. At 6 hours of age he is "breathing hard" and refusing to breast-feed. His respiratory rate is 60 breaths/min with "grunting." His temperature is 96.5°F (35.8°C), and his blood pressure is lower than normal. You ask the nurses to obtain a complete blood count (CBC) while you drive in from home. Upon arrival you confirm that he is in respiratory distress and that his perfusion is poor. The CBC demonstrates a white blood cell (WBC) count of 2500 cells/mm$^3$ with 80% bands. His radiograph is shown in Figure 22–1.

- What is the most likely diagnosis?
- What is the best therapy?

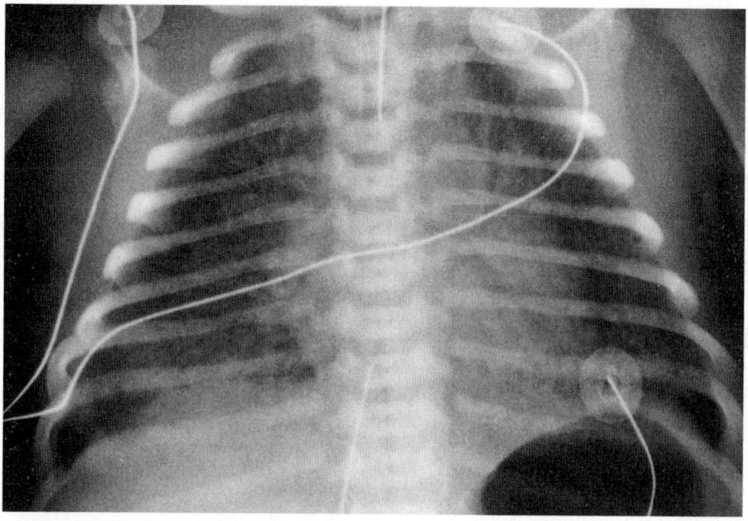

**Figure 22–1.** Chest radiograph of an infant.

# ANSWERS TO CASE 22:
# Group B Streptococcal Infection

*Summary:* A 2800-g infant born by vaginal delivery at 36-weeks' gestation is found to have poor feeding, tachypnea, hypothermia, and poor perfusion at 6 hours of age.

- **Most likely diagnosis:** Group B streptococcus (GBS) infection.
- **Best therapy:** Intravenous (IV) antibiotics (after addressing ABCs).

## ANALYSIS

### Objectives

1. Understand the common presentations of neonatal sepsis.
2. Understand the maternal risk factors for neonatal GBS infection.
3. Appreciate the variety of organisms responsible for neonatal infections.
4. Learn treatment options for the common neonatal infections.

### Considerations

The rapid symptom onset, the low WBC count with left shift, and the chest x-ray findings are typical for GBS pneumonia. At this point, management would include rapid application of the **ABCs** of resuscitation (maintain **A**irway, control **B**reathing, and ensure adequate **C**irculation), followed by rapid institution of appropriate antibiotics once cultures are obtained. Despite these measures, mortality from this infection is high.

# APPROACH TO
# Group B Streptococcal Infection

## DEFINITIONS

**EARLY-ONSET SEPSIS SYNDROME:** Neonatal sepsis occurring in the first 6 days of life. The majority of infection (approximately 85%) occurs in the first 24 hours of life, an additional 5% by approximately 48 hours, and the remainder throughout the next 4 days. The infection source usually is microorganism acquisition from the mother's genitourinary tract.

**GROUP B *STREPTOCOCCUS* (GBS) COLONIZATION:** Infection with GBS limited to mucous membrane sites in a healthy adult; the gastrointestinal (GI) tract is the most common colonization reservoir.

**LATE-ONSET SEPSIS SYNDROME:** Neonatal sepsis usually occurring after approximately 7 days but before approximately 90 days of life. The infection source often is the caregiver's environment.

**INTRAPARTUM ANTIBIOTIC PROPHYLAXIS:** Intravenous penicillin or ampicillin given during labor to prevent newborn GBS disease.

# CLINICAL APPROACH

## Signs and Symptoms of Sepsis

**The signs and symptoms of neonatal sepsis can be subtle and nonspecific,** often overlapping with findings in other conditions, such as respiratory distress syndrome, metabolic disorders, intracranial hemorrhages, and traumatic deliveries. Temperature instability, tachypnea, hypotension, and bradycardia are common findings in sepsis and meningitis. **Overwhelming shock is manifested as pallor and poor capillary refill.** Neurologic findings of impaired level of consciousness, coma, seizures, bulging anterior fontanelle, focal cranial nerve signs, and nuchal rigidity are unusual, but when present hint at meningitis, a condition more commonly seen in late-onset disease. Examination findings seen more frequently with pneumonia (more commonly seen in early-onset disease) include tachypnea, grunting, nasal flaring, retractions (costal or substernal), decreased breath sounds, and cyanosis.

## Evaluation of the Potentially Septic Child

Some neonatal sepsis laboratory findings can be nonspecific, including hypoglycemia, metabolic acidosis, and jaundice. The CBC often is used to help guide therapy, although the sensitivity and specificity of this test are low. Evidence of infection on CBC includes the following:

- Markedly elevated or low WBC counts
- Increased neutrophil count
- Increased immature to total neutrophil (I/T) ratios
- Thrombocytopenia with platelet counts less than 100,000/mm$^3$

The C-reactive protein (an acute phase protein increased with tissue injury) can be elevated in septic infants; some use it as an adjunct to assess for neonatal sepsis.

**A blood culture is crucial for patients with suspected sepsis.** Some argue that the low meningitis incidence, especially in early-onset disease, does not warrant routine cerebral spinal fluid testing; rather, the test should be reserved for documented (positive cultures) or presumed (patients so sick that a full antibiotic course is to be given regardless of culture results) sepsis. Urine cultures usually are included for late-onset disease evaluation. Chest radiologic findings include segmental, lobar, or diffuse reticulogranular patterns, the latter easily confused with respiratory distress syndrome (lack of surfactant).

## Pathogens

The organisms that commonly cause early-onset sepsis colonize in the mother's genitourinary tract and are acquired transplacentally, from an ascending infection or as the infant passes through the birth canal. **Specific organisms include GBS, *Escherichia coli, Haemophilus influenzae,* and *Listeria monocytogenes*.** Late-onset disease occurs when the infant becomes infected in the postnatal environment, such as from the skin, respiratory tract, conjunctivae, gastrointestinal tract, and umbilicus. For the hospitalized infant, bacteria sources include vascular or urinary catheters or contact with health-care workers. Organisms commonly seen to cause late-onset disease include coagulase-negative staphylococci, *Staphylococcus aureus*, *E coli*, *Klebsiella* sp, *Pseudomonas* sp, *Enterobacter* sp, *Candida*, GBS, *Serratia* sp, *Acinetobacter* sp, and anaerobes.

**Group-B *Streptococcus* is the most common cause of neonatal sepsis from birth to 3 months**. Approximately **80% of cases occur as early-onset disease** (septicemia, pneumonia, and meningitis) resulting from vertical transmission from mother to infant during labor and delivery. Respiratory signs (apnea, grunting respirations, tachypnea, or cyanosis) are the initial clinical findings in more than 80% of neonates, regardless of the site of involvement, whereas hypotension is an initial finding in approximately 25% of cases. Other signs are similar to those associated with other bacterial infections described above.

Neonates with GBS meningitis rarely have seizures as a presenting sign, yet 50% develop seizures within 24 hours of infection. The median age at diagnosis of early-onset GBS infection is 13 hours, earlier than for the other bacterial infections described above. Clinical history and findings suggestive of early-onset GBS disease (rather than of a noninfectious etiology for pulmonary findings) include prolonged rupture of membranes, apnea, hypotension in the first 24 hours of life, a 1-minute Apgar score less than 5, and rapid progression of pulmonary disease.

**Factors associated with increased risk for early-onset GBS disease** are **rupture of membranes more than 18 hours before delivery, chorioamnionitis or intrapartum temperature greater than 100.4°F (38°C), previous infant with GBS infection,** mother younger than 20 years, **and low birth weight or prematurity (<37 weeks' gestation).** Mortality as a result of GBS disease is close to 10%. Major neurologic sequelae (cortical blindness, spasticity, and global mental retardation) occur in 12% to 30% of infants who survive meningitis.

The incidence of early-onset GBS infection decreased from 1.7 per 1000 live births in 1993 to 0.6 per 1000 live births in 1998. The decline is largely attributed to the widespread use of GBS risk–reduction guidelines. These guidelines recommend **screening women at 35- to 37-week gestation and offering intrapartum antibiotic prophylaxis to those with risk factors or positive GBS cultures at 35- to 37-week gestation.** Infants born at less than 35-week gestation or born to women who received inadequate intrapartum prophylaxis sometimes undergo a limited evaluation that often includes a CBC and blood culture. The association of early antibiotic use with increased risk of late-onset serious bacterial infections remains under study.

## Treatment

Treatment of suspected early-onset disease includes antibiotics directed at the common pathogens listed above, often consisting of a combination of IV aminoglycosides (gentamicin or tobramycin) and penicillin (often ampicillin). For patients with late-onset disease, therapy often consists of β-lactamase–resistant antibiotics (such as vancomycin) and second- or third-generation cephalosporins. For early- and late-onset disease, antibiotic coverage is adjusted depending on the organism identified and the organism's specific antibiotic sensitivities.

Antibiotics are continued for at least 48 to 72 hours. If cultures are negative and the patient is well, antibiotics often are stopped. For **infants presenting with convincing signs and symptoms of sepsis, antibiotics may be continued even with negative cultures**. For infants with positive cultures, therapy continues for 10 to 21 days depending on the organism and the infection site. Close observation for signs of antibiotic toxicity is important for all infants.

# Comprehension Questions

22.1 A newborn infant was born at home. At 2 days of life he is has puffy, tense eyelids, red conjunctivae, a copious purulent ocular discharge, and chemosis. Which of the following is the most likely diagnosis?

A. Chemical conjunctivitis
B. Chlamydial conjunctivitis
C. Dacryocystitis
D. Gonococcal ophthalmia
E. Pneumococcal ophthalmia

22.2 A term 3500-g female delivered by cesarean section develops a respiratory rate of 70 breaths/min and expiratory grunting at 1 hour of life. She has good tone, good color, and a strong suck. Which of the following is the most likely diagnosis?

A. Intubation and suctioning below the vocal cords
B. Administration of surfactant
C. Initiation of antibiotic therapy
D. Swallow study and upper GI series
E. Observation for a period of several hours

22.3 A term infant is born to a 23-year-old known HIV-positive mother. The mother has been followed closely during the pregnancy, and she has been taking antiretroviral medications for the weeks prior to the delivery. Routine management of the healthy infant should include which of the following?

A. Administration of intravenous immunoglobulin to the baby to decrease the risk of perinatal HIV infection
B. Admission to the neonatal intensive care unit for close cardiovascular monitoring
C. Beginning a course of zidovudine for the infant
D. Chest radiographs to evaluate for congenital *Pneumocystis carinii*
E. HIV enzyme-linked immunosorbent assay (ELISA) on the infant to determine if congenital infection has occurred

22.4 A 2150-g infant is delivered at 34-week gestation. The mother had prenatal care in Mexico and says she had no problems. Her highest temperature during labor was 100.8°F (38.2°C). The amniotic fluid had a brown-stained appearance. At birth the infant had a diffuse erythematous pustular rash, pallor, poor feeding, tachypnea, and cyanosis. His CBC indicates marked monocytosis. He dies at 4 hours of age, soon after initiation of antibiotics. He most likely had which of the following?

A. Congenital syphilis
B. Congenital varicella
C. Disseminated herpes
D. GBS disease
E. Listeriosis

## ANSWERS

22.1 **D.** The time of symptom onset in a neonate with conjunctivitis can be helpful. Chemical conjunctivitis that is self-limited and presents within 6 to 12 hours of birth is the result of ocular silver nitrate or erythromycin prophylaxis irritation. Gonococcal conjunctivitis usually occurs within 2 to 5 days of birth and is the most serious of the bacterial infections; prompt and aggressive topical treatment and systemic antibiotics can prevent serious complications such as corneal ulceration, perforation, and resulting blindness. Parents are treated for gonococcal disease to prevent a child's reinfection. Chlamydial conjunctivitis often presents 5 to 14 days after birth and usually is treated with systemic erythromycin (in part to reduce the infant's risk of chlamydial pneumonia at 2-3 months of age). The risks of oral erythromycin treatment must be weighed against the increased risk of hypertrophic pyloric stenosis, a condition associated with oral erythromycin use in children. Both parents of a child with chlamydial conjunctivitis also are treated.

22.2 **E.** Transient tachypnea of the newborn is a respiratory condition resulting from incomplete evacuation of fetal lung fluid in full-term infants. It occurs more commonly with cesarean deliveries and usually disappears within 24 to 48 hours of life. Often no treatment is indicated unless the infant requires low amounts of supplemental oxygen. Antibiotics would be indicated for a child for whom pneumonia would be suspected; these children usually do not have a vigorous suck as outlined in the question. Intubation and suctioning below the vocal folds hints at meconium aspiration; the intubation would appropriately be accomplished in the delivery room and not hours later. The barium swallow and upper GI series might be helpful to identify a tracheoesophageal fistula. Exogenous surfactant is used for premature infants for whom surfactant deficiency is suspected.

22.3 **C.** HIV transmission from mother to infant has decreased by more than 50% in the past 15 years, probably as a result of perinatal antiretroviral administration to the mother and a zidovudine course to the exposed infant. Transplacentally transmitted maternal HIV antibodies will result in a positive neonatal ELISA; it is not a useful test for determining newborn infection. Intravenous immunoglobulin has not been shown to have a role in decreasing perinatal transmission. Healthy infants born to HIV-infected mothers do not require special monitoring or routine radiographs.

22.4 **E.** Listeria is a gram-positive rod isolated from soil, streams, sewage, certain foods, silage, dust, and slaughterhouses. The food borne transmission of disease is related to soft-ripened cheese, whole and 2% milk, undercooked chicken and hot dogs, raw vegetables, and shellfish. The newborn infant acquires the organism transplacentally or by aspiration or ingestion at delivery. The mortality rate of early-onset disease is approximately 30%.

## Clinical Pearls

- Sepsis in the neonate can present with nonspecific findings of temperature instability, tachypnea, poor feeding, bradycardia, hypotension, and hypoglycemia.
- Early-onset neonatal infection (occurring in the first 6 days of life) usually is caused by organisms of the maternal genitourinary system, including group B *Streptococcus* (GBS), *E coli, H influenzae*, and *L monocytogenes*. Pneumonia and sepsis are common presentations; GBS is the leading cause.
- Late-onset neonatal infection (occurring between 7 and 90 days of life) is often caused by organisms found in the infant's environment, including coagulase-negative staphylococci, *S aureus*, *E coli*, *Klebsiella* sp., *Pseudomonas* sp, *Enterobacter* sp, *Candida*, GBS, *Serratia* sp, *Acinetobacter* sp, and anaerobic bacteria.
- Treatment of early-onset neonatal infection usually includes a penicillin and an aminoglycoside, whereas treatment of late-onset disease consists of with a β-lactamase–resistant antibiotic (such as vancomycin) and often a third-generation cephalosporin.
- The incidence of early-onset GBS infection is decreasing, likely as a result of the widespread implementation of GBS risk–reduction guidelines.

## REFERENCES


Brady MT. Human immunodeficiency virus type 1 infection in infants and children. In: Rudolph CD, Rudolph AM, Hostetter MK, Lister G, Siegel NJ, eds. *Rudolph's Pediatrics*. 21st ed. New York, NY: McGraw-Hill; 2003:1045-1053.

Centers for Disease Control and Prevention. Prevention of perinatal group B streptococcal disease. Revised guidelines from CDC. *MMWR Recomm Rep*. 2002;51(RR-11):1-22.

Edwards MS. Group B streptococcal infections. In: Rudolph CD, Rudolph AM, Hostetter MK, Lister G, Siegel NJ, eds. *Rudolph's Pediatrics*. 21st ed. New York, NY: McGraw-Hill; 2003:999-1001.

Gallagher PG, Baltimore RS. Sepsis neonatorum. In: McMillan JA, Feigin RD, DeAngelis CD, Jones MD, eds. *Oski's Pediatrics: Principles and Practice*. 4th ed. Philadelphia, PA: Lippincott Williams & Wilkins; 2006:482-492.

Glasgow TS, Young PC, Wallin J, et al. Association of intrapartum antibiotic exposure and late-onset serious bacterial infections in infants. *Pediatrics*. 2005;116:696-702.

Lachenauer CS, Wessels MR. Group B *Streptococcus*. In: Kleigman RM, Behrman RE, Jenson HB, Stanton BF, eds. *Nelson Textbook of Pediatrics*. 18th ed. Philadelphia, PA: WB Saunders; 2007:1145-1150.

Moylett EH, Shearer WT. Pediatric human immunodeficiency virus infection. In: McMillan JA, Feigin RD, DeAngelis CD, Jones MD, eds. *Oski's Pediatrics: Principles and Practice*. 4th ed. Philadelphia, PA: Lippincott Williams & Wilkins; 2006:942-952.

Olitsky SE, Hug D, Smith LP. Disorders of the conjunctiva. In: Kleigman RM, Behrman RE, Jenson HB, Stanton BF, eds. *Nelson Textbook of Pediatrics*. 18th ed. Philadelphia, PA: WB Saunders; 2007:2588-2591.

Tong JT. Bacterial conjunctivitis. In: Rudolph CD, Rudolph AM, Hostetter MK, Lister G, Siegel NJ, eds. *Rudolph's Pediatrics*. 21st ed. New York, NY: McGraw-Hill; 2003:2370-2373.

Traboulsi EI. Ophthalmia neonatorum. In: McMillan JA, Feigin RD, DeAngelis CD, Jones MD, eds. *Oski's Pediatrics: Principles and Practice*. 4th ed. Philadelphia, PA: Lippincott Williams & Wilkins; 2006:811-812.

Yogev R, Chadwick E. Acquired immunodeficiency syndrome (human immunodeficiency virus). In: Kleigman RM, Behrman RE, Jenson HB, Stanton BF, eds. *Nelson Textbook of Pediatrics*. 18th ed. Philadelphia, PA: WB Saunders; 2007:1427-1443.

# Case 23

A 3-month-old boy is discovered not breathing in his crib this morning. Cardiopulmonary resuscitation was begun by the parents and was continued by paramedics en route to the hospital. You continue to try to revive the child in the emergency center, but pronounce him dead after 20 minutes of resuscitation. You review the history with the family and examine the child, but you are unable to detect a cause of death.

- How should you manage this situation in the emergency department?
- What is the most likely diagnosis?
- What is the next step in the evaluation?

# ANSWERS TO CASE 23:
# Sudden Infant Death Syndrome

*Summary:* A 3-month-old boy discovered not breathing by his parents.

- **First step:** Tell the boy's parents that despite everyone's best efforts, their son has died. Ask the parents if they would like you to call a friend, family member, religious leader, or other support person. Provide them with a quiet room where they can be left alone.
- **Most likely diagnosis:** Sudden infant death syndrome (SIDS) is the most likely diagnosis, assuming that the parents' story is true. Infanticide must be considered, as well as the possibility of an underlying congenital or metabolic disorder.
- **Next step:** Discuss with the parents that routine protocol is followed after an unexplained infant death. A coroner will perform an autopsy and police investigators will examine the parents' home for clues related to the death. Emphasize that these measures can help to bring closure for the family and may yield important information for preventing future child deaths should the couple have more children.

## ANALYSIS

### Objectives

1. Know the definition of SIDS.
2. Know the factors that are associated with SIDS.
3. Know how to counsel parents about SIDS risk–reducing measures.

### Considerations

Sudden infant death syndrome is one of the most tragic and frustrating medical diagnoses. When the family is in the emergency center, other possible causes of death (eg, child abuse or inherited disorders) cannot be excluded. Your role is to remain objective about these other possibilities yet sympathetic to the parents' grieving. As always, meticulous documentation of the history and physical examination findings is imperative.

# APPROACH TO
# Sudden Infant Death Syndrome

## DEFINITIONS

**APPARENT LIFE-THREATENING EVENT (ALTE):** Observations and events perceived by a caregiver as life-threatening. By definition, the event is observed. Myriad conditions may be responsible, including cardiac, respiratory, central nervous system (CNS), metabolic, infectious, and gastrointestinal causes. In approximately 50% of cases a cause is never known.

**APNEA:** Cessation of breathing for at least 20 seconds that may be accompanied by bradycardia or cyanosis. Recurrent episodes of apnea related to immaturity may occur in premature infants, but usually resolve by 37 weeks postgestational age.

**SUDDEN INFANT DEATH SYNDROME (SIDS):** The sudden death of an infant that cannot be explained by results of a postmortem examination, death scene investigation, and historical information.

## CLINICAL APPROACH

**Sudden infant death syndrome is the most common cause of death in infants between the ages of 1 week and 1 year.** The majority of SIDS deaths occur between 1 and 5 months of age, with a peak incidence between 2 and 4 months of age; it is **more common in winter**. Sudden infant death syndrome is more common among **African-American and Native-American infants**; whether these latter associations result from ethnicity or reflect other environmental factors is unclear.

No cause of SIDS has been identified. Epidemiologic studies suggest that the following are independent SIDS risk factors: **prone sleep position**, sleeping on a soft surface, pre- and postnatal exposure to tobacco smoke, overheating, late or no prenatal care, young maternal age, **prematurity** and/or low birth weight, and **male gender**. The incidence of SIDS has decreased dramatically in areas with public education campaigns targeted at limiting prone sleep positioning. Use of pacifiers, which some believe helps to maintain an infant's respiratory drive, may decrease the incidence of SIDS deaths. The investigation of the unexpected infant death includes a clinical history, a postmortem examination, and a death scene investigation. In some infants, autopsy reveals mild pulmonary edema and scattered intrathoracic petechiae; these findings are supportive but not diagnostic of SIDS.

Explainable causes of sudden infant death can be divided into **congenital and acquired conditions. Congenital conditions** include **cardiac anomalies** (arrhythmia, congenital heart disease), **metabolic disorders, and CNS etiologies.**

**Acquired causes** include **infection** and both **accidental and intentional trauma.** Infants who have experienced an ALTE may be at risk for sudden death. The evaluation of an ALTE infant is guided by the history and physical examination. **A report of feeding difficulties or emesis leads to consideration of swallowing studies, whereas unusual posturing or movements leads to an electroencephalogram**. A complete blood count and serum bicarbonate level obtained close to the time of the event may help to uncover an infectious or metabolic etiology. An electrocardiogram may be considered to look for prolonged QT syndrome or other cardiac anomaly. Documented cardiorespiratory monitoring and polysomnography can be helpful in some cases.

In the past, infants with a history of apnea were thought to be at risk for SIDS, but more recent epidemiologic research has refuted this hypothesis. Siblings of infants who have died of SIDS have been reported to potentially be at increased risk of SIDS themselves, but the role of a possible genetic susceptibility versus environmental factors and unrecognized infanticide in these cases is unclear.

## Comprehension Questions

23.1 Which of the following infants most warrants home cardiorespiratory monitoring?

A. A healthy 3-month-old infant, born at term, whose weight is at the fifth percentile
B. A healthy infant, born at 29-week gestation, whose weight is at the 50th percentile
C. A 5-month-old infant with a history of recurrent bouts of wheezing
D. A premature infant with recurrent apnea and bradycardia
E. A healthy term infant whose older sibling died of SIDS

23.2 A pregnant woman comes to you for a prenatal visit. As her family pediatrician, your advice to her should include which of the following statements about reducing the risk of SIDS?

A. Reduce the infant's exposure to tobacco smoke, and always place the baby in the supine position when she sleeps.
B. Always keep the baby in the prone position, even while awake.
C. Administer supplemental infant vitamins.
D. Attempt to make breast milk the infant's primary source of nutrition.
E. Protect the infant from people who are ill.

23.3 Which of the following statements about SIDS is accurate?
A. Most victims are girls.
B. The incidence is lowest among African Americans and Native Americans.
C. Home monitoring reduces the risk.
D. Most cases are attributable to a metabolic defect.
E. It is the most common cause of death between the ages of 7 and 365 days.

23.4 The investigation of an unexpected infant death includes a history, a postmortem examination, and which of the following?
A. DNA studies
B. An arterial blood gas measurement
C. A venous blood gas measurement
D. A death scene investigation
E. Stool studies

## ANSWERS

23.1 **D.** Home cardiorespiratory monitoring has not been shown to decrease the incidence of SIDS. Monitoring is recommended for symptomatic premature infants (ie, those with apnea and bradycardia), but can safely be discontinued by 43 weeks post-gestational age in most cases. Monitoring may also be warranted for children with certain underlying chronic conditions, such as those with chronic lung disease. It is not recommended for the infants in choices A, B, or C. The occurrence of a genetic susceptibility to SIDS within a family is thought to be exceedingly rare.

23.2 **A.** Although your advice to this woman might also include choices C, D, and E, these measures have not been shown to reduce the infant's risk of SIDS.

23.3 **E.** SIDS is the most common cause of death of infants between 1 week and 1 year of age, and it more commonly affects boys and Native-American and African-American children.

23.4 **D.** A death scene investigation is crucial to rule out trauma, both intentional and accidental.

## Clinical Pearls

- Sudden infant death syndrome (SIDS) is a diagnosis of exclusion assigned only after the postmortem investigation, postnatal history, and crime scene investigation fail to yield another explanation.
- Prone sleep position and exposure to cigarette smoke are significant risk factors for SIDS.
- Apparent life-threatening events (ALTE) are observed occurrences that can be caused by myriad etiologies.
- Apnea of prematurity is not a risk factor for SIDS.

## REFERENCES

American Academy of Pediatrics, Task Force on Infant Sleep Position and Sudden Infant Death Syndrome. Changing concepts of sudden infant death syndrome: implications for infant sleeping environment and sleep position. *Pediatrics*. 2000;105:650-656.

Carroll JL, Loughlin GM. Sudden infant death syndrome. In: McMillan JA, Feigin RD, DeAngelis CD , Jones MD, eds. *Oski's Pediatrics: Principles and Practice*. 4th ed. Philadelphia, PA: Lippincott Williams & Wilkins; 2006:722-728.

Committee on Fetus and Newborn. Apnea, sudden infant death syndrome, and home monitoring. *Pediatrics*. 2003:111;914-917.

Hunt CE, Hauck FR. Sudden infant death syndrome. In: Kliegman RM, Behrman RE, Jenson HB, Stanton BF, eds. *Nelson Textbook of Pediatrics*. 18th ed. Philadelphia, PA: WB Saunders; 2007:1736-1741.

Mitchell EA, Blair PS, L'Hoir MP. Should pacifiers be recommended to prevent sudden infant death syndrome? *Pediatrics*. 2006;117:1755-1758.

National Institutes of Health (NIH). Consensus development conference on infantile apnea and home monitoring. *Pediatrics*. 1987;79:292-299.

Silvestri JM, Wesse-Mayer DE. Apnea and SIDS. In: Rudolph CD, Rudolph AM, Hostetter MK, Lister G, Siegel NJ, eds. *Rudolph's Pediatrics*. 21st ed. New York, NY: McGraw-Hill; 2003:1935-1937.

# Case 24

A 3-month-old boy in respiratory distress presents to the emergency department. It is January, so you suspect the coarse wheezes heard on chest auscultation by the triage nurse are the result of a viral respiratory infection; you approve the administration of an aerosolized albuterol. About 20 minutes later you are able to obtain from the mother a more complete history. She tells you the baby began having intermittent wheezing approximately 4 weeks ago and the episodes have become progressively worse. You then listen to the infant and discover that, in addition to wheezes, a holosystolic murmur can be heard along the left sternal border. The oxygen saturation obtained at triage was normal.

- ➤ What is the most likely diagnosis?
- ➤ What is the treatment for this condition?

# ANSWERS TO CASE 24: Ventricular Septal Defect

*Summary:* A 3-month-old infant presents with respiratory distress, wheezing, and a soft holosystolic heart murmur. His symptoms began 4 weeks ago, and have become progressively worse.

- **Most likely diagnosis:** Ventricular septal defect (VSD).
- **Treatment:** Medical management, and possible eventual surgical closure.

## ANALYSIS

### Objectives

1. Recognize the presenting signs and symptoms of VSD.
2. Know the major acyanotic congenital heart lesions.
3. Be familiar with the fetal circulation (Figure 24–1).

### Considerations

An acyanotic heart lesion is suspected in this child who has a new heart murmur without cyanosis. The fall in pulmonary vascular resistance that occurs in the weeks following birth allows blood to flow from left to right across a VSD, resulting in an audible murmur by 2 to 6 months of life. This child's VSD is of sufficient size to result in congestive heart failure. Unlike the cause of wheezing in most of the other infants presenting to the emergency department in winter, this child's respiratory distress is not due to a viral respiratory infection.

# APPROACH TO Acyanotic Heart Lesions

## DEFINITIONS

**EISENMENGER SYNDROME:** Pulmonary hypertension (HTN) resulting in right-to-left shunting of blood. This may occur with large ventricular septal defects (VSDs), atrioventricular canal lesions, and patent ductus arteriosus (PDA).

**LEFT-TO-RIGHT SHUNT:** Flow of blood from the systemic circulation into the pulmonary circulation across an anomalous connection, such as a PDA. Such lesions result in pulmonary congestion and systemic hypoperfusion, but they typically do not cause cyanosis.

**WIDENED PULSE PRESSURE:** An increase in the difference between systolic and diastolic pressures, resulting in a bounding arterial pulse. Many conditions may cause this finding, including fever, hyperthyroidism, anemia, arteriovenous fistulas, and PDA.

## CLINICAL APPROACH

**Congenital cardiac defects are first categorized according to the presence of cyanosis.** They are then further classified according to chest radiograph findings of increased, normal, or decreased pulmonary vascular markings, and then finally according to ventricular forces indicated on electrocardiography. **The majority of acyanotic lesions result in a change in volume load, usually from the systemic circulation to the pulmonary circulation (so-called left-to-right shunt).** Left untreated, defects that affect volume load can eventually result in increased pulmonary vascular pressure, causing reversal of blood flow across the defect and clinical cyanosis. Other forms of acyanotic defects cause changes in pressure; this group includes pulmonic and aortic valve stenosis and coarctation of the aorta.

**Ventricular septal defect is the most common heart lesion in children**, affecting 3 to 6 of every 1000 live term births. The majority of VSDs occur in the membranous portion of the septum, and small VSDs with minimal left-to-right shunts are the most common. Children with **small VSDs** usually are asymptomatic, and a **harsh, left lower sternal border holosystolic murmur is detected on physical examination.** The **murmur of a large VSD may be less harsh** because of the absence of a significant pressure gradient across the defect; large lesions are accompanied by **dyspnea, feeding difficulties, growth failure, and profuse perspiration**, and they may lead to recurrent infections and **cardiac failure**. Infants with large VSDs generally are not cyanotic, but they may become dusky during feeding or crying. A VSD may not be detected in the first few weeks of life because of high right-sided pressures but become audible as pulmonary vascular resistance drops and left-to-right shunting of blood increases across the defect. In children with significant VSDs, chest radiography shows cardiomegaly and pulmonary vascular congestion, and the electrocardiogram (ECG) shows biventricular hypertrophy.

Most small VSDs close spontaneously by 6 to 12 months of life. Medical management is reserved for infants who are symptomatic from larger VSDs. Medications include diuretics (eg, furosemide, chlorothiazide) and afterload reduction agents (eg, an angiotensin-converting enzyme inhibitor) and sometimes digoxin. When monitoring children with large VSDs one should not be misled by a softening murmur, as this may herald pulmonary vascular disease or infundibular stenosis rather than closure of the defect.

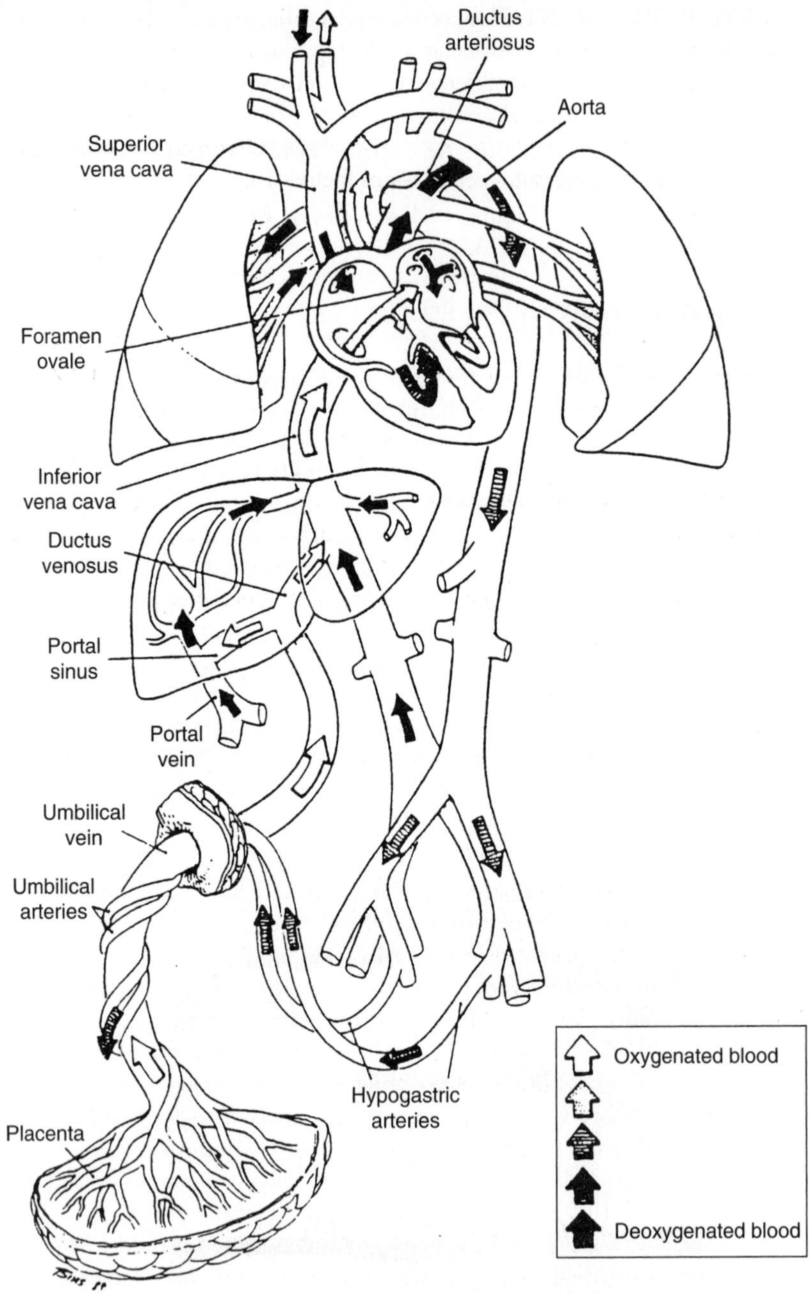


**Figure 24–1.** Fetal circulation. (*Reproduced, with permission, from Cunningham G, Leveno KL, Bloom SL.* Williams Obstetrics. *22nd ed. New York, NY: McGraw-Hill; 2005.)*

Most children with large VSDs develop pulmonary vascular resistance after 1 year of age although it can occur early; children with trisomy 21 are at particular risk of early disease. Children with persistently large shunts after 1 year of age usually undergo surgical closure, as one-third of these children have irreversible pulmonary vascular disease by 2 years of age **(Eisenmenger syndrome).**

Other acyanotic congenital heart lesions include **PDA**, atrial septal defects (ASDs), and atrioventricular septal defects. **Patent ductus arteriosus is most commonly seen in preterm infants,** but it also occurs in nonpremature children. **In utero, the ductus arteriosus shunts blood from the quiescent lungs via the pulmonary artery to the descending aorta.** Shortly after birth, pulmonary resistance begins to fall, and vasoconstriction of the ductus occurs. **Ductus closure in term infants usually occurs within 10 to 15 hours of birth and almost always by 2 days.** Closure is delayed in premature infants, perhaps as a result of impaired vasoconstrictor response to increased oxygen tension. Failure of the ductus to close allows shunting of blood from the systemic circulation to the pulmonary circulation, with resultant myocardial stress, pulmonary vascular congestion, and respiratory difficulty. **A small PDA usually results in no symptoms.** An infant with a **large PDA** typically has a **systolic or continuous "machinery-like" heart murmur,** an active precordium, and a widened pulse pressure. Occasionally, a PDA is present in association with another congenital cardiac lesion and may be difficult to detect. For patients with coarctation or interruption of the aortic arch, a PDA is vital to maintaining blood flow to the systemic circulation. Likewise, a PDA in the presence of an obstructed pulmonic valve is essential for providing blood flow to the lungs (Figure 24–2). Such lesions are called *ductus dependent*.

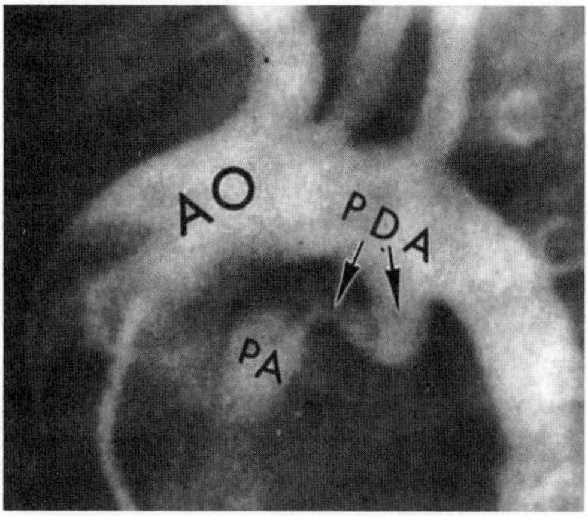


**Figure 24–2.** Angiography of persistent patent ductus arteriosus (PDA). AO, aorta; PA, pulmonary artery. (*Reproduced, with permission, from Rudolph CD, Rudolph AM, Hostetter MK, Lister G, Siegel NJ, eds.* Rudolph's Pediatrics. *21st ed. New York, NY: McGraw-Hill; 2003:1819.)*

**Children with ASDs often are asymptomatic** and are discovered inadvertently on routine physical examination. **Large defects may cause mild growth failure and exercise intolerance** not appreciated except in retrospect after defect closure. Physical findings include **second heart sound splitting that does not vary normally with respiration** ("fixed splitting"), and a systolic murmur at the left upper and midsternal borders caused by high-volume blood flow from the right ventricle into the normal pulmonary artery; the murmur is not blood flowing across the ASD itself. A lower left sternal border diastolic murmur produced by increased flow across the tricuspid valve may be present. The chest radiograph reveals an enlarged right atrium, right ventricle, and pulmonary artery and increased pulmonary vascularity; ECG shows right ventricular hypertrophy and sometimes right-axis deviation. **Atrial septal defects are well tolerated during childhood but can lead to pulmonary HTN in adulthood.** Infective endocarditis is rare; routine prophylaxis is not recommended. An isolated patent foramen ovale usually is not clinically significant and is not considered an ASD.

**Atrioventricular septal defect** (also known as AV canal or endocardial cushion defect) consists of a contiguous atrial and ventricular septal defect as well as abnormal AV (ie, mitral and tricuspid) valves. This acyanotic lesion requires correction in infancy to prevent cardiac failure and associated complications. A systolic murmur of large pulmonary flow is present, and a lower left sternal border diastolic murmur is heard. The second heart sound may be widely split. The chest radiograph and ECG show cardiac enlargement; pulmonary vascularity is increased on the chest film. Left untreated, these children develop **cardiac failure, growth failure, and recurrent pulmonary infections in infancy.** Pulmonary HTN develops with eventual right-to-left shunting and cyanosis. **Surgical correction is performed in infancy**.

## Comprehension Questions

24.1 A 2-month-old girl with Down syndrome is noted to have a systolic and a diastolic heart murmur, and the second heart sound is split. The liver edge is palpable 4 cm below the right costal margin. Her mother reports that lately the baby has been sweaty and sometimes blue around the mouth when she nurses, and she seems to be eating less than previously. Her EKG shows a superiorly oriented QRS frontal plane axis with counterclockwise depolarization pattern and right ventricular hypertrophy. Which of the following is the most likely diagnosis?

A. Atrial septal defect
B. Atrioventricular canal defect
C. Patent ductus arteriosus
D. Patent foramen ovale
E. Ventricular septal defect

24.2 A 29-week-old, 1000-g boy is admitted to the neonatal intensive care unit, where he receives routine care. He does well until day 5 of life, when he develops an increased respiratory rate, mild subcostal retractions, and a widened pulse pressure, but no cyanosis or increased oxygen requirement. A continuous murmur is heard along the left sternal border. Chest radiography shows pulmonary vascular congestion. Which of the following medications may best relieve his symptoms?

A. Albuterol
B. Racemic epinephrine
C. Indomethacin
D. Digoxin
E. Furosemide

24.3 A 12-month-old boy with a stable but moderate-size ventricular septal defect presents to the pediatric dentist for cleaning and management of his multiple caries. Prior to the procedure, he should receive which of the following?

A. Acetaminophen
B. Amoxicillin
C. Digoxin
D. Ditropan
E. None of the above

24.4 A previously healthy term infant suddenly develops respiratory distress on the day 3 of life. An echocardiogram reveals coarctation of the aorta. Which of the following is the most appropriate treatment for immediate stabilization of this infant?

A. Digoxin
B. Furosemide
C. Albuterol
D. Racemic epiniphrine
E. Prostaglandin therapy

## ANSWERS

24.1 **B.** Atrioventricular canal defect is common among children with Down syndrome. This infant's symptoms and clinical findings are most consistent with this diagnosis. While a simple VSD is common in patients with Down syndrome, the multitude of heart murmurs and ECG findings make this answer less likely.

24.2 **C.** A noncyanotic heart lesion is suspected in this child who has a new heart murmur without a corresponding increase in oxygen requirements. The murmur, not heard at birth, becomes evident after the pulmonary vascular resistance falls. His age, history, and physical findings are consistent with a patent ductus arteriosus (PDA). Indomethacin or surgical closure is used to treat this condition.

24.3 **E.** The guidelines for the use of prophylactic antibiotics are updated frequently by the American Heart Association. Among those currently recommended to receive antibiotic prophylactic treatment are patients for whom any heart infection would result in the highest incidence of adverse outcome: previous history of endocarditis, prosthetic valve or material for repair, heart transplant patients, and severe or partially repaired cyanotic congenital heart defects.

24.4 **E.** This infant's symptoms began when his ductus arteriosus began to close. Prostaglandin therapy can reverse this process in the short-term. Surgery or catheterization techniques provide definitive repair.

## Clinical Pearls

- Acyanotic heart lesions are characterized by shunting of blood from the systemic circulation to the pulmonary circulation ("left-to-right shunt").
- The most common congenital acyanotic heart lesion is the ventricular septal defect. Patent ductus arteriosus, atrial septal defect, and arteriovenous canal are other left-to-right shunt lesions.
- Left-to-right shunts eventually can reverse direction (right-to-left) and cause cyanosis if pulmonary hypertension develops (Eisenmenger syndrome).

## REFERENCES

Bernstein D. Acyanotic congenital heart disease: The left-to-right shunt lesions. In: Kliegman RM, Behrman RE, Jenson HB, Stanton BF, eds. *Nelson Textbook of Pediatrics*. 18th ed. Philadelphia, PA: WB Saunders; 2007:1883-1906.

Bernstein D. Evaluation of the infant or child with congenital heart disease. In: Kliegman RM, Behrman RE, Jenson HB, Stanton BF, eds. *Nelson Textbook of Pediatrics*. 18th ed. Philadelphia, PA: WB Saunders; 2007:1881-1883.

Clyman RI. Patent ductus arteriosus in the preterm infant. In: Rudolph CD, Rudolph AM, Hostetter MK, Lister G, Siegel NJ, eds. *Rudolph's Pediatrics*. 21st ed. New York, NY: McGraw-Hill; 2003:135-137.

Hoffman JIE. Left to right shunts. In: Rudolph CD, Rudolph AM, Hostetter MK, Lister G, Siegel NJ, eds. *Rudolph's Pediatrics*. 21st ed. New York, NY: McGraw-Hill; 2003:1782-1795.

Morriss MJH. Coarctation of the aorta. In: McMillan JA, Feigin RD, DeAngelis CD, Jones MD, eds. *Oski's Pediatrics: Principles and Practice*. 4th ed. Philadelphia, PA: Lippincott Williams & Wilkins; 2006:1591-1595.

Wilson W, Taubert KA, Gewitz M, et al. American Heart Association. Prevention of infective endocarditis. *Circulation*. 2007;116:1736-1754.

# Case 25

A term 3700-g infant was delivered vaginally without complications. He breast-feeds well, voids, and passes meconium in the first 12 hours of life. At 15 hours of life he is no longer interested in feeding and appears dusky. His respiratory rate is 65 breaths/min, and capillary refill is 3 seconds. No heart murmur is audible, but a loud single second heart sound is noted.

- What is the most likely diagnosis?
- What is the best management for this condition?

# ANSWERS TO CASE 25:
## Transposition of the Great Arteries

*Summary*: A healthy-appearing term infant suddenly loses interest in feeding and develops cyanosis, poor peripheral perfusion, and tachypnea. Cardiac examination reveals a loud second heart sound and no murmur.

- **Most likely diagnosis:** Cyanotic congenital heart disease (CHD), likely transposition of the great arteries (TGA).
- **Best initial management:** Administer prostaglandin $E_1$ to maintain patency of the ductus arteriosus.

## ANALYSIS

### Objectives

1. Know the major types of cyanotic CHD and their most common clinical presentations.
2. Understand why some types of CHD result in cyanosis whereas others do not.
3. Understand the need to maintain ductus arteriosus patency in some types of CHD.

### Considerations

This child has symptoms consistent with **cyanotic CHD** and likely has **TGA.** In this condition, the cardiac origins of the aorta and the pulmonary artery are switched, thus creating two parallel circuits of blood flow rather than the normal series circuit (Figure 25–1). This situation is **incompatible with life** unless a connection between the pulmonary and systemic circuits exists. During the first hours of life, the **ductus arteriosus and the foramen ovale provide this connection**; symptoms develop when this connection begins to close. Some TGA patients also have a ventricular septal defect (VSD) and may first show signs of disease later in infancy than do babies without VSDs. Management of the infant in this scenario consists of immediate steps to **maintain patency of the ductus arteriosus.** until surgical correction

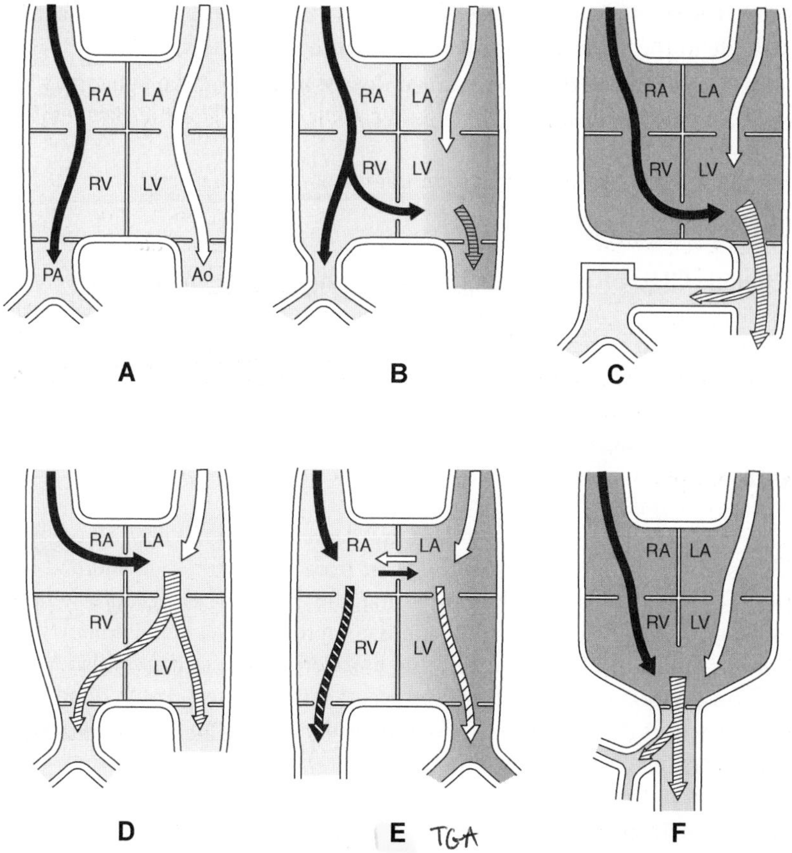


**Figure 25–1.** Schematic drawing of circulation of various cardiac defects: (**A**) Normal circulation; (**B**) tetralogy of Fallot; (**C**) pulmonary artresia; (**D**) tricuspid atresia; (**E**) transposition of the great arteries; (**F**) truncus arteriosus. Black arrows indicate deoxygenated blood; cross-hatched arrows indicate mixed blood; white arrows indicate oxygenated blood. LA, left atrium; LV, left ventricle; RA, right atrium; RV, right ventricle.

# APPROACH TO
# Congenital Cyanotic Heart Disease

## DEFINITIONS

**CYANOSIS:** Bluish discoloration of the skin and mucous membranes caused by insufficient saturation of the blood with oxygen.

**DUCTUS-DEPENDENT LESIONS:** Cardiac defects that are incompatible with life in the absence of a patent ductus arteriosus (PDA).

**RIGHT-TO-LEFT SHUNT:** Abnormal flow of blood from the pulmonary system to the systemic circulation across a cardiac defect. These lesions result in cyanosis.

## CLINICAL APPROACH

**Cyanotic CHD often manifests itself after the PDA begins to close** (ie, ductus dependent). Patency of the ductus maintains a connection between the pulmonary and systemic circulations; closure normally occurs on the first or second day of life in term infants. Previously, neonatal cyanotic CHD management involved emergency surgical repair on very sick infants; the introduction of **prostaglandin $E_1$, an intravenously administered medication that keeps the ductus open,** now allows for infant stabilization prior to more definitive corrections.

**Cyanotic CHD is characterized by decreased pulmonary blood flow.** Unsaturated blood returning to the heart from the periphery is shunted into the systemic circulation, thus bypassing the lungs. This occurs whenever blood flow into the pulmonary system is compromised, as in pulmonary valve stenosis or if the pulmonary artery and aorta origins are switched (TGA).

Transposition of the great arteries occurs in approximately 5% of children with congenital heart disease. **TGA typically causes an "egg-on-a-string" appearance on chest radiography** (Table 25–1), although the appearance may be normal in the first few days of life. Electrocardiography (ECG) shows the normal right-sided dominant pattern of the neonate. Diagnosis is confirmed with echocardiography.

**Initial management of TGA (after prostaglandins) involves creation of an atrial septum** ("atrial septostomy") via cardiac catheterization, which provides immediate symptom palliation. Definitive surgical care often occurs in the first 2 weeks of life; postoperative stenosis at the repair sites is a potential long-term complication.

**Pulmonary valve stenosis, another cyanotic CHD, accounts for approximately 20% to 30% of CHD.** Cyanosis and exercise intolerance, if any, are proportional to the degree of stenosis. Examination reveals an upper left sternal border systolic murmur that radiates to the back and a systolic click. The ECG is normal in mild cases, but greater stenosis causes right-axis deviation and right ventricular hypertrophy. Valvuloplasty is achieved via cardiac catheterization. Pulmonary stenosis may occur in conditions such as glycogen storage disease and Noonan syndrome.

**When pulmonary stenosis occurs with a large VSD, the result is known as tetralogy of Fallot (TOF).** With TOF, the intraventricular septum is displaced anteriorly, resulting in right ventricular outflow obstruction and displacement of the aorta over the right ventricle. Right ventricular hypertrophy

**Table 25–1 TYPICAL RADIOGRAPHIC FINDINGS OF COMMON HEART LESIONS**

| HEART ANOMALY | RADIOGRAPHIC APPEARANCE |
|---|---|
| Tetralogy of Fallot | "Boot-shaped" heart and decreased pulmonary vascularity |
| Pulmonary atresia (with intact ventricular septum) | Decreased pulmonary vascularity |
| Tricuspid atresia (with normally related great vessels) | Decreased pulmonary vascularity |
| Epstein anomaly | Heart size may be normal to massive, with normal or decreased pulmonary vascularity |
| Transposition of the great arteries | "Egg-on-a-string" (narrow mediastinum) with normal to increased pulmonary vascularity |
| Truncus arteriosus | Cardiomegaly and increased pulmonary vascularity |
| Total anomalous pulmonary venous return | "Snowman" (supracardiac shadow caused by anomalous pulmonary veins entering the innominate vein and persistent left superior vena cava), and increased pulmonary vascularity |
| Hypoplastic left heart syndrome | Cardiomegaly and increased pulmonary vascularity |

develops as a result of the hemodynamic changes caused by the other abnormalities. The characteristic finding on chest radiograph is a **boot or wooden shoe appearance** ("coeur en sabot," Table 25–1). If pulmonary stenosis is mild at birth, neonates have normal color (so-called pink tetralogy), but by early childhood most become cyanotic as a result of stenosis progression. **Many children with TOF also experience hypercyanotic spells ("tetralogy spells")** caused by a sudden increase in right-to-left shunting of blood. These spells may be brought on by activity or agitation, or they may occur without apparent precipitant. Such children can be seen assuming a squatting posture, which compresses peripheral blood vessels, thus increasing pulmonary blood flow and systemic arterial oxygen saturation. With current surgical management, 90% of patients with TOF survive to adulthood.

**Cyanosis is a hallmark of children who have tricuspid valve abnormalities of tricuspid atresia** or **Ebstein anomaly**. In tricuspid atresia, no outlet exists between the right atrium and the right ventricle, forcing systemic venous return to enter the left atrium via the foramen ovale or an associated atrial septal defect; a VSD also is often present. The tricuspid valve of Ebstein anomaly usually is regurgitant and often obstructs ventricular outflow because of a large anterior leaflet. Both conditions often are "ductal dependent" in the neonate, and both require surgical correction.

## Comprehension Questions

25.1 A 12-year-old boy requires a sports physical examination. He denies chronic health problems, including adverse exertion symptoms. The clinician notes a I–II/VI left upper sternal border systolic murmur that does not radiate. The second heart sounds splits normally, and no audible click is appreciated. Peripheral perfusion is normal, and the fingers are not clubbed. Which of the following is the best recommendation?

A. He should not play strenuous sports.
B. He can participate in sports without restrictions.
C. A chest radiograph and an ECG before further recommendation can be made.
D. A cardiology evaluation.
E. He may participate in sports, but he should seek immediate medical attention for dyspnea or other adverse symptoms.

25.2 A term, 3700-g infant is born vaginally without complications. At 24 hours of age, a II/VI systolic murmur is noted in the mitral area that radiates to the back. A similar murmur is noted in the right axilla. The infant is pink and breathing easily, and his bedside chart shows that he has been taking 30 cc of formula approximately every 2 hours. Initial management should include which of the following?

A. Chest radiography, ECG, and four extremity blood pressures.
B. Immediate administration of prostaglandin $E_1$.
C. Transfer to a neonatal intensive care unit.
D. Consultation by a pediatric cardiologist.
E. Discharge home with follow-up in the pediatric clinic at 3 days of life.

25.3 A 4-year-old boy presents for a well-child visit. His mother notes that he breathes fast and his lips turn "dusky" when he runs or plays hard. The symptoms resolve once he stops the activity. On examination, he has a II/VI left upper sternal border systolic murmur that radiates to the back; a faint click is heard. Which of the following is the most likely cause of this child's exercise intolerance?

A. Asthma
B. Atrial septal defect
C. Pulmonary valve stenosis
D. Tricuspid atresia
E. Ventricular septal defect

25.4 A 15-month-old girl is playing quietly in your waiting room. The skin around her mouth is faintly blue, but she appears comfortable. She arises from her squatting position to run after her brother, and she suddenly becomes dyspneic and cyanotic. She returns to a squatting position and soon is breathing comfortably with only slight perioral cyanosis. Which of the following would you expect to see on her chest radiograph?

A. A "boot-shaped" heart
B. An "egg on a string"
C. Lung hyperinflation
D. Pneumonia
E. Pulmonary congestion

## ANSWERS

25.1 **B.** This child has a benign pulmonary flow murmur, differentiated from a pathologic pulmonary murmur in that it does not radiate, no click is heard, and no signs and symptoms of cardiac disease (digital clubbing, cyanosis, exercise intolerance) are found.

25.2 **E.** This infant has peripheral pulmonic stenosis, a benign childhood murmur. Other frequently encountered benign childhood murmurs are the venous hum (a low-pitched murmur heard at the sternal notch only when the child is upright) and the Still vibratory murmur (a high-pitched "musical" systolic murmur heard best at the left sternal border in the supine position). Although it may be difficult to diagnose the multitude of pathologic heart sounds, clinicians certainly should know the characteristics of the common benign childhood murmurs.

25.3 **C.** Although pulmonary stenosis and tricuspid atresia are cyanotic heart lesions, exercise-induced cyanosis and systolic murmur are characteristic of pulmonary stenosis.

25.4 **A.** This child has TOF; she experiences improvement when squatting and "tet" (hypercyanotic) spells when running. The "boot-shaped" heart is a characteristic chest radiographic finding.

## Clinical Pearls

- Cyanotic congenital heart disease is characterized by decreased pulmonary blood flow (right-to-left shunt). Transposition of the great arteries and defects of the tricuspid valve and pulmonary outflow tract are examples of cyanotic heart defects.
- Lesions of congenital heart disease incompatible with life except in the presence of a PDA are termed "ductus dependent."
- Prostaglandin $E_1$ is often used in infants with cyanotic congenital heart disease to maintain the patent ductus arteriosus until more definitive surgical correction can be attempted.
- The heart defects in tetralogy of Fallot are (1) ventricular septal defect, (2) pulmonic stenosis, (3) overriding aorta, and (4) right ventricular hypertrophy.

## REFERENCES

Bernstein D. Cyanotic congenital heart lesions: lesions associated with decreased pulmonary blood flow. In: Kliegman RM, Behrman RE, Jenson HB, Stanton BF, eds. *Nelson Textbook of Pediatrics*. 18th ed. Philadelphia, PA: WB Saunders; 2007:1906-1918.

Bernstein D. Cyanotic congenital heart lesions: lesions associated with increased pulmonary blood flow. In: Kliegman RM, Behrman RE, Jenson HB, Stanton BF, eds. *Nelson Textbook of Pediatrics*. 18th ed. Philadelphia, PA: WB Saunders; 2007:1918-1930.

Neches WH, Park SC, Ettedgui JA. Transposition of the great arteries. In: McMillan JA, Feigin RD, DeAngelis CD, Jones MD, eds. *Oski's Pediatrics: Principles and Practice*. 4th ed. Philadelphia, PA: Lippincott Williams & Wilkins; 2006:1537-1539.

Teitel DF. Right-to-left shunts. In: Rudolph CD, Rudolph AM, Hostetter MK, Lister G, Siegel NJ, eds. *Rudolph's Pediatrics*. 21st ed. New York, NY: McGraw-Hill; 2003:1814-1826.

# Case 26

A 3-year-old boy has a 20-day history of high fevers that spike twice daily. He was diagnosed with otitis media on the fifth day of fever and was prescribed amoxicillin, but the fever persisted. The fever is associated with a faint rash on the trunk and proximal extremities and complaints of "body aches." A chest radiograph is normal, but a complete blood count (CBC) shows a hemoglobin of 9.8 mg/dL, a hematocrit of 29.9%, a white blood cell count of 18,000/$mm^3$ and a platelet count of 857,000/$mm^3$. He has developed an aversion to bearing weight and continues to have fevers to 102.5°F (39.2°C), but otherwise he has normal vital signs. His examination is remarkable for scattered lymphadenopathy, hepatosplenomegaly, and mild swelling of his interphalangeal joints and knees.

- ➤ What is the most likely diagnosis?
- ➤ What is the best diagnostic test for this disorder?
- ➤ What is the treatment for this condition?

# ANSWERS TO CASE 26:
# Juvenile Rheumatoid Arthritis

*Summary:* A 3-year-old boy has 20 days of high-spiking fevers and a rash and "body aches" that wax and wane with the fevers. He also has a 1-day history of refusal to bear weight. His examination is significant for lymphadenopathy, organomegaly, and joint swelling. His chest radiograph is negative, but the CBC reveals leukocytosis, thrombocytosis, and anemia.

- **Most likely diagnosis:** Systemic-onset juvenile rheumatoid arthritis (JRA; Still disease).
- **Best diagnostic test:** No laboratory studies are diagnostic for JRA, but a history plus a CBC, blood cultures, erythrocyte sedimentation rate (ESR), rheumatoid factor (RF), antinuclear antibody (ANA), and synovial fluid assessment can aid in establishing or eliminating this diagnosis.
- **Treatment:** Nonsteroidal anti-inflammatory drugs (NSAIDs), methotrexate, and glucocorticoids can be used to control symptoms. Physical and occupational therapy are important for preserving function and preventing deformity.

## ANALYSIS

### Objectives

1. Know the three forms of JRA and their most common presenting signs and symptoms.
2. Recognize systemic-onset JRA as an important consideration in the evaluation of childhood fever of unknown origin (FUO).

### Considerations

The **differential diagnosis for childhood FUO** is long and includes **infectious, hematologic, and rheumatologic causes**. The fever pattern can sometimes aid in narrowing the diagnostic possibilities. In this case, the **daily high-spiking fevers associated with a characteristic rash are suggestive of systemic JRA.** Organomegaly and lymphadenopathy also are characteristic of systemic JRA. Arthritis may develop after other symptoms begin, as in this case, sometimes appearing months or even years into the disease course. For cases where arthritis first appears late in the disease course, leukemia may be a consideration.

# APPROACH TO
## Juvenile Rheumatoid Arthritis

## DEFINITIONS

**ARTHRALGIA:** Any pain that affects a joint.

**ARTHRITIS:** Swelling or effusion or the presence of two or more of the following signs: limited range of motion, tenderness or pain on motion, and increased heat in one or more joints.

**SYSTEMIC-ONSET JRA:** Characterized by arthritis with prominent visceral involvement, including visceromegaly, serositis, and lymphadenopathy.

**PAUCIARTICULAR JUVENILE RHEUMATOID ARTHRITIS (OLIGO-ARTHRITIS):** JRA with involvement of one to four joints.

**POLYARTICULAR JUVENILE RHEUMATOID ARTHRITIS (POLY-ARTHRITIS):** JRA with involvement of five or more joints.

## CLINICAL APPROACH

**Juvenile rheumatoid arthritis is the most common rheumatologic disorder in children.** The diagnosis specifies onset prior to age 16 years and symptom duration of 6 weeks or longer. Other causes of arthritis in children (infectious and other rheumatologic causes) must be excluded; in the **sexually active adolescent, gonococcal arthritis must be considered.** Three diverse entities fall under the JRA rubric, classified according to symptoms occurring in the first 6 months of illness: **(1) systemic-onset disease, (2) polyarticular disease, and (3) pauciarticular disease.**

Systemic symptoms dominate the clinical scene in systemic-onset JRA, making the diagnosis difficult if frank arthritis is not present. **Daily high-spiking fevers, a rash and arthralgias that wax and wane with the fever, lymphadenopathy, and organomegaly are characteristic of systemic-onset disease.** Pericarditis, hepatitis, pleural effusion, and encephalopathy also may occur.

**Polyarticular disease** is diagnosed when **five or more joints are involved** and systemic signs and symptoms are mild or absent. This disease is more common in girls and usually occurs in the teen years, but it may appear as early as 8 years of age. Patients are stratified by RF: RF-negative patients generally have a better prognosis, although 5% to 10% progress to severe joint destruction. More than half of RF-positive patients progress to chronic disease; they are believed to be nearly identical to the adult entity of rheumatoid arthritis.

**Pauciarticular JRA** involves fewer than five joints; it is divided into early- and late-onset categories. Early-onset disease occurs predominantly in females, and serum ANA analysis often is positive. Half of the children with early-onset disease develop iridocyclitis (iris and ciliary body inflammation;

also called "anterior uveitis") that often is asymptomatic. Eye disease does not parallel the arthritis activity. Late-onset disease primarily affects boys older than 8 years. Late-onset JRA can progress to lumbar and sacral joint involvement (ankylosing spondylitis).

The initial laboratory evaluation for the child with suspected systemic JRA includes a CBC, ESR, and blood cultures. **Leukocytosis, thrombocytosis, and anemia support the diagnosis of systemic JRA.** The ESR is elevated, and blood cultures are negative. **Evaluation of synovial fluid** may be necessary to rule out septic arthritis, particularly in the presence of exquisitely tender joints or when only a single joint is involved. Rheumatoid factor and ANA usually are negative in systemic JRA.

**Medications** for JRA include **NSAIDs, steroids, methotrexate**, and other immunosuppressive agents. Physical and occupational therapy are vital for maintaining joint function and preventing further deformities. **Routine slit-lamp ophthalmic examinations to monitor for uveitis** are indicated. Approximately 50% of systemic JRA patients eventually recover completely, but 25% develop chronic and destructive arthritis. **Death can occur, usually from overwhelming infection.**

## Comprehension Questions

26.1 A 14-year-old girl has a 3-day history of swollen "neck nodes" and a diffuse salmon-colored rash. On review of systems, she reports a sore throat and a cough with low-grade fever 5 days ago; these symptoms resolved 2 days ago. On examination, she has enlarged posterior auricular and suboccipital lymph nodes and tender swelling of multiple large and small joints. Which of the following is the most likely diagnosis?

A. Pauciarticular JRA
B. Polyarticular JRA
C. Rubella
D. Systemic lupus erythematosus
E. Systemic-onset JRA

26.2 A 5-year-old girl is referred to a pediatric rheumatologist with a 4-week history of mild swelling and decreased range of motion in the left knee and right elbow. She is afebrile and appears otherwise well. Positive findings on which of the following evaluations will be most helpful in establishing her diagnosis?

A. Arthrocentesis
B. Complete blood count
C. Computerized tomographic scan of the involved joints
D. Slit-lamp examination of her eyes
E. Bone scan

26.3 An obese 12-year-old African-American boy complains of right knee pain. He denies trauma to the right leg. He has a notable limp favoring the right lower extremity. Initial evaluation of his condition should include which of the following?
A. Antinuclear antibody
B. Complete blood count
C. Magnetic resonance imaging of both knees
D. Range of motion of the right hip
E. Rheumatoid factor

26.4 A 3-year-old boy with suspected systemic-onset JRA develops tachycardia and dyspnea on the fifth hospital day. He complains that his chest hurts. Heart auscultation reveals a "friction rub" sound. Which of the following is the next best step in management?
A. Give him a nebulized albuterol treatment.
B. Give him a dose of furosemide.
C. Give him some acetaminophen.
D. Check his oxygenation status via pulse oxymetry, obtain a stat electrocardiogram, and consult with a pediatric cardiologist.
E. Check his oxygenation status via pulse oxymetry, obtain a stat chest x-ray, and initiate intravenous antibiotics.

## ANSWERS

26.1 **C.** The differential diagnosis for childhood arthritis includes infectious and rheumatologic disorders. Her signs and symptoms are typical of rubella. Vaccination is given at age 1 year and again at school entry. The major reason for vaccination is to prevent congenital rubella syndrome, a devastating neonatal condition; the disease usually is mild in non-neonates.

26.2 **D.** JRA is the most common cause of uveitis in children. Uveitis onset may be insidious, and may be the only initial manifestation of JRA. The disease is more common in young girls. Slit-lamp findings include calcific band keratopathy, posterior synechiae, and cataracts. Children with JRA should have periodic slit-lamp examinations in order to detect eye disease early. Consideration may be given to obtaining the tests suggested in the other answer choices, but positive results on these tests are unlikely to be specific for JRA.

26.3 **D.** Careful attention is paid to the hips when evaluating knee complaints; pain from a hip problem can be referred to the knee. Slipped capital femoral epiphysis occurs most commonly in obese African-American boys. JRA rarely affects the hip in the initial disease course.

26.4 **D.** A friction rub is characteristic of pericarditis, which is a common and serious complication of JRA. The friction rub is a "grating" or "creaking" sound that often is best heard along the left sternal border. Patients typically complain of chest pain that is relieved when the patient is asked to lean forward, and worsened by deep inspiration or coughing; pain is not always present, however. Rarely, pericarditis in JRA may precede the development of arthritis by months or even years. Low voltage QRS complexes and ST-segment elevation may be seen on the electrocardiogram. Treatment consists of salicylates or steroids.

## Clinical Pearls

- The spectrum of juvenile rheumatoid arthritis comprises three entities: (1) systemic-onset disease, (2) polyarticular disease, and (3) pauciarticular disease.
- Systemic-onset juvenile rheumatoid arthritis is an important consideration in the differential diagnosis of childhood fever of unknown origin.
- The diagnosis of juvenile rheumatoid arthritis is based on clinical criteria and by the exclusion of other possibilities; no single laboratory test confirms the diagnosis.

## REFERENCES

Cassidy JT. Juvenile rheumatoid arthritis. In: McMillan JA, Feigin RD, DeAngelis CD , Jones MD, eds. *Oski's Pediatrics: Principles and Practice*. 4th ed. Philadelphia, PA: Lippincott Williams & Wilkins; 2006:2538-2543.

Miller KM, Apt L. Anterior uveitis. In: Rudolph CD, Rudolph AM, Hostetter MK, Lister G, Siegel NJ, eds. *Rudolph's Pediatrics*. 21st ed. New York, NY: McGraw-Hill; 2003: 2382-2384.

Miller ML, Cassidy JT. Juvenile rheumatoid arthritis. In: Kliegman RM, Behrman RE, Jenson HB, Stanton BF, eds. *Nelson Textbook of Pediatrics*. 18th ed. Philadelphia, PA: WB Saunders; 2007:1001-1011.

Wallace CA, Sherry DD. Juvenile rheumatoid arthritis. In: Rudolph CD, Rudolph AM, Hostetter MK, Lister G, Siegel NJ, eds. *Rudolph's Pediatrics*. 21st ed. New York, NY: McGraw-Hill; 2003:836-840.

# Case 27

A 2-year-old girl, born at 32 weeks' gestation, comes to your office for an initial visit. Her 1-month stay in the neonatal intensive care unit was complicated by necrotizing entercolitis (NEC), requiring surgical removal of a small section of her intestine that included the ileocecal valve. She had an uncomplicated postoperative course, and, per her mother, has been developing normally and gaining weight. Her mother reports that the child has a healthy appetite, a varied diet, and no history of abnormal stooling. She is concerned, though, that her daughter has been getting progressively paler since her last clinic visit with another provider 6 months ago. Physical examination reveals an overall healthy-appearing toddler with normal vital signs. She has pallorous skin and conjunctivae and a well-healed abdominal surgical scar. The remainder of her physical examination is normal. You order a complete blood count and a reticulocyte count and find that the hemoglobin is 7 g/dL, the mean corpuscular volume is 110 fL, and the reticulocyte count is 2%.

➤ What is the most likely cause of this child's anemia?

➤ How should she be treated?

# ANSWERS TO CASE 27: Macrocytic (Megaloblastic) Anemia Secondary to Vitamin $B_{12}$ Deficiency

*Summary:* A 2-year-old former premature infant with history of NEC and intestinal resection presenting with pallor and anemia.

- **Most likely cause:** Vitamin $B_{12}$ deficiency secondary to terminal ileal resection and compromised intestinal absorption.
- **Treatment:** Monthly intramuscular vitamin $B_{12}$ supplementation.

## ANALYSIS

### Objectives

1. Describe the typical findings in macrocytic anemia.
2. List the potential causes of macrocytic anemia.
3. Understand the treatment options for macrocytic anemia.

### Considerations

Evaluation of a child with suspected anemia involves performing thorough personal and family histories and a comprehensive physical examination. Anemia can result from a variety of disorders, including defective red blood cell production, hemolysis, or blood loss. The clinician's goal, therefore, is to gather historical clues (atypical patient or family dietary histories, family history of blood dyscrasias) and examination findings (splenomegaly, flow murmur, hematochezia) that are important in guiding appropriate diagnostic and therapeutic plans.

# APPROACH TO Macrocytic Anemia

## DEFINITIONS

**MEAN CORPUSCULAR VOLUME (MCV):** Average size of a red blood cell; large cells are macrocytic; small cells are microcytic.

**RETICULOCYTE COUNT:** Percentage of red blood cells that are immature (new).

**INTRINSIC FACTOR:** Glycoprotein secreted in the stomach that binds to vitamin $B_{12}$; the intrinsic factor-vitamin $B_{12}$ complex then attaches to receptors in the distal ileum and is absorbed.

## CLINICAL APPROACH

**Anemia typically is distinguished by the size of the red blood cells.** Children with **iron deficiency develop a microcytic anemia and typically have a low MCV**; their red blood cells are smaller than normal because of the decreased amount of hemoglobin in each cell. Children who quickly lose a large amount of blood usually have a normocytic anemia; the cells are normal, but there are fewer of them.

Various conditions may result in **macrocytic anemia, usually associated with an elevated MCV. Hypothyroidism, trisomy 21, vitamin $B_{12}$ deficiency, and folate deficiency** often are associated with macrocytic anemia and a low reticulocyte count, as a result of inadequate bone marrow production. A macrocytic anemia also may be seen with active hemolysis, but usually this anemia is accompanied by an elevated reticulocyte count.

Vitamin $B_{12}$-mediated macrocytic anemia can occur as a result of dietary deficiency, malabsorption, or inborn errors of metabolism. Vitamin $B_{12}$, an important factor in DNA synthesis, is available in many foods (meats, fish, eggs). A pure dietary deficiency is rare in children, but diets devoid of all animal products may result in a deficiency. **Breast-fed infants of mothers who adhere to a strict vegan diet are at risk for vitamin $B_{12}$ deficiency.** Malabsorption can occur when the terminal ileum is absent, as in this case scenario, or when infectious or inflammatory conditions compromise intestinal function.

Children with the rare condition "juvenile pernicious anemia" are unable to secrete intrinsic factor and become vitamin $B_{12}$ deficient between the ages of 1 and 5 years, when the supply of vitamin $B_{12}$ passed transplacentally from mother to child is exhausted. These children will exhibit worsening irritability, loss of appetite, and decreased activity. Children affected with this condition are at risk for permanent neurologic damage resulting from spinal cord demyelinization. Therapy is intramuscular vitamin $B_{12}$ replacement. High-dose oral replacement *may* be corrective (limited, inconclusive studies at present) in patients with intrinsic factor deficiency or severe dietary deficiency that cannot be corrected with dietary modification.

A variety of other more unusual causes of vitamin $B_{12}$ deficiency can be listed. The fish tapeworm *Diphyllobothrium latum* uses vitamin $B_{12}$, and intestinal infestation can result in macrocytic anemia. Similarly, any intestinal infectious or inflammatory process, such as parasitic infection or inflammatory bowel disease, could promote vitamin $B_{12}$ deficiency. Infants exclusively fed goat's milk, nutritionally deficient in both vitamin $B_{12}$ and folate, are at risk not only for vitamin $B_{12}$ deficiency but also brucellosis if the milk is unpasteurized. For infants feed goat's milk, vitamin and mineral supplementation is required.

Treatment for $B_{12}$ deficiency is guided by the underlying disorder. Eradicating or suppressing a gastrointestinal infection or inflammatory disorder should promote sufficient mucosal repair to permit adequate vitamin $B_{12}$ absorption and further vitamin $B_{12}$ therapy may not be required. For patients with an inability to produce intrinsic factor and for those with absence or permanent dysfunction of the gastric antrum or terminal ileum (the site of intrinsic factor production and absorption, respectively) monthly parenteral vitamin $B_{12}$ therapy is indicated.

For patients with macrocytosis but normal $B_{12}$ and folate levels, consideration for atypical bone marrow pathology (such as leukemia or myelodysplasia) must be entertained. Referral to a pediatric hematologist would be warranted.

## Comprehension Questions

27.1 You are called to the bedside of a mother who just delivered a healthy term infant and has a question regarding her infant's nutrition. The mother was fed goat's milk as a child and wants to do the same for her infant. Under which of the following conditions is goat's milk acceptable as infant nutrition?

A. Goat's milk proteins are hydrolyzed before feeds.
B. Infants are provided supplemental vitamins and minerals.
C. Goat's milk is freshly obtained from goats.
D. Infants of mothers with milk intolerance should preferentially receive goat's milk.
E. Goat's milk is diluted with water.

27.2 You receive the results of a CBC you performed in your clinic on a pallorous 9-month-old boy. Other than pallor, no historical or physical examination concerns were noted during the patient's visit. The laboratory technician reports a hemoglobin of 8.6 g/dL, an MCV of 105 fL, and platelet count of 98,000/mm$^3$. You are also told that the white blood cell count is 8500/mm$^3$ and the differential reveals 47% neutrophils and 42% lymphocytes, and that no atypical lymphocytes are seen. Which of the following is the most appropriate next step in this child's care?

A. Measurement of serum iron and total iron binding capacity levels.
B. Initiate oral iron supplementation.
C. Measurement of vitamin $B_{12}$ and folate levels.
D. Begin oral vitamin $B_{12}$ and folate supplementation.
E. Obtain a STAT referral to pediatric hematologist.

27.3 The parents of a previously healthy 3-year-old girl bring the child to your office because she is complaining that her tongue hurts. The parents also report she has appeared weak and listless over the last several months, and has not been eating well. Recently she has exhibited trouble walking. The family usually eats a regular diet, including meats and vegetables. On physical examination, her tongue is smooth, red, and tender. She is pale and tachycardic. Her complete blood count reveals a macrocytic anemia. Which of the following is the most likely diagnosis in this child?

A. Folate deficiency
B. Iron deficiency
C. Vitamin D deficiency
D. Zinc deficiency
E. Vitamin $B_{12}$ deficiency

27.4 You are working at a Native American clinic in Alaska. A 16-year-old adolescent female comes to your office for an evaluation of lethargy. Her father notes that recently she has looked pale. She eats a regular diet and has no significant past medical history. Her menses are regular and have not been excessive. During the last few years, she has helped her mother in the family seafood restaurant after school, but is increasingly tired and unable to complete all of her work. Her complete blood count reveals a megaloblastic anemia. Which of the following is the next appropriate study?

A. Folate level
B. Stool for rotavirus
C. Iron level
D. Stool for ova and parasites
E. Transcobalamin level

## ANSWERS

27.1 **B.** Infants drinking goat's milk must have nutritional supplementation with vitamin $B_{12}$, folate, and iron. Several goat's milk–based formulas including these nutrients are available. Fresh, unpasteurized goat's milk can contain *Brucella ovis* and cause brucellosis. Diluting milk will only serve to dilute the caloric content.

27.2 **C.** This infant has hematologic parameters consistent with macrocytic anemia. The mild thrombocytopenia reported is periodically seen in patients with vitamin $B_{12}$ deficiency, and is thought to be related to impaired DNA synthesis and ineffective thrombopoiesis. The results reported are not typical for iron deficiency and neither an iron panel nor iron supplementation is warranted. At this point, your workup should include checking folate and $B_{12}$ levels; supplementation of these compounds is not yet justified. Myelodysplasia or leukemia is in the differential, but is probably less likely with a normal white blood cell count and differential (no atypical cells); referral to Pediatric Hematology may ultimately be required, but some preliminary data can be gathered first.

27.3 **E.** This is the typical presentation for juvenile pernicious anemia, a rare autosomal recessive condition in which the child is not able to secrete intrinsic factor and cannot absorb vitamin $B_{12}$. Supplies of vitamin $B_{12}$ passed to the fetus from the mother typically are sufficient for at least the first 1 to 2 years of life. A deficiency in transcobalamin results in megaloblastic anemia in infancy because transcobalamin is required for $B_{12}$ transport and utilization; therefore, vitamin $B_{12}$ provided by the mother cannot be used effectively.

27.4 **D.** The fish tapeworm *Diphyllobothrium latum* uses vitamin $B_{12}$ for growth and egg production; as many as one million eggs per day may be produced. The parasite also inactivates the vitamin $B_{12}$–intrinsic factor complex, inhibiting absorption in the terminal ileum. The fish tapeworm is the longest tapeworm to infect humans, sometimes growing to more than 10 m in length. Most infestations are asymptomatic, with megaloblastic anemia occurring in 2% to 9% of tapeworm infections. Risk factors include eating raw or undercooked fish. In North America, it is most commonly seen in the northern United States, Alaska, and Canada. Eggs have a unique morphology and are easily found in stool samples.

## Clinical Pearls

- Vitamin $B_{12}$ dietary deficiency is rare; infants breast-fed by vegan mothers are at risk to become vitamin $B_{12}$ deficient and should receive supplementation.
- Infants drinking goat's milk must be supplemented with vitamin $B_{12}$, folate, and iron.
- Vitamin $B_{12}$ deficiency related to gastric antrum or ileal resection requires parenteral vitamin $B_{12}$ supplementation.
- Vitamin $B_{12}$ deficiency can lead to permanent neurologic damage.

## REFERENCES

Allen R, Kamen BA. The megaloblastic anemias. In: Rudolph CD, Rudolph AM, Hostetter MK, Lister G, Siegel NJ, eds. *Rudolph's Pediatrics*. 21st ed. New York, NY: McGraw-Hill; 2003:1529-1531.

Blanton R. Adult tapeworm infections. In: Kliegman RM, Behrman RE, Jenson HB, Stanton BF, eds. *Nelson Textbook of Pediatrics*. 18th ed. Philadelphia, PA: WB Saunders; 2007:1512-1514.

Glader B. Megaloblastic anemias. In: Kliegman RM, Behrman RE, Jenson HB, Stanton BF, eds. *Nelson Textbook of Pediatrics*. 18th ed. Philadelphia, PA: WB Saunders; 2007:2011-2014.

Martin PL. Nutritional anemias. In: McMillan JA, Feigin RD, DeAngelis CD, Warshaw JB, eds. *Oski's Pediatrics: Principles and Practice*. 4th ed. Philadelphia, PA: Lippincott Williams & Wilkins; 2006:1692-1696.

# Case 28

A 3-year-old boy arrives to the emergency center after having suffered a seizure. The family reports that they had moved to Baltimore from the Midwest 3 months ago. The child was the product of a normal pregnancy and delivery, and he had experienced no medical problems until the move. The parents report that he has developed emotional lability, abdominal pain, "achy bones," and intermittent vomiting and constipation. They initially attributed his behavior to the move and to the chaos in their house, which is being extensively renovated.

- ➤ What is the most likely diagnosis?
- ➤ What is the best test to diagnose this condition?
- ➤ What is the best therapy?

# ANSWERS TO CASE 28: Lead Toxicity

*Summary:* A 3-year-old, previously healthy child now living in a home undergoing extensive renovations has developed seizures, neurologic changes, and abdominal complaints.

- **Most likely diagnosis:** Lead toxicity.
- **Best test:** Blood lead level (BLL).
- **Best therapy:** Remove child from lead source and initiate chelation therapy.

## ANALYSIS

### Objectives

1. Understand the signs, symptoms, and treatment of lead poisoning.
2. Be familiar with the environmental sources of lead.
3. Understand the sources of other environmental exposures.

### Considerations

This child is demonstrating evidence of lead poisoning. He may have been exposed to dust in the environment, or he may have displayed pica (the eating of nonfood substances such as paint chips, dirt, or clay). Therapy can be initiated immediately while awaiting the blood lead level. During the evaluation and treatment, other children in the home must be screened for elevated lead levels as well.

*Note:* Lead exposure sources vary across the United States. In the northeastern United States, older homes undergoing renovation are common sources of exposure. Leaded paint is far less common in other parts of the country. An investigation includes a travel history and an accounting of lead exposures through hobbies (such as stained glass), home renovation, and similar activities.

# APPROACH TO Lead Poisoning

## DEFINITIONS

**CHELATING AGENT:** A soluble compound that binds a metal ion (in this case lead) so that the new complex is excreted in the urine.

**PLUMBISM:** Alternate name for lead poisoning.

## CLINICAL APPROACH

The incidence of lead poisoning in the United States has decreased dramatically over the last 20 years. Previous sources (gasoline, foods, beverage cans) have been eliminated; **lead-containing paint in older homes is the major source.** Rarer sources include foodstuffs from countries where regulations are not strict, **unglazed lead-containing dishes, ingestion of leaded items (jewelry, fishing equipment), and exposure through burning of lead-containing batteries or through hobbies involving lead smelting.** Several lines of toys were recalled in 2007 when they were found to be coated with lead-based paint.

The signs and symptoms vary from none (especially at lower lead levels) to those listed in this case. However, symptoms may be seen at low blood lead levels (BLLs), and a child with very high BLLs occasionally may be asymptomatic. **Anorexia, hyperirritability, altered sleep pattern, and decreased play are commonly seen. Developmental regression, especially with speech, can be seen.** Abdominal complaints (occasional vomiting, intermittent pain, and constipation) are sometimes noted. **Persistent vomiting, ataxia, altered consciousness, coma, and seizures are signs of encephalopathy.** Permanent, long-term consequences include learning and cognitive deficits and aggressive behavior; with less lead in the environment and decreasing average lead levels, these more subtle findings are more common than acute lead encephalopathy.

The BLL is the diagnostic test of choice, and demonstrates recent ingestion; however, a significant amount of lead is stored in other tissue, most notably bone. BLL, then, does not accurately reflect total body lead load. Other tests (free erythrocyte protoporphyrin, basophilic stippling, glycosuria, hypophosphatemia, long bone "lead lines," and gastrointestinal tract radiopaque flecks) in symptomatic patients are less specific.

**Treatment varies depending on the BLL and the patient's symptoms. Admission to the hospital, stabilization, and chelation are appropriate for symptomatic patients.** Therapy for asymptomatic patients could involve simple investigation of the child's environment, outpatient chelation, or immediate hospitalization (Table 28–1). Close contact with local health agencies is important; they usually are charged with ensuring that the child's environment is lead-free.

**Chelation** in an asymptomatic child may consist of intramuscular calcium disodium ethylenediaminetetraacetic acid (CaEDTA) or more commonly oral meso-2,3-dimercaptosuccinic acid (DMSA, succimer). Hospitalized symptomatic patients are often treated with 2, 3-dimercaptopropanol (British anti-Lewisite [BAL]) and CaEDTA. Fluid balance is tricky; urine output is maintained because CaEDTA is renally excreted, but encephalopathy may be exacerbated with overhydration.

Newer research has cast doubt on the utility of chelation therapy in children with lead levels less than 45 μg/dL. Lead levels do decrease acutely with

**Table 28–1 SUMMARY OF RECOMMENDATIONS FOR CHILDREN WITH CONFIRMED (VENOUS) ELEVATED BLOOD LEAD LEVELS**

| BLOOD LEAD LEVEL (μG/DL) | | | | |
|---|---|---|---|---|
| 10-14 | 15-19 | 20-44 | 45-69 | ≥70 |
| Lead education<br>• Dietary<br>• Environmental<br>Follow-up blood lead monitoring | Lead education<br>• Dietary<br>• Environmental<br>Follow-up blood lead monitoring<br>Proceed according to actions for 20-44 μg/dL if:<br>• A follow-up BLL is in this range at least 3 months after initial venous test<br>or<br>• BLLs increase | Lead education<br>• Dietary<br>• Environmental<br>Follow-up blood lead monitoring<br>Complete history and physical exam<br>Lab work:<br>• Hemoglobin or hematocrit<br>• Iron status<br>Environmental investigation<br>Lead hazard reduction<br>Neurodevelopmental monitoring<br>Abdominal x-ray (if particulate lead ingestion is suspected) with bowel decontamination if indicated | Lead education<br>• Dietary<br>• Environmental<br>Follow-up blood lead monitoring<br>Complete history and physical exam<br>Complete neurological exam<br>Lab work:<br>• Hemoglobin or hematocrit<br>• Iron status<br>• Free erythrocyte protoporphyrin (FPP) or zine protoporphyrin (ZPP)<br>Environmental investigation<br>Lead hazard reduction<br>Neurodevelopmental monitoring<br>Abdominal X-ray with bowel decontamination if indicated<br>Chelation therapy | Hospitalize and commence chelation therapy<br>Proceed according to actions for 45-69 μg/dL |

***The following actions are NOT recommended at any blood lead level:***

- Searching for gingival lead lines
- Testing of neurophysiologic function
- Evaluation of renal function (except during chelation with EDTA)
- Testing of hair, teeth, or fingernails for lead
- Radiographic imaging of long bones
- X-ray fluorescence of long bones

*(Reproduced from the Centers for Disease Control and Prevention, www.cdc.gov.)*

chelation therapy, but affected children do not show improvement in long-term cognitive testing.

Targeted BLL screening of at-risk children rather than universal screening is recommended. Questionnaires to assess the risk of lead exposure query the age of the home or day care center, the possibility of exposure to high-lead environments (battery recycling plant, lead smelter, etc), or environments in which others (siblings, playmates, etc) with elevated BLLs have been identified. Some state and federal programs, such as Early Periodic Screening, Diagnosis, and Treatment and Healthy Kids, provide further guidance on lead screening.

## Comprehension Questions

28.1 A developmentally normal two-year-old child is in your inner city office for a well-child check. As part of the visit, you obtain a blood lead level and a hemoglobin level in accordance with your state's Medicaid screening guidelines. The following week, the state lab calls your office to report the child's blood lead level is 14 Ìg/dL. Appropriate management of this level should include which of the following actions?

A. Initiate chelation therapy.
B. Perform long bone radiographs.
C. Reassure the parents that no action is required.
D. Repeat the blood lead level in three months.
E. Report to the local health department for environmental investigation.

28.2 While evaluating the family in the previous question, you discovered a three-year-old sibling with a lead level of 50 µg/dL. You reported the case to the local authorities and initiated chelation therapy. All lead sources in the home have since been removed (verified by dust wipe samples), and the parents do not work in occupations prone to lead exposure. After a course of outpatient chelation therapy, the three-year-old's lead level dropped to 5 µg/dL. Today, however, the child's three month followup blood lead level is 15 µg/dL. At this point, appropriate management includes which of the following actions?

A. Initiate a course of inpatient parenteral chelation therapy.
B. Perform long bone radiographs.
C. Reassure the parents and repeat a blood lead level in three months.
D. Recommend the family move to another home.
E. Repeat a course of outpatient chelation therapy.

28.3 A term newborn infant is admitted to the Neonatal ICU after having a seizure in the Well Baby Nursery. Your examination reveals a microcephalic infant with low birth weight who does not respond to sound. In your discussions with the family, you discover this is the parents' first child. They recount odd symptoms that have developed in the both of them in the last few months, including fine tremors in their upper extremities and blurry vision. They also note that they both can no longer smell their food and that it "tastes funny." The mother notes that she has had trouble walking straight in the last few weeks, but she attributes that to her pregnancy. Which of the following environmental toxins is most likely to have caused these findings?

A. Inorganic arsenic salts
B. Lead
C. Methyl mercury
D. Orellanine
E. Polychlorinated biphenyls

28.4 A previously healthy two-year-old boy is brought to the emergency department by ambulance after having a generalized tonic-clonic seizure at home. The mother reports that she put him to bed early the night before because she was having some friends over for a Bunco party. This afternoon when she awoke she found him wandering around the house, seemingly off balance, and he was "not acting right." She called EMS as soon as he had his seizure. The responding paramedic reported that the child's initial blood glucose was 15 mg/dL; after administration of lorazepam and a bolus of D10W he stopped seizing. Upon examination you find a heart rate of 110 beats per minute, a respiratory rate of 20 breaths per minute, a temperature of 37°C (98.6°F), and a blood pressure of 89/43 mm Hg. His pupils are reactive, and his funduscopic examination is normal. The rest of his examination is benign. Which of the following is the most likely cause of the seizure?

A. 3,4-methylenedioxymethamphetamine (MDMA; 'Ecstasy') ingestion
B. Brain tumor
C. Ethanol ingestion
D. Exogenous insulin administration
E. Head trauma

## ANSWERS

28.1 **D.** The patient's lead screen is mildly elevated. Appropriate management includes educating the parents about potential lead exposures in the environment as well as in the diet. A repeat level should be performed in three months. Chelation therapy is currently advised for patients with a blood lead level of 45 μg/dL and above. Environmental investigation is recommended in patients with a blood lead level of 20 μg/dL and above, or if levels remain elevated despite educational efforts. Long bone radiographs are not recommended at any blood lead level.

28.2 **C.** In this case, reassurance is appropriate. Lead deposits in bone, and chelation does not remove all lead from the body. After chelation is complete, lead levels tend to rise again; the source is thought to be the redistribution of lead stored in bone. Repeat chelation is only recommended if the blood lead level rebounds to 45 μg/dL or higher. Moving to another home is not necessary, assuming the health department successfully remediated their current home. Long bone radiographs are not recommended at any blood lead level.

28.3 **C.** Infants exposed in utero to methyl mercury may display low birthweight, microcephaly, and seizures. They also display significant developmental delay and can have vision and hearing impairments. Symptoms in children and adults include ataxia, tremor, dysarthria, memory loss, altered sensorium (including vision, hearing, smell, and taste), dementia, and ultimately death. Acute ingestion of arsenic causes severe gastrointestinal symptoms; chronic exposure causes skin lesions and can cause peripheral neuropathy and encephalopathy. Orellanine is a toxin found in the Cortinarius species of mushroom that causes nausea, vomiting, and diarrhea; renal toxicity may occur several days later. Polychlorinated biphenyls (PCBs) cross the placenta and accumulate in breast milk; exposure in utero is thought to cause behavioral problems in later life.

28.4 **C.** While all of the answers are situations or conditions that can be associated with seizure, ethanol ingestion is the most likely based on the history of a toddler with hypoglycemia poorly supervised with presumed access to alcohol after an adult party. An ingestion of MDMA can certainly cause seizure in a toddler but is usually associated with hypertension, dilated pupils, and hyperthermia. There was no evidence of trauma on exam, and the funduscopic exam did not suggest increased intracranial pressure. If insulin was in the home and Munchausen by Proxy was suspected, simultaneous evaluation of serum insulin level and C peptide during an episode of hypoglycemia may help make the diagnosis.

## Clinical Pearls

- Lead-containing paint in older homes is the major source of lead exposure in the United States.
- Behavioral signs of lead toxicity include hyperirritability, altered sleep patterns, decreased play activity, loss of developmental milestones (especially speech), and altered state of consciousness. Physical symptoms include vomiting, intermittent abdominal pain, constipation, ataxia, coma, and seizures.
- Chelation therapy in an asymptomatic child with elevated lead levels consists of intramuscular calcium disodium ethylenediaminetetraacetic acid (CaEDTA) or oral meso-2,3-dimercaptosuccinic acid (succimer). Hospitalized patients with symptomatic disease are often treated with 2,3-dimercaptopropanol (BAL) and CaEDTA.

## REFERENCES

American Academy of Pediatrics. Lead exposure in children: prevention, detection, and management. *Pediatrics*. 2005;116:1036-1046.

Centers for Disease Control and Prevention. Recommendations for blood lead screening of young children enrolled in Medicaid: targeting a group at high risk. Advisory Committee on Childhood Lead Poisoning Prevention (ACCLPP). *MMWR* 2000; 49(No. RR-14):1-13.

Chisolm JJ. Lead poisoning. In: McMillan JA, Feigin RD, DeAngelis CD, Jones MD, eds. *Oski's Pediatrics: Principles and Practice*. 4th ed. Philadelphia, PA: Lippincott Williams & Wilkins; 2006:767-772.

Landriagan PJ, Forman JA. Chemical pollutants. In: Kliegman RM, Behrman RE, Jenson HB, Stanton BF, eds. *Nelson Textbook of Pediatrics*. 18th ed. Philadelphia, PA: Saunders Elsevier; 2007:2906-2908.

Mahajan PV. Heavy metal intoxication. In: Kliegman RM, Behrman RE, Jenson HB, Stanton BF, eds. *Nelson Textbook of Pediatrics*. 18th ed. Philadelphia, PA: Saunders Elsevier; 2007:2909-2912.

Markowitz M. Lead poisoning. In: Kliegman RM, Behrman RE, Jenson HB, Stanton BF, eds. *Nelson Textbook of Pediatrics*. 18th ed. Philadelphia, PA: Saunders Elsevier; 2007:2913-2917.

Sperling MA. Hypoglycemia. In: Kliegman RM, Behrman RE, Jenson HB, Stanton BF, eds. *Nelson Textbook of Pediatrics*. 18th ed. Philadelphia, PA: Saunders Elsevier; 2007:666.

Tenenbein M. Toxic ingestions and exposures. In: Rudolph CD, Rudolph AM, Hostetter MK, Lister G, Siegel NJ, eds. *Rudolph's Pediatrics*. 21st ed. New York, NY: McGraw-Hill; 2003:354-379.

# Case 29

A 14-year-old Hispanic male presents with a 3-day complaint of "brown urine." He has been your patient since birth and has experienced no major illnesses or injuries, is active in band and cross-country, and denies drug use or sexual activity. Two weeks ago he had 2 days of fever and a sore throat, but he improved spontaneously and has been well since. His review of systems is remarkable only for his slightly puffy eyes, which he attributes to late-night studying for final examinations. On physical examination he is afebrile, his blood pressure is 135/90 mm Hg, he is active and nontoxic in appearance, and he has some periorbital edema. The urine dipstick has a specific gravity of 1.035 and contains 2+ blood and 2+ protein. You spin the urine, resuspend the sediment, and identify red blood cell casts under the microscope.

- What is the most likely cause of this patient's hematuria?
- What laboratory tests would support this diagnosis?
- What is the prognosis of this condition?

# ANSWERS TO CASE 29:
## Acute Poststreptococcal Glomerulonephritis

*Summary:* A healthy adolescent male with a preceding pharyngitis has periorbital edema and mild hypertension, and has developed tea-colored urine that on microscopy reveals red blood cells.

- **Most likely diagnosis:** Acute poststreptococcal glomerulonephritis (APSGN).
- **Laboratory studies:** $C_3$ (low in 90% of cases), $C_4$ (usually normal); antistreptolysin-O (ASO) enzyme antibodies and antideoxyribonuclease B (anti-DNase B) antibodies provide evidence of recent streptococcal infection.
- **Prognosis:** Excellent; 95% to 98% of affected children recover completely.

## ANALYSIS

### Objectives

1. Recognize the typical presentation of APSGN.
2. Know the different diagnostic possibilities for a patient with dark urine.
3. Discuss appropriate follow-up care for the patient with APSGN.

### Considerations

This patient is otherwise healthy, had pharyngitis, and now has hematuria, proteinuria, edema, and hypertension. Although APSGN is likely, other possibilities must be considered. Strenuous activity can cause rhabdomyolysis and dark urine, but patients with these conditions often will have muscle aches, fatigue, nausea and vomiting, and fever. Immunoglobulin A (Berger) nephropathy is characterized by recurrent painless hematuria, usually preceded by an upper respiratory tract infection. Henoch-Schönlein purpura (HSP) is a relatively common cause of nephritis in pediatrics, but most cases occur in younger children, peaking in incidence between 4 and 5 years of age. Lupus nephritis (systemic lupus erythematosus [SLE]) can present as described and is considered if the hematuria does not resolve or if the $C_3$ level does not normalize in 6 to 12 weeks.

# APPROACH TO
# Acute Poststreptococcal Glomerulonephritis

## DEFINITIONS

**GLOMERULONEPHRITIS:** Glomerular inflammation resulting in the triad of hematuria, proteinuria, and hypertension.

**RED CELL CASTS:** Injured glomeruli have increased permeability and leak red cells and proteins into the proximal convoluted tubule; the material subsequently clumps in the distal convoluted tubule and in the collecting ducts. When passed, these cell clumps retain the shape of the tubule in the urine. Red cell casts are markers for glomerular injury.

## CLINICAL APPROACH

**Acute poststreptococcal glomerulonephritis (APSGN) is the most common of the postinfectious nephritides,** comprising 80% to 90% of cases. Other bacteria, viruses, parasites, and fungi also have been implicated. Males are more commonly affected; it is most common in children between the ages of 5 and 15 years and is rare in toddlers and infants. The group A β-hemolytic *Streptococcus* (GABHS) infection can be in the form of either pharyngitis ("strep throat") or a superficial skin lesion (impetigo). Not all GABHS infections result in APSGN; certain GABHS strains are "nephritogenic" and are more likely to result in APSGN. Rheumatic fever only rarely occurs concomitantly with APSGN. **Antibiotic use during the initial GABHS infection may reduce the subsequent rheumatic fever risk**, yet has **not been shown to prevent APSGN.** The nephritis risk after infection with a nephritogenic strain of GABHS remains 10% to 15%.

**Generally the interval between GABHS pharyngitis and APSGN is 1 to 2 weeks;** the interval between GABHS impetigo and APSGN is 3 to 6 weeks. Symptom onset is abrupt. Although almost all patients have **microscopic hematuria,** only 30% to 50% develop gross hematuria. In addition, 85% present with edema and 60% to 80% develop hypertension.

The **most important laboratory test** in patients with APSGN is measurement of **serum $C_3$ and $C_4$ levels. $C_3$ is low in 90% of APSGN cases, whereas $C_4$ usually is normal.** If both levels are low, an alternate diagnosis is considered. Urinalysis typically reveals high specific gravity, low pH, hematuria, proteinuria, and red cell casts. Documentation of a recent streptococcal infection is helpful; **serum markers include the presence of ASO enzyme antibodies and anti-DNase B antibodies.** ASO antibodies are found in 80% of children with recent GABHS pharyngitis but in less than 50% of children with recent GABHS skin infection. ASO titers are positive in 16% to 18% of normal children.

**Anti-DNase B antibodies assays are more reliable**; they are present in almost all patients after GABHS pharyngitis and in the majority of patients after GABHS skin infection. Antibodies to other streptococcal antigens (nicotamide adenosine dinucleotide glycohydrolase [NADase], hyaluronidase, and streptokinase) may also be assayed. Renal biopsy is no longer routine. Treatment is generally supportive. Fluid balance is crucial; diuretics, fluid restriction, or both may be necessary. Sodium and potassium intake may require restriction. **Hypertension** usually is easily controlled with **calcium-channel blockers**. Strict bed rest and corticosteroid medications are not helpful. Dialysis is rarely required.

**Resolution usually is rapid and complete**. The edema resolves in 5 to 10 days, and patients usually are normotensive within 3 weeks. $C_3$ levels usually normalize in 2 to 3 months; a persistently low $C_3$ level is uncommon and suggests an alternate diagnosis. Urinalysis may be persistently abnormal for several years.

## Comprehension Questions

29.1 A 16-year-old adolescent male complains of intermittent cola-colored urine of several years' duration, usually when he has a "cold." He is otherwise well and has no medical complaints. When the dark-colored urine is present, he has no dysuria. None of his family members has similar complaints or renal disease. On physical examination he is normotensive and appears healthy. Which of the following is the most likely cause of his intermittent hematuria?

A. Acute poststreptococcal glomerulonephritis
B. Henoch-Schönlein purpura nephritis
C. IgA nephropathy
D. Recurrent kidney stones
E. Rapidly progressive glomerulonephritis

29.2 The parents of a healthy 12-year-old girl bring her to you for a physical examination required for summer camp. They have no complaints, and the girl denies any problems. Her last menses was normal 2 weeks prior. The camp requires a urine screen. To your surprise, the clean-catch urine screen has significant hematuria. Red cell casts are noted. You tell the findings to the parents, and they respond that "everyone on dad's side of the family has blood in their urine and they are all doing well." The family history is negative for deafness and for renal failure. Microscopy of renal tissue from this patient or from her father will most likely reveal which of the following?

A. Endothelial cell swelling and fibrin in the subendothelial space
B. Immune complex deposition in the mesangium
C. Large numbers of crescentic glomeruli
D. Renal cell carcinoma
E. Thinning of the basement membrane

29.3 A 17-year-old adolescent female has joint tenderness for 2 months; the pain has affected her summer job as a lifeguard. In the morning, she awakens with bilateral knee pain and swelling and right hand pain. The pain eases during the day but never completely resolves. Nonsteroidal anti-inflammatory drugs help slightly. She also wants a good "face cream" because "her job has worsened her acne." On physical examination you notice facial erythema on the cheeks and nasolabial folds. She has several oral ulcers that she calls cold sores, bilateral knee effusions, and her right distal interphalangeal joints on her hand are swollen and tender. Her liver is palpable 3 cm below the costal margin. She has microscopic hematuria and proteinuria. Which of the following is the most likely cause of this young woman's arthritis?

A. Juvenile rheumatoid arthritis
B. Lyme disease
C. Osteoarthritis
D. Postinfectious arthritis
E. Systemic lupus erythematosus

29.4 You are not surprised to see one of your most challenging patients, a 16-year-old adolescent female who has been seen several times per week over the last 2 months complaining of cough, occasional hemoptysis, malaise, and intermittent low-grade fever. Thus far you have identified a microcytic, hypochromic anemia for which she has been taking iron (without response) and migratory patchy infiltrates on chest radiograph that seem unaffected by antibiotic treatment. She has no tuberculosis (TB) exposure risks, and her TB skin test was negative. Today she also complains of facial edema and tea-colored urine. You suddenly realize her symptoms can be grouped as which of the following syndromes?

A. Alport syndrome
B. Denys-Drash syndrome
C. Goodpasture syndrome
D. Hemolytic-uremic syndrome
E. Nephrotic syndrome

## ANSWERS

29.1 **C.** Recurrent painless gross hematuria, frequently associated with an upper respiratory tract infection, is typical of IgA nephropathy. These patients may develop chronic renal disease over decades. If proteinuria, hypertension, or impaired renal function were found, a biopsy would be necessary. The other options are not consistent with the asymptomatic, intermittent nature of this patient's problem.

29.2 **E.** This history is consistent with benign familial hematuria, an autosomal dominant condition that causes either persistent or intermittent hematuria without progression to chronic renal failure. Biopsy reveals a thin basement membrane; in some cases the biopsy is normal. Immune complex deposition with immunoglobulin (Ig)A in the mesangium is seen in HSP and IgA nephropathy; endothelial cell swelling with fibrin deposition is seen in hemolytic-uremic syndrome, and crescentic glomeruli are seen in rapidly progressive glomerulonephritis.

29.3 **E.** Systemic lupus erythematosus affects more women than men, and nephritis is a common presenting feature. Her rash, photosensitivity, oral ulcers, hepatomegaly, arthritis, and nephritis combine to make this a likely diagnosis. A positive antinuclear antibody test and low $C_3$ and $C_4$ levels would help to confirm the diagnosis.

29.4 **C.** Goodpasture syndrome is the clinical diagnosis when patients exhibit nephritis and pulmonary hemorrhage. It can be caused by a number of conditions, including SLE and HSP. Alport syndrome is a genetic defect in collagen synthesis that leads to abnormal basement membrane formation; patients will develop hematuria, proteinuria, and renal failure. Denys-Drash syndrome is a group of findings composed of Wilms tumor, gonadal dysgenesis, and nephropathy.

## Clinical Pearls

- Post streptococcal glomerulonephritis is the most common postinfectious nephritis and has a good prognosis.
- Confirming the diagnosis of APSGN requires evidence of invasive streptococcal infection such as a elevated anti-DNAase B titer.

## REFERENCES

Brewer ED. Glomerulonephritis and nephrotic syndrome. In: McMillan JA, Feigin RD, DeAngelis CD, Jones MD, eds. *Oski's Pediatrics: Principles and Practice*. 4th ed. Philadelphia, PA: Lippincott Williams & Wilkins; 2006:1854-1862.

Davis ID, Avner ED. Acute poststreptococcal glomerulonephritis. In: Kliegman RM, Behrman RE, Jenson HB, Stanton BF, eds. *Nelson Textbook of Pediatrics*. 18th ed. Philadelphia, PA: Saunders Elsevier; 2007:2173-2175.

Davis ID, Avner ED. Conditions particularly associated with hematuria. In: Kliegman RM, Behrman RE, Jenson HB, Stanton BF, eds. *Nelson Textbook of Pediatrics*. 18th ed. Philadelphia, PA: Saunders Elsevier; 2007:2168-2188.

Eddy AA. Glomerular disorders. In: Rudolph CD, Rudolph AM, Hostetter MK, Lister G, Siegel NJ, eds. *Rudolph's Pediatrics*. 21st ed. New York,NY: McGraw-Hill; 2003a: 1677-1681.

Eddy AA. Henoch-Schönlein purpura nephritis. In: Rudolph CD, Rudolph AM, Hostetter MK, Lister G, Siegel NJ, eds. *Rudolph's Pediatrics*. 21st ed. New York, NY: McGraw-Hill; 2003b:1688-1689.

Kashtan CE. Denys-Drash syndrome. In: Rudolph CD, Rudolph AM, Hostetter MK, Lister G, Siegel NJ, eds. *Rudolph's Pediatrics*. 21st ed. New York, NY: McGraw-Hill; 2003:1701-1702.

Schleiss MR. Group A *Streptococcus*. In: Rudolph CD, Rudolph AM, Hostetter MK, Lister G, Siegel NJ, eds. *Rudolph's Pediatrics*. 21st ed. New York, NY: McGraw-Hill; 2003:998.

Silverman ED. Pediatric systemic lupus erythematosus. In: Rudolph CD, Rudolph AM, Hostetter MK, Lister G, Siegel NJ, eds. *Rudolph's Pediatrics*. 21st ed. New York, NY: McGraw-Hill; 2003:847-851.

# Case 30

Parents bring their 5-year-old daughter to your clinic because she has developed breast and pubic hair over the past 3 months. Physical examination reveals a girl whose height and weight are above the 95th percentile, Tanner stage II breast and pubic hair development, oily skin, and facial acne.

- What is the most likely diagnosis?
- What is the best next step in the evaluation?

# ANSWERS TO CASE 30:
# Precocious Puberty

*Summary:* A 5-year-old girl has breast and pubic hair development, tall stature, and facial acne.

- **Most likely diagnosis:** Idiopathic central precocious puberty.
- **Next step in the evaluation:** Inquire about birth history, illnesses, hospitalizations, medications, siblings' health status, and family history of early puberty and diseases. Serum follicle-stimulating hormone (FSH) and luteinizing hormone (LH) levels and bone age radiographs are helpful.

## ANALYSIS

### Objectives

1. Understand the underlying causes of precocious puberty.
2. Describe laboratory and radiologic tests that are helpful in determining the etiology of precocious puberty.
3. Establish the treatment and follow-up necessary for a child with precocious puberty.

### Considerations

This 5-year-old girl has precocious puberty signs (breast and pubic hair development and tall stature). She may have true (central) precocious puberty or precocious (noncentral) pseudopuberty. A central nervous system (CNS) cause of true precocious puberty must be ruled out because she is younger than 6 years, and must be ruled out in boys at any age.

# APPROACH TO
# Precocious Puberty

## DEFINITIONS

**DELAYED PUBERTY:** No signs of puberty in girls by age 13 years or in boys by age 14 years. May be caused by gonadal failure, chromosomal abnormalities (Turner syndrome, Klinefelter syndrome), hypopituitarism, chronic disease, or malnutrition.

**PRECOCIOUS PUBERTY:** Secondary sexual characteristic onset before age 8 years in girls and 9 years in boys. Children in different ethnic groups undergo puberty differently; African-American girls often do so earlier than Caucasian girls.

**TRUE (CENTRAL) PRECOCIOUS PUBERTY:** Gonadotropin-dependent. Hypothalamic-pituitary-gonadal activation leading to secondary sex characteristics.

**PRECOCIOUS PSEUDOPUBERTY:** Gonadotropin-independent. No hypothalamic-pituitary-gonadal activation. Hormones usually are either exogenous (birth control pills, estrogen creams) or from adrenal/ovarian tumors.

**PREMATURE ADRENARCHE:** Early activation of adrenal androgens (typically in girls ages 6 to 8 years), with gradually increasing pubic/axillary hair development and body odor.

**PREMATURE THELARCHE:** Early breast development (typically in girls ages 1 to 4 years), without pubic/axillary hair development or linear growth acceleration.

## CLINICAL APPROACH

**More common in girls, true precocious puberty** stems from **secretion of hypothalamic GnRH** with normal-appearing, but early, progression of pubertal events. Sexual precocity is **idiopathic** in **more than 90% of girls**, whereas a **structural CNS abnormality is present in 25% to 75% of boys**.

Girls with gonadotropin-independent, precocious pseudopuberty have an independent source of estrogens causing their pubertal changes. An exogenous source of estrogen (birth control pills, hormone replacement) or an **estrogen-producing tumor of the ovary or adrenal gland** must be considered. **Central nervous system lesions** causing precocious puberty without neurologic symptoms are rarely malignant and seldom require neurosurgical intervention.

A detailed history offers important clues regarding the onset of puberty. Three main patterns of precocious pubertal progression can be identified, particularly in girls. Most girls who are younger than 6 years at onset have rapidly progressing sexual precocity, characterized by early physical and osseous maturation with a loss of ultimate height potential. Girls older than 6 years typically have a slowly progressing variant with parallel advancement of osseous maturation and linear growth and preserved height potential. In a small percentage of girls, there is spontaneous regression or unsustained central precocious puberty at a young age, with normal pubertal development at an expected age.

A neurologic history may identify past hydrocephalus, head trauma, meningoencephalitis, or the presence of headaches, visual problems, or behavioral changes. The type, sequence, and age at which pubertal changes were first noticed (breast and pubic/axillary hair development, external genitalia maturation, menarche) give valuable information regarding the etiology of the problem. Important questions include the following:

- Has the child been rapidly outgrowing shoes and clothes (evidence of linear growth acceleration)?
- Has the child's appetite increased?
- Has the child developed body odor?
- Was the child possibly exposed to an exogenous source of sex steroids (oral contraceptives, hormone replacement, anabolic steroids)?
- At what ages did parents and siblings undergo puberty?
- Is there a known or suspected family history of congenital adrenal hyperplasia?

Physical examination offers further important information (Figures 30–1 and 30–2). Serial height measurements are critical for determining the child's growth velocity. The skin should be examined for café-au-lait spots (neurofibromatosis, McCune-Albright disease), oiliness, and acne. The presence of axillary hair and body odor, the amount of breast tissue, and whether the nipples and areolae are enlarging and thinning is documented. The amount, location, and character of pubic hair should be noted. The abdomen is palpated for masses. Boys are examined for enlargement of the penis and testes (>2.5 cm in precocious puberty) and thinning of the scrotum (prepubertal scrotum is thick and nonvascular). If the testes are different in size and consistency, a unilateral mass is considered. Testicular transillumination may be helpful. In girls, the clitoris, labia, and vaginal orifice are examined to identify vaginal secretions, maturation of the labia minora, and vaginal mucosa estrogenization (dull, gray-pink, and rugaed rather than shiny, smooth, and red). A neurologic examination also is performed.

In precocious puberty, serum sex hormone concentrations usually are appropriate for the observed stage of puberty, but inappropriate for the child's chronologic age. Serum estradiol concentration is elevated in girls, and serum testosterone level is elevated in boys with precocious puberty. Because LH and FSH levels fluctuate, single samples often are inadequate. An immunometric assay for LH is more sensitive than the radioimmunoassay when using random blood samples; with this test, serum LH is undetectable in prepubertal children, but is detectable in 50% to 70% of girls (and an even higher percentage of boys) with central precocious puberty. A gonadotropin-releasing hormone (GnRH) stimulation test, measuring response time and peak values of LH and FSH after intravenous administration of GnRH, is a helpful diagnostic tool.

**Bone age radiographs are advanced beyond chronologic age in precocious puberty**. Organic CNS causes of central sexual precocity are ruled out by computerized tomography (CT) or magnetic resonance imaging (MRI), particularly in girls younger than 6 years and in all boys. Pelvic ultrasonography is indicated if gonadotropin-independent causes of precocious puberty (ovarian tumors/cysts, adrenal tumors) are suspected based on examination.

The goal of treating precocious puberty is to prevent premature closure of the epiphyses, allowing the child to reach full adult growth potential. Gonadotropin-releasing hormone agonists are used for treatment of central precocious puberty. These analogues desensitize the gonadotropic cells of the pituitary to the stimulatory effect of GnRH produced by the hypothalamus. Nearly all boys and

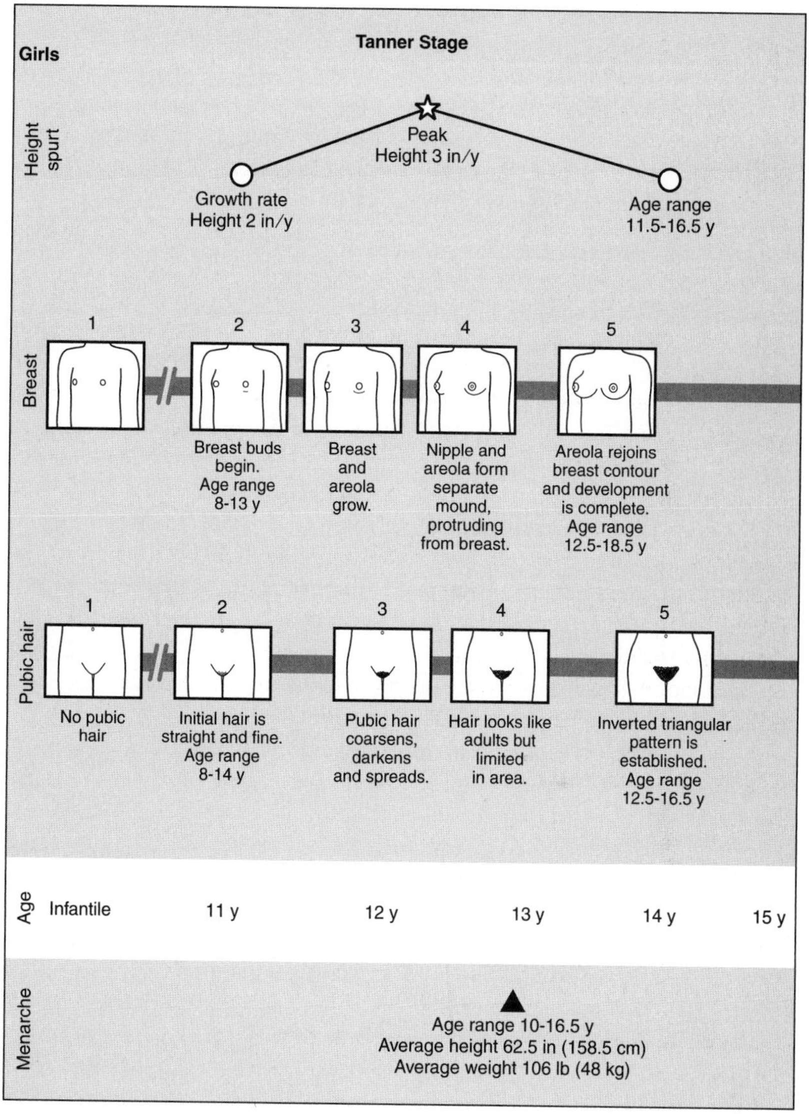


**Figure 30–1.** Female Tanner staging.

most girls with rapidly progressive precocious puberty are candidates for treatment. Girls with slowly progressive puberty do not seem to benefit from GnRH agonist therapy in adult height prognosis. A pediatric endocrinologist should evaluate children considered for GnRH agonist treatment.

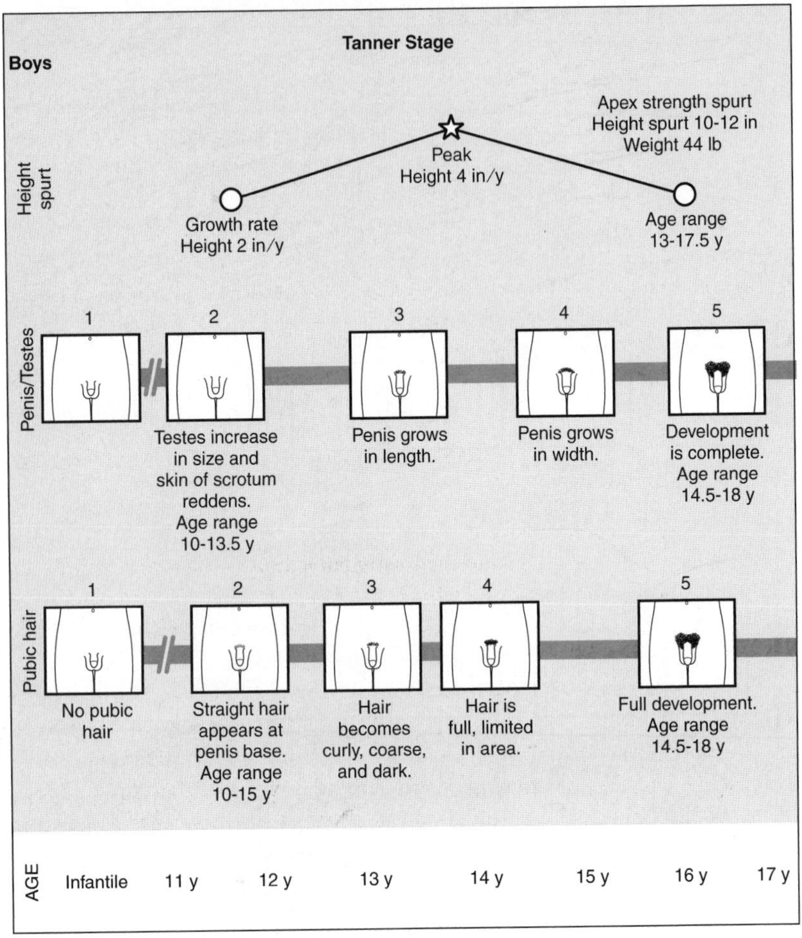


**Figure 30–2.** Male Tanner staging.

## Comprehension Questions

30.1 A 5-year-old girl has bilateral breast development that was first noticed 6 months ago. She takes no medications, and no source of exogenous estrogen is present in the home. Family history is unremarkable. Physical examination reveals a girl who is at the 50th percentile for height and weight, with normal blood pressure, normal skin without oiliness, Tanner stage II breasts, soft abdomen without palpable masses, no body odor, no pubic/axillary hair, and mild estrogenization of the vagina. Which of the following is the most likely explanation for the child's breast development?

A. Adrenal tumor
B. Central precocious puberty
C. Congenital adrenal hyperplasia
D. Premature adrenarche
E. Premature thelarche

30.2 A 4-year-old boy has started growing pubic hair and has recently exhibited aggressive "bullying" behavior at his preschool. History reveals the boy to be a term infant without postnatal complications. The child takes no medications. Family history is unremarkable. He has one younger sister who is well. Physical examination reveals height and weight above the 95th percentile, marked muscular development, Tanner stage II pubic hair development, scant axillary hair, prepubertal testicular size, a masculine voice, and oily skin. The abdominal examination is normal. The child's bone age is 6 years. Which of the following is the most appropriate next step in management?

A. Brain MRI
B. Dexamethasone challenge test
C. Reassure the family that no studies are needed
D. Serum 17$\alpha$ -hydroxyprogesterone level
E. Testicular ultrasound

30.3 A mother brings to your office her 13-year-old daughter who is "falling behind" in growth and who has not yet exhibited pubertal changes. Physical examination reveals a height less than the fifth percentile, no signs of secondary sexual characteristics, a small mandible, low posterior hairline, prominent ears, and a broad chest. Which of the following is the most appropriate next step in management?

A. Abdominal ultrasound
B. Bone age radiograph
C. Chromosome analysis
D. Reassure the family and recommend height measurement in 6 months
E. Treat with growth hormone injections

30.4 A father brings his 14-year-old son to your clinic because his teacher has concerns about his poor school performance and maladjusted behavior. He has poor grades in all subjects, is extremely shy, and has always had difficulty in adjusting socially. On examination, he is at the 95th percentile for height and 5th percentile for weight. It is very difficult to engage him in conversation. The testes are prepubertal, he has mild hypospadias, and he has no secondary sexual characteristics. Which of the following is the most likely cause of his pubertal delay?

A. Hypopituitarism
B. Klinefelter syndrome
C. Marfan syndrome
D. Noonan syndrome
E. Testicular tumor

## ANSWERS

30.1 **E.** All of this child's findings are estrogen related. She has no virilization. Postulated premature thelarche causes include ovarian cysts and transient gonadotropin secretion. No treatment is necessary.

30.2 **D.** Boys with congenital adrenal hyperplasia have virilization despite prepubertal testicles. This results from a disorder of steroid synthesis, leading to a deficiency of cortisol and an overproduction of androgenic intermediary metabolites such as 17α-hydroxyprogesterone.

30.3 **C.** This child has Turner syndrome (45, XO). Other features include webbed neck, high arched palate, increased nevi, renal anomalies, increased arm-carrying angle, and edema of the hands and feet. Treatment includes recombinant human growth hormone and estrogen replacement therapy.

30.4 **B.** Klinefelter syndrome (47, XXY) usually comes to attention because of gynecomastia and small testes. These males usually are clinically normal at birth. Treatment involves replacement therapy with a long-acting testosterone beginning at age 11 to 12 years.

## Clinical Pearls

- True precocious puberty is the onset of secondary sexual characteristics before age 8 years in girls and 9 years in boys. It stems from secretion of hypothalamic gonadotropin-releasing hormone and is more common in girls.
- Precocious puberty is idiopathic in more than 90% of girls, and a structural central nervous system abnormality is noted in 25% to 75% of boys.
- When compared to norms, the serum estradiol level is elevated in girls and the testosterone level is elevated in boys with precocious puberty. Bone age radiographs are advanced beyond chronologic age.
- The goal of treating precocious puberty is to prevent premature closure of the epiphyses, allowing the child to reach full adult growth potential.

## REFERENCES

Garibaldi L. Disorders of pubertal development. In: Kliegman RM, Behrman RE, Jenson HB, Stanton BF, eds. *Nelson Textbook of Pediatrics*. 18th ed. Philadelphia, PA: WB Saunders; 2007:2309-2316.

Plotnick LP, Long DN. Puberty and gonadal disorders. In: McMillan JA, Feigin RD, DeAngelis CD, Jones MD, eds. *Oski's Pediatrics: Principles and Practice*. 4th ed. Philadelphia, PA: Lippincott Williams & Wilkins; 2006:2079-2084.

Styne DM, Cuttler L. Normal pubertal development. In: Rudolph CD, Rudolph AM, Hostetter MK, Lister G, Siegel NJ, eds. *Rudolph's Pediatrics*. 21st ed. New York, NY: McGraw-Hill; 2003:2093-2105.

White PC. Congenital adrenal hyperplasia and related disorders. In: Kliegman RM, Behrman RE, Jenson HB, Stanton BF, eds. *Nelson Textbook of Pediatrics*. 18th ed. Philadelphia, PA: WB Saunders; 2007:2360-2368.

# Case 31

A 3740-g infant is delivered vaginally after an uncomplicated 38-week gestation. Health-care providers have immediate difficulty in determining whether the infant is a boy or girl. There appear to be small scrotal sacs that resemble enlarged labia and no palpable testes with either a microphallus and hypospadias or an enlarged clitoris. No vaginal opening is apparent. The remainder of the examination is normal.

- What is the most likely diagnosis?
- What is the next step in evaluation?

# ANSWERS TO CASE 31:
# Ambiguous Genitalia

*Summary:* A full-term newborn has ambiguous genitalia.

➤ **Most likely diagnosis:** Congenital adrenal hyperplasia (CAH).

➤ **Next step in evaluation:** Karyotype, serum electrolyte levels, and serum 17α-hydroxyprogesterone level.

## ANALYSIS

### Objectives

1. Understand the underlying causes of ambiguous genitalia.
2. Describe factors that influence gender assignment in infants with ambiguous genitalia.
3. Describe the treatment and follow-up of infants after gender assignment.

### Considerations

**This neonate with sexual ambiguity represents a psychosocial emergency.** Upon proper gender assignment for rearing and appropriate medical management, individuals born with ambiguous genitalia should be able to lead well-adjusted lives and satisfactory sex lives. Making a correct diagnosis as early as possible is critical. **Gender assignment** in the neonate born with sexual ambiguity should be influenced by the possibility of achieving **unambiguous and sexually useful genital structures.** Clear and comprehensive discussions with the parents, focusing on their understanding, anxieties, and religious, social, and cultural beliefs, are critical for an appropriate gender assignment. Once gender is assigned, it should be reinforced by appropriate surgical, hormonal, and psychological measures.

# APPROACH TO
# Child with Ambiguous Genitalia

## DEFINITIONS

**CONGENITAL ADRENAL HYPERPLASIA (CAH):** Autosomal recessive disorder of adrenal steroid production with an enzymatic deficiency (usually 21-hydroxylase) causing inadequate production of cortisol, excessive production of androgenic intermediary metabolites, and virilization.

**HERMAPHRODITISM:** Discrepancy between gonad morphology and external genitalia.

**INTERSEX STATE:** Infant with ambiguous genitalia.

**MICROPHALLUS:** Penis size below the fifth percentile for age; neonate with a stretched penile length of less than 2 cm.

**VIRILIZATION:** Masculinization where infant girls exhibit clitoromegaly, labial fusion, and labial pigmentation; infant boys usually appear normal.

## CLINICAL APPROACH

Evaluation of the infant with ambiguous genitalia must occur rapidly to alleviate family anxiety. An endocrinologist, clinical geneticist, urologist, and psychiatrist are essential members of the intersex evaluation team. The **goals of the evaluation** are to determine the **etiology** of the intersex problem, **assign gender**, and **intervene with surgical or other treatment** as soon as possible.

Intersex abnormalities include **female pseudohermaphroditism, male pseudohermaphroditism, true hermaphroditism,** and **mixed gonadal dysgenesis.**

**Female pseudohermaphroditism:** 46,XX karyotype; largest neonatal group with ambiguous genitalia; predominant etiology is CAH; rarer etiologies include exposure to maternal androgens/progestins and congenital vaginal absence with uterine absence or abnormality; degree of masculinization depends on stage of development at time of androgenic stimulation and potency and duration of exposure.

**Male pseudohermaphroditism:** 46,XY karyotype; etiologies include testosterone dyssynthesis, 5α-reductase/dihydrotestosterone deficiency, and decreased androgen binding to target tissues (androgen insensitivity syndrome most common form of male pseudohermaphroditism); phenotypically normal females with functioning testicular tissue, variable incomplete virilization of genitalia, and short, pouchlike vaginas; typically diagnosed at puberty when primary amenorrhea noted; maintain as females and offer vaginoplasty.

**True hermaphroditism:** About 70% 46,XX and remainder 46,XY or mosaic; comprises less than 10% of all intersex cases; bilateral ovotestes or ovary and testis on opposite sides; testicular tissue determines virilization degree; gender assignment based on genitalia appearance (approximately 75% assigned male gender); contradictory reproductive structures removed in older patients with assigned gender.

**Mixed gonadal dysgenesis:** Most 46,XY/45,XO karyotype; testis with Sertoli and Leydig cells, but no germinal elements, on one side and streak gonad on other; hypospadias, partial labioscrotal fusion, and undescended testes most common (incompletely virilized male appearance); usually assigned female gender and undergo gonadectomy (25% of streak gonads develop malignancy); assign as male if testes descended.

## Assessment

After obtaining a careful history, a family pedigree should be constructed to identify consanguinity and to document cases of genital ambiguity, infertility, unexpected pubertal changes, or inguinal hernias. Physical findings could support a genetically transmitted intersex condition. The history of an unexplained neonatal death may suggest a family history of CAH. Maternal exposure to endogenous or exogenous androgens should be investigated.

A thorough physical examination is crucial in determining the diagnosis and making the most reasonable gender assignment. A critical physical finding is the presence or absence of a testis in a labioscrotal compartment. Other physical findings include hyperpigmentation of the labioscrotal folds (common in infants with CAH); phallic size and location of urethral opening; palpation of a uterus on bimanual examination; evidence of failure to thrive (failure to regain birth weight, progressive weight loss, vomiting); and dehydration. **Phallic size is the most important factor in determining an infant's sex assignment.**

**Karyotype analysis using activated lymphocytes is an important first step in the laboratory evaluation of infants with ambiguous genitalia.** Results with a high degree of accuracy can be available in less than 72 hours. To determine mosaicism, repeat studies on multiple tissues may be necessary. If CAH is suspected, biochemical studies might include a **serum 17α-hydroxyprogesterone level.** Plasma testosterone levels alone usually are not helpful. Urinary steroids and plasma androgens, measured before and after administration of corticotropin (adrenocorticotropic hormone [ACTH]) and human chorionic gonadotropin (hCG), help to determine whether a block in testosterone synthesis or 5α-reductase deficiency exists.

An ultrasonogram or pelvic magnetic resonance imaging (MRI), urogenital sinus x-ray after contrast injection, and fiberoptic endoscopy may also aid in the evaluation. Laparoscopy usually is not necessary in the newborn because primary emphasis is placed on the external genitalia and the possibilities for adequate sexual function in assigning gender.

## Treatment

The major treatment consideration for infants with ambiguous genitalia is the possibility of achieving cosmetically and functionally normal external genitalia by surgical and hormonal means. **Because the presence of ambiguous external genitalia may reinforce doubt about the sexual identity of the infant, reconstructive surgery is performed as early as medically and surgically feasible, usually before 6 months of age.** Feminizing genitoplasty is the most common surgical procedure performed in female pseudohermaphrodites, in true hermaphrodites, and in male pseudohermaphrodites reared as females. The goal of this surgery is to reduce the size of the clitoris while maintaining vascularity and innervation, feminizing the labioscrotal folds, and ultimately creating a vagina. Because of the high incidence of gonadal tumors in individuals with certain forms of gonadal dysgenesis, gonadectomy performed concurrently with the initial repair of the external genitalia is mandatory. **A male with hypospadias often requires multiple procedures to create a phallic urethra. Circumcision is avoided** in these individuals because the foreskin tissue is commonly used for reconstruction.

If steroid production is the underlying etiology of the intersex problem, treatment is provided to prevent further virilization. **Administration of hydrocortisone to individuals with CAH helps to inhibit excessive production of androgens and further virilization.** Hormone substitution therapy in hypogonadal patients is prescribed so that secondary sexual characteristics develop at the expected time of puberty. Oral estrogenic hormone substitution is initiated in females, and repository injections of testosterone are given to males. With the exception of some female pseudohermaphrodites and true hermaphrodites reared as females, disorders that cause ambiguous genitalia usually lead to infertility.

## Comprehension Questions

31.1 A 3650-g term infant has ambiguous genitalia, including an enlarged clitoris/microphallus and one palpable testis in the labioscrotal folds. Sonogram reveals a uterus and ovaries. Which of the following is the most likely explanation for the child's ambiguous genitalia?

A. Aromatase deficiency
B. Congenital adrenal hyperplasia
C. Female pseudohermaphroditism
D. Male pseudohermaphroditism
E. True hermaphroditism

31.2 A mother brings in her 1-week-old son who has vomited four times over the last 24 hours. He has no fever or diarrhea. The infant is breast-feeding poorly and is "floppy" per the mother. He has had only one wet diaper in the last 12 hours. Physical examination reveals a lethargic infant who has lost 250 g since birth, with pulse of 110 bpm, dry oral mucosa, and no skin turgor. Which of the following tests would be reasonable to consider after stabilization and electrolyte measurement?

A. Serum cortisol level
B. Urine cortisol level
C. Serum 21-hydroxylase level
D. Serum 17α-hydroxyprogesterone level
E. Serum testosterone level

31.3 A mother brings in her 15-year-old daughter because she has never started her periods. She otherwise is healthy and takes no medications. Her past medical history is unremarkable except for inguinal hernia repair as an infant. Family history is unremarkable. She is at the 75th percentile for height and weight, has Tanner stage IV breast development, and no pubic or axillary hair development. Her anogenital examination reveals a short, pocketlike vaginal opening. Which of the following is the most likely explanation for her amenorrhea?

A. Adrenal tumor
B. Congenital adrenal hyperplasia
C. Pituitary tumor
D. Testicular feminization
E. Turner syndrome

31.4 You examine a full-term 3780-g newborn in the nursery and notice that he has marked hypotonia, a very small penis, and unilateral cryptorchidism. Which of the following is the most likely explanation for these findings?

A. Congenital adrenal hyperplasia
B. Male pseudohermaphroditism
C. Maternal treatment with steroids
D. Mixed gonadal dysgenesis
E. Prader-Willi syndrome

## ANSWERS

31.1 **E.** The gonad in the labioscrotal fold suggests a testis, but a uterus and an ovary on sonography are highly suggestive of a true hermaphrodite. Gender assignment in this case should be based on the possibility of surgical correction of the external genitalia. Assignment of female sex and an attempt to preserve ovarian tissue is appropriate.

31.2 **D.** Male infants with salt-losing CAH develop clinical symptoms similar to pyloric stenosis, intestinal obstruction, heart disease, cow's milk intolerance, and other causes of failure to thrive. Their genitalia appear normal. A serum 17α-hydroxyprogesterone level typically is elevated. Without appropriate treatment (hydrocortisone, mineralocorticoid, and sodium supplementation), cardiovascular collapse and death may occur within a few weeks. Many states have neonatal screening programs for CAH, yet infants with salt-losing CAH (21-hydroxylase deficiency) can become very ill and die before the screening results are known.

31.3 **D.** Testicular feminization results from decreased androgen binding to target tissues or androgen insensitivity. Patients have 46,XY karyotypes yet appear as phenotypically normal females with a short or

present as 1° amenorrhea

atretic vagina. Androgen insensitivity is the most common form of male pseudohermaphroditism. Maintaining female gender assignment is appropriate, and vaginoplasty is frequently needed after puberty.

31.4 **E.** Although severe hypotonia, failure to thrive, and hypogonadism characterize Prader-Willi syndrome in early life, hyperphagia, obesity, mental retardation, and the appearance of bizarre behavior manifest by age 6 years. Morbid obesity, limited sexual function, and severe behavioral abnormalities may occur. Mixed gonadal dysgenesis is a reasonable choice given the unilateral cryptorchidism and hypogonadism, but severe hypotonia usually is not a finding in that disorder.

## Clinical Pearls

- The goal of evaluating a neonate with sexual ambiguity is to determine the etiology of the intersex problem, assign gender, and intervene with surgical or other treatment as soon as possible.
- Treatment of sexual ambiguity is directed toward achieving cosmetically and functionally normal external genitalia by surgical and hormonal means.
- Reconstructive surgery for a patient with ambiguous genitalia is performed as early as medically and surgically feasible, usually before age 6 months.

## REFERENCES

Diamond DA. In: Wein AJ, Kavassi LR, Novick AC, et al. *Campbell's Urology*. 9th ed. Philadelphia, PA: WB Saunders; 2007:3799-3829.

Grumbach MM. Abnormalities of sex determination and differentiation. In: Rudolph CD, Rudolph AM, Hostetter MK, Lister G, Siegel NJ, eds. *Rudolph's Pediatrics*. 21st ed. New York, NY: McGraw-Hill; 2003:2079-2101.

Laufer MR, Goldstein DP. Pediatric and adolescent gynecology—Part I. In: Ryan KJ, Berkowitz RS, Barbieri RL, Dunaif A, eds. *Kistner's Gynecology and Women's Health*. 7th ed. St. Louis: Mosby; 1999:233-259.

Rapaport R. Disorders of sex development (intersex). In: Kliegman RM, Behrman RE, Jenson HB, Stanton BF, eds. *Nelson Textbook of Pediatrics*. 18th ed. Philadelphia, PA: WB Saunders; 2007:2394-2403.

Rapaport R. Hypofunction of the testes. In: Behrman RE, Kliegman RM, Jenson HB, Stanton BF, eds. *Nelson Textbook of Pediatrics*. 18th ed. Philadelphia, PA: WB Saunders; 2007:2379-2384.

White PC. Disorders of the adrenal glands. In: Kliegman RM, Behrman RE, Jenson HB, eds. *Nelson Textbook of Pediatrics*. 18th ed. Philadelphia, PA: WB Saunders; 2007:2349-2355.

# Case 32

A 15-year-old adolescent male presents to your clinic with 3 days of burning upon urination. He denies urinary frequency, change in urine appearance, penile discharge, or genital lesions. He reports no significant past medical history. He is sexually active and infrequently uses condoms. His examination is normal, other than slight erythema of the urethral orifice with scant mucoid discharge. The urinalysis is positive only for trace leukocytes and leukocyte esterase.

- ➤ What is the most likely diagnosis?
- ➤ What is the next step in evaluation?

# ANSWERS TO CASE 32:
# Urethritis

*Summary:* An adolescent with dysuria, penile discharge, and urinalysis consistent with urethritis and possible sexually transmitted disease (STD).

➤ **Most likely diagnosis:** Urethritis.

➤ **Next step in evaluation:** Obtain a thorough history and review of systems, focusing on sexual history and symptoms consistent with possible extragenital infection. Perform a focused examination for oropharyngeal, abdominal, genitourinary (GU), joint, or skin abnormalities. Send urine for routine culturing and nucleic acid amplification testing for gonorrhea (GC) and chlamydia.

## ANALYSIS

### Objectives

1. Describe the various etiologies of urethritis.
2. Describe the workup and treatment of urethritis.
3. Understand other disorders presenting similarly to urethritis.

### Considerations

This adolescent with urinary symptoms represents a typical presentation for STD. Presenting symptoms and examination findings may permit narrowing the list of possible pathogens, but STDs frequently coexist and physical signs often overlap. An accurate diagnosis without testing is difficult. Basic investigations include checking urine or urethral secretions for specific infections (GC, chlamydia). Additional studies should be selectively considered.

# APPROACH TO
## Adolescent with Urethritis

## DEFINITIONS

**GONOCOCCAL URETHRITIS:** Urethral infection due to *Neisseria gonorrhoeae*; incubation period 2 to 5 days; dysuria and mucopurulent urethral discharge possible; extragenital infection possible including oropharynx and skin; diagnose by nucleic acid amplification of urine or traditional culturing of GU secretions on Thayer-Martin agar.

**NONGONOCOCCAL URETHRITIS:** Urethral infection usually due to *Chlamydia trachomatis*; incubation period 5 to 10 days; dysuria and mucoid urethral discharge possible; diagnose by nucleic acid amplification of urine or traditional tissue culturing of GU secretions.

**NUCLEIC ACID (DNA, PCR) AMPLIFICATION:** Technique for detecting bacterial nucleic acid; high sensitivity and specificity; can be performed on urine or urethral secretions.

**URINE NITRITE:** End-product of *Enterobacter* growth; typically indicative of urinary tract infection (UTI); colony count greater than $10^5$ usually required for positive nitrite test.

**URINE LEUKOCYTE ESTERASE:** Product of inflammatory response associated with pyuria on urinalysis; typically positive in urethritis.

**CONDYLOMA:** Caused by human papillomavirus (HPV); small papular to large pedunculated lesions usually seen on genitalia, in perianal areas, or on surrounding skin; asymptomatic or associated with local inflammatory reaction marked by tenderness or burning.

**BALANITIS:** Inflammation of the glans penis; etiologies include infectious and traumatic.

## CLINICAL APPROACH

Evaluation of the **adolescent with dysuria** should commence with a **sexual** and **GU history** of both the patient and sexual partner(s), if known. Multiple partners, early sexual activity, inconsistent condom use, and use of drugs and alcohol are known STD risk factors. **Gonorrheal and chlamydial acquisition rates** historically increase as adolescents age, and recurrence rates can be **as high as 40%.**

The timing and constellation of GU signs and symptoms can be helpful in narrowing the differential diagnosis and prompting appropriate laboratory studies and treatment. Questions should include whether **dysuria, frequency, discharge, or changes in urine appearance** have been noted. One should inquire about **lesions on the genitalia**, around the anus, or on the skin of the lower abdomen, groin, or inner thighs. Rashes elsewhere on the body also should be investigated; the transient, **pustular rash associated with disseminated gonococcal infection** or the macular rash on the palms of patients with secondary syphilis could be identified. Importantly, more than 60% of urethritis patients are asymptomatic, and only about one-third will have frank dysuria or discharge. Annual GC and chlamydia urine screening in sexually active adolescents is recommended by some.

Dysuria in an otherwise healthy, sexually active male should raise suspicion for an underlying STD. **Chlamydial urethritis** tops the differential diagnosis; other possibilities include gonococcal urethritis and *Ureaplasma urealyticum* or *Mycoplasma genitalium* infections. Dysuria caused by an inflammatory process involving the penile epidermis, rather than mucosa, should be included in the differential diagnosis (candidal balanitis, inflamed condyloma). In both sexes, typical GU infections may present atypically; gonorrhea may not present with a purulent urethral discharge, and herpes infection could be associated with mucoid urethral discharge.

Initial evaluation of a patient with GU complaints would include **urine dipstick analysis** for leukocytes, leukocyte esterase, and/or nitrite, routine urine culturing, and **urine PCR testing for GC and chlamydia.** Urine PCR testing has largely replaced urethral swabs for culture because the sensitivity of urine PCR testing is nearly equivalent and it is a less invasive alternative. PCR testing sometimes is not accepted in courts, so if the patient is a possible **victim of abuse, urethral swabs** are often required. A vaginal swab for culture is included if a pelvic examination already is planned to evaluate the female patient. Urinary tract infection typically is differentiated from urethritis, with the former usually associated with positive nitrite, positive urine culture with an expected organism, and negative STD screening.

Standard therapies for specific infections are widely available and should be consulted as sensitivity patterns change. Current treatment regimens for **GC** include a **single intramuscular dose of ceftriaxone (Rocephin)** or oral cefixime (Suprax). **Chlamydia** therapy choices include one dose of **azithromycin (Zithromax)** or a 1-week course of doxycycline (Vibramycin) or erythromycin (E.E.S.). Patients with GC infection are treated for possible chlamydial coinfection. In both sexes, treatment can be appropriate, before results return, for classic symptoms, an abnormal GU examination, intercourse with an infected partner, or for compliance and follow-up concerns.

Appropriate screening and timely treatment of STD-associated urethritis is important because an asymptomatic carrier state is a possibility. Tubo-ovarian scarring and infertility in the female patient are possible, even when she is asymptomatic. **Prior chlamydial infection carries a twofold increased risk for ectopic pregnancy.**

## Comprehension Questions

32.1 A 16-year-old adolescent female presents with a 1-day history of stabbing left groin pain, and white vaginal discharge and mild dysuria for the past week. There has been no abnormal vaginal bleeding, with her last menses approximately 3 weeks ago. She reports one UTI since menarche, but no STDs. She has been sexually active for the past year and takes an oral contraceptive. Her partners irregularly use condoms. She is afebrile, but has left lower quadrant and suprapubic abdominal pain on deep palpation and minimal guarding. Which of the following is the most appropriate next step?

A. Request emergent surgery consultation.
B. Perform urinalysis and urine pregnancy testing.
C. Order pelvic ultrasonography.
D. Perform pelvic examination and Pap smear.
E. Order follicle-stimulating hormone and luteinizing hormone.

32.2 For the past few days, a 12-year-old boy has been complaining of an irritated and itchy penis and burning on urination. He has not had frequency or change in urine appearance. His mother noted a whitish-yellow staining of his underwear yesterday when she was doing the laundry. His past medical history is unremarkable. He is an uncircumcised boy without penile or scrotal lesions, other than marked erythema of the glans penis with whitish coronal exudate upon foreskin retraction. Urinalysis is unremarkable. Which of the following is the most likely diagnosis?

A. Gonococcal urethritis
B. Candidal balanitis
C. Nongonococcal urethritis
D. Urinary tract infection
E. Herpes genitalis

32.3 A 17-year-old adolescent female presents with severe pain in the right upper quadrant and has some pain in her right shoulder. She has nausea, fever, and chills. The abdominal pain increases with movement or Valsalva activities. On physical examination, you confirm pain over the gallbladder, but also notice that she has right lower quadrant abdominal pain. Her pelvic examination is significant for discharge from the cervical os and pain upon cervical motion. Which of the following is the most likely etiology for her complaint?

A. Appendicitis
B. Ectopic pregnancy
C. Fitz-Hugh-Curtis syndrome
D. Gallbladder disease
E. Right lower quadrant pneumonia

32.4 A 15-year-old adolescent female has burning on urination, but no fever, urinary frequency, hematuria, vaginal discharge, GU lesions, or abdominal pain. She has regular cycles. Her abdominal examination is normal. Her GU examination reveals erythema surrounding the vaginal introitus, but no vaginal discharge, tenderness, or masses during the pelvic examination. Her urinalysis is benign. Which of the following is the most important historical clue to be gathered?

A. Miscarried last year
B. Douching twice daily over the past month
C. Treated for UTI last year
D. Treated for chlamydia last year
E. Receiving contraceptive injections quarterly

## ANSWERS

32.1 **B.** STD is a concern in this patient with pyuria and abdominal pain; a surgical evaluation at this time does not seem necessary. In addition to pelvic inflammatory disease (PID), possible etiologies include UTI, ovarian torsion, ovarian cyst, and ectopic pregnancy. The first step in evaluation should be urinalysis and pregnancy testing. A pelvic examination and testing for GC and chlamydia should be included in the evaluation of this sexually active female, but a Pap smear is not likely to identify the etiology of her symptoms. Pelvic ultrasonography may be required if the physical examination proves equivocal.

32.2 **B.** This patient's examination is most consistent with candidal balanitis. The potential for bacterial or fungal overgrowth in the uncircumcised male is approximately 30% greater than for circumcised males. In balanitis and other conditions causing irritated skin, dysuria without other evidence of urethritis or UTI may occur. In this patient with candidiasis, a topical treatment with an antifungal (clotrimazole) would be reasonable.

32.3 **C.** This girl likely has Fitz-Hugh-Curtis syndrome. This disease can be seen in both sexes, but is more prevalent in girls and usually is associated with evidence of acute PID. Evidence of PID may be absent, however. The right upper quadrant pain results from ascending pelvic infection and inflammation of the liver capsule and diaphragm. It can mimic other abdominal emergencies and must be considered in sexually active adolescents as a diagnosis of exclusion. This condition was once thought to be caused only by *N gonorrhoeae*; *C trachomatis* infection probably is more common. The acute phase is described above and in the question; a chronic phase of persistent right upper quadrant pain or complete resolution of symptoms can also be seen.

32.4 **B.** Chemical urethritis as a result of frequent douching is likely in this patient. Other possible etiologies for this benign urethritis include chemical irritants (soaps), fabrics (rayon), and drying agents (powders). Past pregnancy and a history of GU disorder are important, but have less relevance in this case, especially given her benign pelvic examination and urinalysis. Treatment typically entails eliminating the offending agent and waiting for symptoms to subside.

## Clinical Pearls

- The goals of evaluating urethritis are to diagnose and treat infections that can threaten the viability of reproductive organs or cause extragenital or systemic infection.
- Typical sexually transmitted diseases may present atypically or in combination, making patient and partner history, focused examination, and case-specific testing important tools.
- Dysuria does not always indicate urethritis or urinary tract infection. Irritated genitourinary lesions or chemical urethritis can promote dysuria with scant or no findings on examination or urinalysis.

## REFERENCES


Jenkins RR. Sexually transmitted diseases. In: Kliegman RM, Behrman RE, Jenson HB, Stanton BF, eds. *Nelson Textbook of Pediatrics*. 18th ed. Philadelphia, PA: WB Saunders; 2007:855-863.

Matson SC, Ehrman W. Adolescents and sexually transmitted diseases. In: Osborn LM, DeWitt TG, First LR, Zenel JA, eds. *Pediatrics*. Philadelphia, PA: Elsevier Mosby; 2005:1446-1454.

Orr DP, Blythe MJ. Sexually transmitted diseases. In: McMillan JA, Feigin RD, DeAngelis CA, Jones MD, eds. *Oski's Pediatrics: Principles and Practice*. 4th ed. Philadelphia, PA: Lippincott Williams & Wilkins; 2006:584-592.

Shafer MA, Moscicki A-B. In: Rudolph CD, Rudolph AM, Hostetter MK, Lister G, Siegel NJ, eds. *Rudolph's Pediatrics*. 21st ed. New York, NY: McGraw-Hill; 2003: 260-270.

# Case 33

A 6-year-old boy without significant past medical history complains of a persistently runny nose. His family has tried over-the-counter cold remedies with only marginal and temporary success. His mother reports the symptoms are worse in the spring and summer. His complaints include sneezing paroxysms, an itchy throat, and eye tearing. His mother notes persistent mouth breathing and loud snoring. His examination reveals dark circles under his eyes and a crease across the bridge of his nose. His nasal turbinates are pale blue, boggy, and coated with clear drainage.

➤ What is the most likely diagnosis?

➤ What is the best management for this condition?

# ANSWERS TO CASE 33: Allergic Rhinitis

*Summary:* A 6-year-old boy with clear rhinorrhea and allergic symptoms including itchy throat, tearing eyes, an allergic crease, and allergic shiners.

- ➤ **Most likely diagnosis:** Allergic rhinitis.
- ➤ **Best management:** Allergen avoidance, systemic antihistamines, nasal steroids.

## ANALYSIS

### Objectives

1. Describe the physiology of allergic rhinitis.
2. Become familiar with the differential diagnosis of persistent rhinitis.
3. Contrast the possible treatments of allergic rhinitis.

### Considerations

This patient's symptoms are consistent with allergic disease. The **nasal bridge crease** results from the **"allergic salute,"** a characteristic upward nose rubbing. His **allergic "shiners"** are caused by nasal mucosal edema interfering with venous drainage resulting in venous pooling under the eye.

# APPROACH TO Allergic Rhinitis

## DEFINITIONS

**ALLERGIC CREASE:** A horizontal skinfold across the nasal bridge from chronic nose rubbing (an "allergic salute").

**RHINITIS:** Inflammation of the nasal mucosa.

**SINUSITIS:** Mucous membrane inflammation of a sinus cavity.

## CLINICAL APPROACH

Allergic rhinitis, which occurs in 20% to 40% of children and increases in prevalence with age, must be distinguished from other causes of rhinitis. Viral and bacterial upper respiratory tract infections (URIs) usually cause congestion and mucopurulent drainage. A nasal foreign body can cause unilateral purulent, foul-smelling, and sometimes bloody drainage. Persistent clear drainage, especially after head trauma, can indicate a cerebrospinal fluid leak; it can be identified by demonstrating glucose in the drainage. Cocaine abuse can lead to chronic clear or bloody rhinitis. Malignancy can cause a persistent bloody discharge.

Diagnostic testing usually is unnecessary; the diagnosis of allergic rhinitis is made by history and examination alone. **Eosinophils in a Hansel stain of nasal drainage support the diagnosis**; sinus imaging is rarely needed. Allergy testing may be helpful in patients with severe symptoms; the results are useful if the inciting allergen(s) can be removed from the environment or if immunotherapy (allergy injections) is contemplated.

Rhinitis management depends on the etiology. **Viral URIs require no treatment**; the disease is self-limited. Bacterial sinusitis usually improves with antibiotic therapy for upper respiratory tract pathogens such as *Moraxella catarrhalis*, *Streptococcus pneumoniae*, nontypeable *Haemophilus influenza*, and, less commonly, *Staphylococcus aureus*, *Streptococcus viridans*, and anaerobes. **Vasomotor rhinitis, with symptoms similar to allergic rhinitis but more related to weather changes, physical stimuli, or emotion in patients lacking atopic histories or nasal smear eosinophilia, requires no treatment**; however, a topical antihistamine such as azelastine (Astelin) may be helpful in older children. Medication-caused nasal congestion (oral contraceptives, reserpine, α-blockers, methyldopa [Aldomet], aspirin, nonsteroidal anti-inflammatory drugs, and decongestant nasal spray overuse) are treated by elimination of the offending agent.

**The principal treatment of allergic rhinitis is allergen avoidance**. If the allergen is unidentified or environmentally pervasive (eg, tree pollen), medications may be useful. **Antihistamines** can control many symptoms, such as sneezing, itching, and nasal drainage. Some agents, such as diphenhydramine, are sedating, thus limiting their usefulness in the school-aged child; newer antihistamines, such as loratadine, are nonsedating and are preferable alternatives.

**Decongestants**, indicated for significant nasal obstruction, are given alone or in conjunction with antihistamines. Pseudoephedrine is the most commonly used pediatric decongestant; side effects include hypertension, agitation, insomnia, and occasionally hallucinations. Topical decongestant nasal sprays (Afrin), useful initially for significant obstruction, should be used for only a few days at a time because chronic use leads to rebound edema (rhinitis medicamentosa). Over-the-counter decongestants intended for use in children under 2 are no longer available; there was no evidence supporting efficacy, and dosing errors caused morbidity and occasional mortality.

**Nasal steroids are effective for treatment of allergic rhinitis**. Adverse effects may include epistaxis, irritation, and burning; in general, nasal steroids are well tolerated. Little or no systemic effect is expected, but studies have suggested a slightly decreased growth rate but normal final height in patients who chronically use nasal or inhaled steroids.

## Comprehension Questions

33.1 A 4-year-old boy has nasal drainage for 2 months. His mother has asthma and his father has eczema. On examination, you find foul-smelling, blood-tinged left-sided nasal drainage; he is completely obstructed on that side. His other nostril is without drainage or edema. Which of the following is the best next step in managing this patient?

A. Computerized tomography of the sinuses
B. Nasal steroids and oral antihistamines
C. Oral antibiotics
D. Otolaryngology evaluation for possible foreign body
E. Reassurance that his condition is benign and requires observation only

33.2 A 16-year-old adolescent female reports frequent URIs for the last few years. She said her last doctor always prescribed antibiotics and she would eventually improve. She reports clear nasal drainage with congestion, itchy eyes and nose, and cough. Which of the following is the best next step in managing this patient?

A. Computerized tomography of the sinuses
B. Evaluation for possible foreign body
C. Nasal steroids and oral antihistamines
D. Oral antibiotics
E. Reassurance that her condition is benign and requires observation only

33.3 A 4-year-old boy has a 3-month history of bilateral purulent nasal drainage but no fever or other complaints. Examination reveals several small, shiny, gray, pedunculated masses partially occluding both nasal meatus. A diagnostic workup should include which of the following?

A. Complete blood count with peripheral smear
B. Nasal smear for eosinophilia
C. Nitroblue tetrazolium (NBT) test
D. Sweat chloride test
E. Total immunoglobulin levels

CF → nasal polyps < 10-12yo

33.4 A 10-year-old girl complains of left-sided nasal congestion for 5 months. Decongestants and antihistamines have not helped. She denies placing any object in her nose. Today her mother noticed increasing left-sided facial swelling and tenderness. Examination of the girl reveals a pink, nontender, fleshy mass in her left nares that completely occludes the airway. Initial management should include which of the following?

A. Facial magnetic resonance imaging
B. Foreign-body removal with alligator forceps
C. Nasal steroids with antihistamines
D. Reassurance that her condition is benign and requires observation only
E. Sweat chloride test

## ANSWERS

33.1 **D.** This boy has unilateral purulent nasal discharge, likely due to a foreign body; it should be removed as soon as possible. A malignancy is possible, as is sinusitis, but a foreign body is more likely. The nasal symptoms of allergic rhinitis symptoms are typically bilateral.

33.2 **C.** This patient has a classic allergic rhinitis history. Patients may believe they have recurrent URIs when in fact they have allergic symptoms. Although allergic rhinitis occasionally is difficult to distinguish from other cause of rhinitis, a history and physical examination usually are diagnostic. Imaging is not necessary to diagnose allergic rhinitis, and antibiotics are not effective. While the symptoms are not life-threatening, allergic rhinitis does cause significant morbidity and lost school (and work) days, so treatment is appropriate.

33.3 **D.** Nasal polys can result from the chronic inflammation of allergic rhinitis and chronic sinusitis, but a child with polyps who is younger than 10 to 12 years should be tested for cystic fibrosis (CF); approximately 25% of CF patients have nasal polyps. The child in this case has no other CF symptoms, but his age and the polyps indicate testing is a priority. Immotile cilia syndrome (Kartagener syndrome: situs inversus, chronic sinusitis/otitis media, airway disease) is a possibility in this boy, but the test to confirm this diagnosis (cilia electron microscopy) was not listed in the question. Nasal eosinophils are suggestive of allergic disease but not diagnostic. A positive NBT test suggests a phagocytic defect, and low total immunoglobulin levels suggest a humoral immunodeficiency.

33.4 **A.** Rhabdomyosarcoma is the most common pediatric soft-tissue sarcoma, and approximately half of these tumors are located in the head and neck region. The tumor typically presents as a sometimes tender mass, causing symptoms from normal structure displacement. When arising from nasal tissue, it can obstruct the nares and extend into the skull (causing cranial nerve involvement). The first step in the evaluation is computerized tomography or magnetic resonance imaging to determine tumor size and location. A completely resectable tumor has the best prognosis. Chronic allergic rhinitis can result in nasal polyps, but the description suggests a single mass larger than a typical polyp. Attempting to remove a fleshy mass in the office with alligator forceps is not appropriate.

## Clinical Pearls

- Allergic rhinitis is allergen mediated; thus, allergen avoidance is the best treatment.
- Nasal steroids are the most effective chronic allergic rhinitis medications, often used with antihistamines.
- Nasal polyps can be sequelae of chronic inflammation and allergic rhinitis, but younger patients with polyps must be screened for cystic fibrosis.

## REFERENCES

Arndt CAS. Soft tissue sarcomas. In: Kliegman RM, Behrman RE, Jenson HB, Stanton BF, eds. *Nelson Textbook of Pediatrics*. 18th ed. Philadelphia, PA: Saunders Elsevier; 2007:2144-2146.

Bacharier L. Allergic rhinitis and conjunctivitis. In: Rudolph CD, Rudolph AM, Hostetter MK, Lister G, Siegel NJ, eds. *Rudolph's Pediatrics*. 21st ed. New York, NY: McGraw-Hill; 2003:817-818.

Breitfeld PP, Grier HE. Rhabdomyosarcoma. In: Rudolph CD, Rudolph AM, Hostetter MK, Lister G, Siegel NJ, eds. *Rudolph's Pediatrics*. 21st ed. New York, NY: McGraw-Hill; 2003:1612-1614.

Haddad J, Turner RB, Hayden GF, Pappas DE, Hendley JO. Disorders of the upper respiratory tract. In: Kliegman RM, Behrman RE, Jenson HB, Stanton BF, eds. *Nelson Textbook of Pediatrics*. 18th ed. Philadelphia, PA: Saunders Elsevier; 2007:1742-1756.

Long SS. The common cold. In: McMillan JA, Feigin RD, DeAngelis CD, Jones MD, eds. *Oski's Pediatrics: Principles and Practice*. 4th ed. Philadelphia, PA: Lippincott Williams & Wilkins; 2006:1467-1470.

Milgrom H, Yeung DYM. Allergic rhinitis. In: Kliegman RM, Behrman RE, Jenson HB, Stanton BF, eds. *Nelson Textbook of Pediatrics*. 18th ed. Philadelphia, PA: Saunders Elsevier; 2007:949-952.

Orenstein DM. Cystic fibrosis. In: Rudolph CD, Rudolph AM, Hostetter MK, Lister G, Siegel NJ, eds. *Rudolph's Pediatrics*. 21st ed. New York, NY: McGraw-Hill; 2003:1967-1980.

Shott SR. Olfactory disorders. In: Rudolph CD, Rudolph AM, Hostetter MK, Lister G, Siegel NJ, eds. *Rudolph's Pediatrics*. 21st ed. New York, NY: McGraw-Hill; 2003:1264.
Simons FER. Allergic rhinitis and associated disorders. In: McMillan JA, Feigin RD, DeAngelis CD, Jones MD, eds. *Oski's Pediatrics: Principles and Practice*. 4th ed. Philadelphia, PA: Lippincott Williams & Wilkins; 2006:2428-2432.
Wald ER. Paranasal sinusitis. In: McMillan JA, Feigin RD, DeAngelis CD, Jones MD, eds. *Oski's Pediatrics: Principles and Practice*. 4th ed. Philadelphia, PA: Lippincott Williams & Wilkins; 2006:1470-1476.

# Case 34

A 16-year-old adolescent male, a resident at the local police department's boot camp, was in his normal state of health until this morning, when he developed a headache and a fever of 105.8°F (41°C). Over the next 2 hours, he developed a stiff neck and began vomiting. He was brought to the emergency department (ED) when he developed altered mental status. No one else in the facility is ill. In the ED, his heart rate is 135 bpm, blood pressure 120/70 mm Hg, respiratory rate 25 breaths/min, and temperature 104°F (40°C). He is combative, unaware of his surroundings, and does not follow instructions. Kernig and Brudzinski signs are present.

- What is the most likely diagnosis?
- How would you confirm the diagnosis?
- What treatment is indicated?
- What are possible complications?

# ANSWERS TO CASE 34:
# Bacterial Meningitis

*Summary:* A 16-year-old adolescent male has fever, headache, stiff neck, and altered mental status. He is tachycardic but normotensive.

- ➤ **Most likely diagnosis:** Bacterial meningitis.
- ➤ **Confirm diagnosis:** Lumbar puncture (LP).
- ➤ **Treatment:** Intravenous antibiotics.
- ➤ **Complications:** Deafness, cranial nerve palsies, and, rarely, hemiparesis or global brain injury.

## ANALYSIS

### Objectives

1. Describe the typical presentation of bacterial meningitis.
2. Describe how a patient's age affects the presentation and outcome of bacterial meningitis.
3. List typical pathogens and appropriate treatment strategies by age group.

### Considerations

This teen has the typical triad of meningitis symptoms: fever, headache, and a stiff neck; his altered mental status is another typical finding. Other causes of mental status changes include viral meningoencephalitis, trauma, intentional or accidental ingestion, and hypoglycemia. Of these alternatives, only viral meningitis would likely explain the fever and stiff neck.

# APPROACH TO
# Bacterial Meningitis

## DEFINITIONS

**BRUDZINSKI SIGN:** A physical finding consistent with meningitis; while the patient is supine, the neck is passively flexed resulting in involuntary knee and hip flexion.

**ENCEPHALITIS:** Brain parenchyma inflammation causing brain dysfunction.

**KERNIG SIGN:** A physical finding consistent with meningitis; while the patient is supine, the legs are flexed at the hip and knee at 90° angle resulting in pain with leg extension.

**MENINGITIS:** Leptomeningeal inflammations, typically infectious, but may also be caused by foreign substances.

## CLINICAL APPROACH

**The microbiology and clinical presentation of meningitis varies based on the patient's age.** The incidence of **neonatal meningitis** is between 0.2 and 0.5 cases per 1000 live births, most commonly due to ***Escherichia coli* and group B *Streptococcus*** (*Streptococcus agalactiae*). ***Listeria monocytogenes*** and other organisms (*Citrobacter* sp, *Staphylococcus* sp, group D streptococci, and *Candida* sp) are less common. Infants at increased risk for meningitis include low-birth-weight and preterm infants, and those born to mothers with chorioamnionitis, after a prolonged rupture of the amniotic membranes, or by traumatic delivery. Most neonatal bacterial meningitis occurs by hematogenous spread. Clinical symptoms in infants are nonspecific and not the typical triad of headache, fever, and stiff neck; instead, infants may have thermal instability (often hypothermia), poor feeding, emesis, seizures, irritability, and apnea. **Infants may have a bulging fontanelle**, and they may be either hypotonic or hypertonic.

**Bacterial meningitis in older children** is usually caused by ***Streptococcus pneumoniae*** **or *Neisseria meningitidis;*** vaccination has essentially eliminated *Haemophilus influenza* type B. Other rarer causes in this age group include *Pseudomonas aeruginosa*, *Staphylococcus aureus*, *Staphylococcus epidermidis*, *Salmonella* sp, and *Listeria monocytogenes*.

The incidence of pneumococcal meningitis is 1 to 6 cases per 100,000 children per year, more commonly occurring in the winter. It is an **encapsulated pathogen**; children with a **poorly functioning or absent spleen are at higher risk.** Children with **sickle cell disease** have an infection incidence 300 times greater than in unaffected children. Other risk factors include sinusitis, otitis media, pneumonia, and head trauma with subsequent cerebrospinal fluid (CSF) leak.

*Neisseria meningitidis* colonizes the upper respiratory tract in approximately 15% of normal individuals; carriage rates up to 30% are seen during invasive disease outbreaks. Disease appears to be caused by "new" infection rather than long-term carriage. In the United States, most disease is caused by serotypes B and C. Family members and day care workers in close contact with children having meningitis are at 100- to 1000-fold increased risk for contracting disease. A plethora of other bacterial, viral, fungal, and mycobacterial agents can cause meningitis.

The **classic symptoms of meningitis seen in older children and adults** may be accompanied by **mental status changes, nausea, vomiting, lethargy, restlessness, ataxia, back pain, Kernig and Brudzinski signs, and cranial nerve**

**palsies.** Approximately one quarter to one-third of patients have a **seizure** during the illness course. Patients with *N meningitidis* can have a petechial or purpuric rash (purpura fulminans), which is associated with septicemia. Patients with septicemia due to *N meningitidis* often are gravely ill and may or may not have associated meningitis.

The **test of choice for suspected meningitis is an LP**, which usually can be performed safely in children with few complications. **Contraindications** include a **skin infection over the planned puncture site,** evidence of or clinical concern for **increased intracranial pressure**, and a critically ill patient who may not tolerate the procedure. **Cerebrospinal fluid analysis includes Gram stain and culture, white and red blood cell counts, and protein and glucose analysis.** Bacterial antigen screens can be performed in patients already receiving antibiotics before the LP; these antigens may persist for several days, even when the culture is negative. Typical bacterial meningitis findings include an elevated opening pressure, several hundred to thousands of white blood cells with polymorphonuclear cell predominance, and elevated protein and decreased glucose levels.

Treatment strategies vary by patient age, likely pathogens, and local resistance patterns. A **CSF Gram stain can guide the decision-making process.** In the neonatal period, ampicillin often is combined with a third-generation cephalosporin or an aminoglycoside to cover infections caused by group B *Streptococcus*, *L monocytogenes*, and *E coli*. Neonates in an intensive care unit may be exposed to nosocomial infections; prevalent pathogens in that nursery must be considered.

In some locales, more than half of the pneumococcal isolates are intermediately or highly penicillin resistant; 5% to 10% of the organisms are cephalosporin resistant. Thus, **in suspected pneumococcal meningitis, a third-generation cephalosporin combined with vancomycin is often recommended.** Most *N meningitidis* strains are susceptible to penicillin or cephalosporins.

**Acute meningitis complications** may include **seizures, cranial nerve palsies, cerebral infarction, cerebral or cerebellar herniation, venous sinus thrombosis, subdural effusions**, syndrome of inappropriate (secretion) of antidiuretic hormone **(SIADH)** with hyponatremia, and central diabetes insipidus. The **most common long-term sequela is hearing loss** (up to 30% of patients with pneumococcus); patients with bacterial meningitis usually have a hearing evaluation at the conclusion of antibiotic treatment. Mental retardation, neuropsychiatric and learning problems, epilepsy, behavioral problems, vision loss, and hydrocephalus are less commonly seen.

## Comprehension Questions

34.1 A 13-year-old boy has a 1-day history of fever and lethargy, and was unable to be awoken this morning. In the emergency department his respiratory rate is 7 breaths/min, heart rate 55 bpm, temperature 105.8°F (41°C), and blood pressure (BP) 60/40 mm Hg. He has altered mental status, a stiff neck, and a purpuric rash over his trunk. Which of the following is the most appropriate next step in the management of this patient?

A. Computerized tomography of the head
B. Intravenous antibiotics
C. Intubation
D. Lumbar puncture
E. Serum chemistries

34.2 An 8-year-old girl has persistent fever and headaches. Her parents report that for the 2 weeks prior she has complained of frontal headache that was significant enough to keep her from school. She has had intermittent temperature elevations to 101°F (38.3°C), and she started vomiting a nonbloody, nonbilious fluid a few days ago. She has had frequent otitis media and sinusitis episodes, but her last episode of otitis media occurred approximately 5 weeks ago. On examination, you find a lethargic girl in no respiratory distress. She has a temperature of 100°F (37.7°C), heart rate 109 bpm, and blood pressure (BP) 100/60 mm Hg. She has nuchal rigidity and frontal sinus tenderness. Which of the following is the most appropriate next step in the management of this patient?

A. Computerized tomography of the head
B. Intravenous promethazine for emesis
C. Lumbar puncture
D. Sinus radiographs
E. Trial of subcutaneous sumatriptan for migraine

34.3 A 2-week-old infant develops a temperature to 102°F (38.9°C). Pregnancy and delivery were uncomplicated. The irritable, fussy infant has a heart rate of 170 bpm and respiratory rate 40 breaths/min. The anterior fontanelle is full, but he has no nuchal rigidity; the rest of the examination is unremarkable. Which of the following is the most appropriate management of this infant?

A. Encourage oral fluids and office follow-up in 24 hours.
B. Order computerized tomography of the head followed by an LP.
C. Perform an LP, blood culture, urine culture, and admit to the hospital.
D. Prescribe intramuscular ceftriaxone and office follow-up in 1 week.
E. Prescribe oral amoxicillin and office follow-up in 1 week.

34.4 A 14-year-old boy complains of fever and stiff neck for 2 days. He has a sore throat and has been unable to eat for 1 day because of the pain. On examination, he is alert and oriented, but he has nuchal rigidity and posterior pharyngeal midline fullness. He drools to avoid the pain of swallowing. Which of the following is the best next step in the management of this patient?

A. Order computerized tomography of the head.
B. Order lateral neck radiographs.
C. Perform a lumbar puncture.
D. Prescribe intramuscular antibiotics.
E. Prescribe oral antibiotics.

## ANSWERS

34.1 **C.** This patient in the question has meningococcemia; he is in shock, and he is about to die. The ABCs of airway, breathing, and circulation should always take precedence over diagnostic studies. *N meningitidis* can present as meningococcemia with purpura and shock; in some cases patients will also have meningitis. The LP should be deferred, however, until he is clinically stable. Intravenous fluids to support his cardiovascular status and antibiotics should be administered immediately.

34.2 **A.** This girl's history of sinusitis and a prolonged headache with worsening emesis and nuchal rigidity suggest an intracranial abscess due to her sinusitis. In her case, CNS imaging (with contrast) is performed prior to an LP. Performing an LP when a mass lesion might be causing increased intracranial pressure can result in herniation of the brain and patient death. Sinus films would show sinusitis but would not reveal an intracranial abscess. Merely treating her symptoms with promethazine or sumatriptan would delay the diagnosis of her underlying problem.

34.3 **C.** This infant potentially has a serious bacterial infection, and an evaluation including a LP is performed. Infants do not reliably demonstrate a Kernig or Brudzinski sign; a lack of nuchal rigidity should not preclude an LP. Computerized tomography scan before an LP in an infant with an open anterior fontanelle is rarely necessary; brain herniation is exceedingly rare. A course of oral antibiotics, or a single dose of ceftriaxone, is not sufficient to treat meningitis or septicemia.

34.4 **B.** A retropharyngeal abscess is causing this boy's neck stiffness; he does not have meningitis. He has a normal mental status, dysphagia, and fullness in his oropharynx. Lateral neck films are a simple way to confirm this diagnosis. Prescribing antibiotics without identifying the diagnosis would not be appropriate in this case.

## Clinical Pearls

- The typical meningitis presentation in older children consists of fever, headache, and nuchal rigidity.
- Nuchal rigidity is not a reliable finding of meningitis until 12 to 18 months of age.
- Pneumococcal disease (including meningitis) is more common in patients with functional or anatomic asplenia.
- Approximately one-third of meningitis patients have a seizure at some point in the disease.
- Typical cerebrospinal fluid findings of bacterial meningitis include elevated protein level, reduced glucose concentration, and several hundred to thousands of white blood cells per cubic millimeter.

## REFERENCES

Feigin RD. Bacterial meningitis beyond the newborn period. In: McMillan JA, Feigin RD, DeAngelis CD, Jones MD, eds. *Oski's Pediatrics: Principles and Practice*. 4th ed. Philadelphia, PA: Lippincott Williams & Wilkins; 2006:924-933.

Goldstein NA, Hammerschlag MR. Deep neck abscesses. In: McMillan JA, Feigin RD, DeAngelis CD, Jones MD, eds. *Oski's Pediatrics: Principles and Practice*. 4th ed. Philadelphia, PA: Lippincott Williams & Wilkins; 2006:1492-1496.

Haslem RHA. Brain abscess. In: Kliegman RM, Behrman RE, Jenson HB, Stanton BF, eds. *Nelson Textbook of Pediatrics*. 18th ed. Philadelphia, PA: Saunders Elsevier; 2007:2524-2525.

Lebel MH. Meningitis. In: McMillan JA, Feigin RD, DeAngelis CD, Jones MD, eds. *Oski's Pediatrics: Principles and Practice*. 4th ed. Philadelphia, PA: Lippincott Williams & Wilkins; 2006:493-496.

Prober CG. Acute bacterial meningitis beyond the neonatal period. In: Kliegman RM, Behrman RE, Jenson HB, Stanton BF, eds. *Nelson Textbook of Pediatrics*. 18th ed. Philadelphia, PA: Saunders Elsevier; 2007:2513-2521.

Tureen J. Meningitis. In: Rudolph CD, Rudolph AM, Hostetter MK, Lister G, Siegel NJ, eds. *Rudolph's Pediatrics*. 21st ed. New York, NY: McGraw-Hill; 2003:900-904.

# Case 35

You receive a call from the mother of a previously healthy 2-year-old boy. Yesterday, he developed a temperature of 104°F (40°C), cramping abdominal pain, emesis, and frequent watery stools. The mother assumed he had the same gastroenteritis like his aunt or many other children in his day care center. However, today he developed bloody stools with mucus and seemed more irritable. While you are asking about his current hydration status, the mother reports that he is having a seizure. You tell her to call the ambulance and then notify the local hospital's emergency center of his imminent arrival.

- What is the most likely diagnosis?
- How can you confirm this diagnosis?
- What is the best management for this illness?
- What is the expected course of this illness?

# ANSWERS TO CASE 35:

## Bacterial Enteritis

*Summary*: This child was exposed in his day care center and at home to gastrointestinal (GI) illnesses. He has fever, abdominal pain, and watery diarrhea that progressed to bloody diarrhea with mucus. He had a new-onset seizure.

- **Most likely diagnosis:** Bacterial enteritis with neurologic manifestations.
- **Diagnostic tools:** Fecal leukocytes, fecal blood, and stool culture.
- **Management:** Varies with age and suspected organism; hydration and electrolyte correction is a priority. *Salmonella* infections are self-limited and generally are not treated except in patients younger than 3 months or in immunocompromised individuals; *Shigella* infections, although self-limited, are generally treated to shorten the illness and decrease organism excretion. Antimotility agents are not used.
- **Course:** Left untreated, most GI infections in healthy children will spontaneously resolve. Extraintestinal infections are more likely in immunocompromised individuals.

## ANALYSIS

### Objectives

1. Describe the typical clinical presentation of bacterial enteritis.
2. List potential pathogens for gastroenteritis, considering the patient's age.
3. Discuss treatment options and explain when treatment is necessary.
4. Discuss potential complications of bacterial enteritis.

### Considerations

Bloody stools can be caused by many diseases, not all of which are infectious. In this child, GI bleeding also could be caused by Meckel diverticulum, intussusception, Henoch-Schönlein purpura, hemolytic uremic syndrome, *Clostridium difficile* colitis, and polyps. The description is most consistent, however, with infectious enteritis typical of *Shigella* or *Salmonella*.

# APPROACH TO
# Bacterial Enteritis

## DEFINITIONS

**COLITIS:** Inflammation of the colon.

**DIARRHEA:** Frequent passage of unusually soft or watery stools.

**DYSENTERY:** An intestinal infection resulting in severe bloody diarrhea with mucus.

**ENTERITIS:** Inflammation of the small intestine, usually resulting in diarrhea; may be a result of infection, immune response, or other causes.

## CLINICAL APPROACH

***Salmonella* organisms** are aerobic gram-negative rods and can survive as facultative anaerobes. They are motile and do not ferment lactose. Infection is **more common in warmer months.** *Salmonella* infections can be separated into nontyphoidal disease (gastroenteritis, meningitis, osteomyelitis, and bacteremia) and typhoid (or enteric) fever, caused primarily by *Salmonella typhi.* Outbreaks usually occur sporadically but can be food related and occur in clusters. Many animals harbor ***Salmonella***. Exposure to **poultry and raw eggs probably is the most common source of human infection**; sources may also include iguanas and turtles. Infection requires the ingestion of many organisms; person-to-person spread is uncommon.

Gastroenteritis is the most common nontyphoidal disease presentation. Children usually have sudden onset of nausea, emesis, cramping abdominal pain, and watery or bloody diarrhea. Most develop a low-grade fever; some have **neurologic symptoms** (confusion, headache, drowsiness, and seizures). Between 1% and 5% of patients with *Salmonella* infection develop transient bacteremia, with subsequent extraintestinal infections (osteomyelitis, pneumonia, meningitis, and arthritis); these findings are more common in immunocompromised patients and in infants.

***Shigella* organisms are small gram-negative bacilli**. They are nonlactose fermenting facultative anaerobes, and have recently been shown to be motile. Four *Shigella* species cause human disease: *S dysenteriae*, *S boydii*, *S flexneri*, and *S sonnei*. Infections most commonly occur in warmer months and in the first 10 years of life (peaking in the second and third years). Infection usually is transmitted **person to person** but may occur via food and water. Relatively few *Shigella* organisms are required to cause disease. Typically, children have fever, cramping abdominal pain, watery diarrhea (often progressing to small bloody stools), and anorexia; they appear ill. Untreated, diarrhea typically lasts 1 to 2 weeks and then resolves. **Neurologic findings** may include headache, confusion, seizure, or hallucinations. *Shigella* meningitis is infrequent. Uncommon complications include rectal prolapse, cholestatic hepatitis, arthritis, conjunctivitis, and cystitis. Rarely, *Shigella* causes a rapidly progressive sepsis-like presentation (Ekiri syndrome) that quickly results in death.

*Salmonella* or *Shigella* tests include a **stool culture**, although results frequently are negative even in infected test subjects. **Fecal leukocytes usually are positive**, but this nonspecific finding only suggests colonic inflammation. An occult blood assay often is positive. In ***Shigella* infection**, the peripheral white count usually is normal, but a **remarkable left shift** is often seen with more bands than polymorphonuclear cells. *Salmonella* infection usually results in a mild leukocytosis.

**Treatment focuses on fluid and electrolyte balance correction. Antibiotic treatment** of *Salmonella* **usually is not necessary**; it does not shorten the GI disease course and **may increase the risk of hemolytic-uremic syndrome (HUS).** Infants younger than 3 months of age and immunocompromised individuals often are treated for GI infection, as they are at increased risk for disseminated disease. *Shigella* is self-limited as well, but antibiotics shorten the illness course and decrease the duration organisms are shed. Antimotility agents are indicated for neither *Salmonella* nor *Shigella.*

In addition to the above organisms, enteroinvasive *Escherichia coli*, *Campylobacter* sp, and *Yersinia enterocolitica* can cause dysentery, with fever, abdominal cramps, and bloody diarrhea. *Yersinia* can cause an "acute abdomen"-like picture. Enterohemorrhagic (or Shigatoxin-producing) *E coli* can cause bloody diarrhea but usually no fever. Infection with *Vibrio cholera* produces vomiting and profuse, watery, nonbloody diarrhea with little or no fever.

**Hemolytic-uremic syndrome, the most common cause of acute childhood renal failure, develops in 5% to 8% of children with diarrhea caused by enterohemorrhagic *E coli* (O157:H7)**; it is seen less commonly after *Shigella*, *Salmonella*, and *Yersinia* infections. It usually is seen in children younger than 4 years. The underlying process may be microthrombi, microvascular endothelial cell injury causing microangiopathic hemolytic anemia, and consumptive thrombocytopenia. Renal glomerular deposition of an unidentified material leads to capillary wall thickening and subsequent lumen narrowing. The typical presentation occurs 1 to 2 weeks after a diarrheal illness, with acute onset of pallor, irritability, decreased or absent urine output, and even stroke; children may also develop petechiae and edema. Treatment is supportive; some children require dialysis. Most children recover and regain normal renal function; all are followed for hypertension and chronic renal failure.

## Comprehension Questions

35.1 A 2-year-old boy developed emesis and intermittent abdominal pain yesterday, with several small partially formed stools. His parents were not overly concerned because he seemed fine between the pain episodes. Today, however, he has persistent bilious emesis and has had several bloody stools. Examination reveals a lethargic child in mild distress; he is tachycardic and febrile. He has a diffusely tender abdomen with a vague tubular mass in the right upper quadrant. Which of the following is the most appropriate next step in managing this condition?

A. Computerized tomography of the abdomen
B. Contrast enema
C. Intravenous antibiotics for *Shigella*
D. Parental reassurance
E. Stool cultures

35.2 A previously healthy 2-year-old girl had 3 days of bloody diarrhea last week that spontaneously resolved. Her mother now thinks she looks pale. On examination, you see that she is afebrile, her heart rate is 150 bpm, and her blood pressure is 150/80 mm Hg. She is pale and irritable, has lower-extremity pitting edemas, and has scattered petechiae. After appropriate laboratory studies, initial management should include which of the following?

A. Careful management of fluid and electrolyte balance
B. Contrast upper GI series with small bowel delay films
C. Intravenous antibiotics and platelet transfusion
D. Intravenous steroids and aggressive fluid resuscitation
E. Intubation and mechanical ventilation

35.3 A family reunion picnic went awry when the majority of attendees developed emesis and watery diarrhea with streaks of blood. Unaffected attendees did not eat the potato salad. A few ill family members are mildly febrile. They come as a group to your office, seeking medications. Which of the following is the most appropriate management for their condition?

A. Antimotility medication
B. Hydration and careful follow-up
C. Intramuscular ceftriaxone
D. Oral amoxicillin
E. Oral metronidazole

35.4 You are asked to see a 1-month-old infant to provide a second opinion. During a brief, self-limited, and untreated diarrheal episode last week, his primary physician ordered a stool assay for *Clostridium difficile* toxin; the result is positive. The infant now is completely asymptomatic, active, smiling, and well hydrated. His physician said treatment was not necessary, but the mother wants treatment. Which of the following is the most appropriate response?

A. *Clostridium difficile* commonly colonizes the intestine of infants; treatment is not warranted.
B. The infant should take a 7-day course of oral metronidazole.
C. The infant should take a 10-day course of oral vancomycin.
D. The infant should be admitted to the hospital for intravenous metronidazole
E. A repeat study to look for the C *difficile* organism is warranted.

## ANSWERS

35.1 **B.** This child has an intussusception. He has bloody stools, but he also has bilious emesis, colicky abdominal pain, and a right upper quadrant mass. In experienced hands, a contrast enema procedure may be diagnostic and therapeutic. Ensure that a surgeon and a prepared operating room are available should the reduction via contrast enema fail or result in intestinal perforation. While a CT may diagnose intussusception, an enema is preferred as it can be therapeutic as well as diagnostic.

35.2 **A.** Hemolytic-uremic syndrome may be seen after bloody diarrhea, presenting with anemia, thrombocytopenia, and nephropathy. The child in question is hypertensive and has edema, so large amounts of fluids may be counterproductive. Steroids typically are not helpful. The thrombocytopenia is consumptive; unless the patient is actively bleeding, platelet transfusion is not helpful. Most of the care for such patients is supportive, concentrating on fluids and electrolytes. Early dialysis may be needed. Hypertensive patients should have appropriate control of their blood pressure.

35.3 **B.** This family probably has *Salmonella* food poisoning. Antibiotics are not indicated for this healthy family, and antimotility agents may prolong the illness. Frequent handwashing should be emphasized.

35.4 **A.** *Clostridium difficile* colonizes approximately half of normal healthy infants in the first 12 months. In this infant without a history of antibiotic treatment or current symptoms, treatment is unnecessary. C *difficile* colitis rarely occurs without a history of recent antibiotic use.

## Clinical Pearls

- In normal children older than 3 months, isolated intestinal *Salmonella* infections do not require antibiotic treatment; antibiotics do not shorten the course of illness.
- Suspected *Shigella* intestinal infections usually are treated to shorten the illness course and to decrease organism shedding.
- Hemolytic-uremic syndrome, a potential sequela of bacterial enteritis, is the most common cause of acute renal failure in children.

## REFERENCES

Bhutta ZA. Acute gastroenteritis in children. In: Kliegman RM, Behrman RE, Jenson HB, Stanton BF, eds. *Nelson Textbook of Pediatrics*. 18th ed. Philadelphia, PA: Saunders Elsevier; 2007:1605-1617.

Brandt M. Intussusception. In: McMillan JA, Feigin RD, DeAngelis CD, Jones MD, eds. *Oski's Pediatrics: Principles and Practice*. 4th ed. Philadelphia, PA: Lippincott Williams & Wilkins; 2006:1938-1940.

Eddy AA. Hemolytic uremic syndrome. In: Rudolph CD, Rudolph AM, Hostetter MK, Lister G, Siegel NJ, eds. *Rudolph's Pediatrics*. 21st ed. New York, NY: McGraw-Hill; 2003:1696-1698.

Pavia AT. *Salmonella, Shigella,* and *Escherichia coli* infections. In: Rudolph CD, Rudolph AM, Hostetter MK, Lister G, Siegel NJ, eds. *Rudolph's Pediatrics*. 21st ed. New York, NY: McGraw-Hill; 2003:981-990.

Pickering LK. *Salmonella* infections. In: McMillan JA, Feigin RD, DeAngelis CD, Jones MD, eds. *Oski's Pediatrics: Principles and Practice*. 4th ed. Philadelphia, PA: Lippincott Williams & Wilkins; 2006:1112-1116.

Sheth RD. Hemolytic-uremic syndrome. In: McMillan JA, Feigin RD, DeAngelis CD, Jones MD, eds. *Oski's Pediatrics: Principles and Practice*. 4th ed. Philadelphia, PA: Lippincott Williams & Wilkins; 2006:2600-2602.

Stevenson RJ. Intussusception. In: Rudolph CD, Rudolph AM, Hostetter MK, Lister G, Siegel NJ, eds. *Rudolph's Pediatrics*. 21st ed. New York, NY: McGraw-Hill; 2003: 1407-1408.

# Case 36

A 15-year-old adolescent female has periumbilical pain that began 8 hours ago; since then she has vomited once and has had one small, loose, bowel movement. Her last meal was 12 hours ago, and she is not hungry. She denies dysuria, urinary frequency, and sexual activity; her last menses 1 week ago was normal. On examination, she is moderately uncomfortable and has a low-grade fever 101.5°F (38.6°C); her other vital signs are normal. Her abdominal examination reveals few bowel sounds, rectus muscle rigidity, and tenderness to palpation, particularly periumbilically. Breath sounds are clear; she has no rashes. Her pelvic examination shows no vaginal discharge, but there is some abdominal tenderness with gentle bimanual palpation. She has pain with digital rectal examination.

- What is the most likely diagnosis?
- What is the next step in the management of this patient?

# ANSWERS TO CASE 36: Appendicitis

*Summary:* A 15-year-old adolescent female with periumbilical pain of 8-hour duration, followed by anorexia, emesis, and a loose bowel movement. She has no dysuria or sexual activity, and the pain appears unrelated to her menses. Her physical examination shows a quiet, rigid, tender abdomen, and pain with digital rectal examination.

- **Most likely diagnosis:** Appendicitis.
- **Next step in management:** A surgeon should be consulted once the diagnosis of appendicitis is suspected. Abdominal ultrasound has high sensitivity for diagnosis of appendicitis in experienced pediatric centers, but abdominal CT is more generally used. Urinalysis is useful to eliminate a urinary tract infection (UTI) as a cause and a complete blood count (CBC) often shows leukocytosis. Despite this adolescent's denial of sexual activity, a urine pregnancy test should be obtained.

## ANALYSIS

### Objectives

1. Recognize the presenting clinical signs for appendicitis.
2. Know the differential diagnosis for appendicitis.
3. Recognize the need to maintain a high index of suspicion for appendicitis to prevent possible complications.

### Considerations

The definitive diagnosis of appendicitis may not be made until surgery. For this patient, the initial **abdominal pain followed by anorexia and vomiting** suggests appendicitis. **The pain of appendicitis classically begins periumbilically and then migrates to the right lower quadrant.** The pain can occur laterally (retrocecal appendix), or it can be more diffuse (perforated appendix with resultant generalized peritonitis). The utility of rectal examinations for children with suspected appendicitis is debatable; they can be helpful for localizing the pain source in a female adolescent.

The adolescent female in this case is early in her disease process and arguably might be safely observed for a few hours if the diagnosis remains in question. Once the appendicitis is strongly considered, however, surgical management should occur in a timely fashion; perforation rates exceed 65% if diagnosis is delayed beyond 36 to 48 hours from symptom onset. Possible appendicitis complications (wound infection, abscess formation, intestinal obstruction, adhesions) are rare following uncomplicated appendectomy but occasionally occur with appendiceal perforation.

# APPROACH TO
# Appendicitis

## DEFINITIONS

**APPENDICITIS:** Appendix inflammation occurs after luminal obstruction. If the appendix is not removed, appendiceal wall necrosis results in perforation and peritoneal contamination.

**MCBURNEY'S POINT:** The junction of the lateral and middle third of the line joining the right anterior superior iliac spine and the umbilicus (Figure 36–1); typically this area is of greatest discomfort in acute appendicitis.

**PSOAS SIGN:** Irritation of the psoas muscle caused by passive hip extension in patients with appendicitis.

**OBTURATOR SIGN:** Irritation of the obturator muscle caused by passive internal rotation of the thigh in patients with appendicitis.

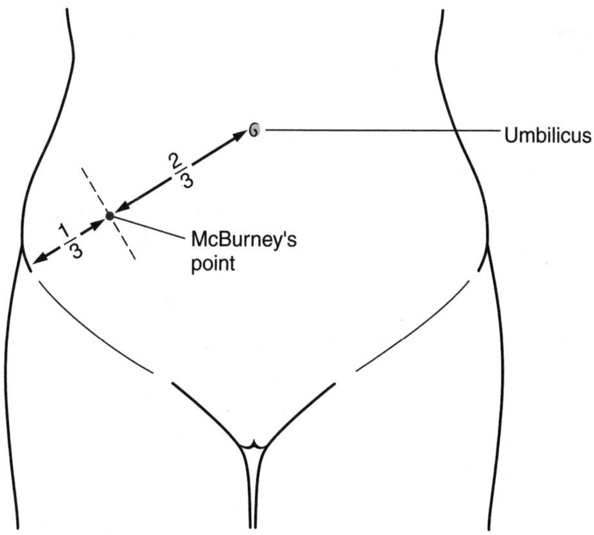


**Figure 36–1.** McBurney's point.

## CLINICAL APPROACH

A person's lifetime risk of appendicitis has been estimated at 6% to 20%, with the **peak incidence in adolescence.** Intrinsic appendiceal obstruction, inspissated fecal material (appendicolith), is found in 30% to 50% of patients at the time of surgery. Extrinsic compression usually is caused by enlarged lymph nodes associated with bacterial or viral infections. The obstruction causes vascular thrombosis, ischemia, and, ultimately, perforation.

The differential diagnosis for acute abdominal pain in childhood is long (Table 36–1). Worsening abdominal pain in the periumbilical area, which then migrates to the right lower quadrant, is characteristic of acute appendicitis. Likewise, anorexia, nausea, and vomiting that begin after the onset of pain is strongly indicative of the diagnosis.

A gentle abdominal examination can provide meaningful data while not frightening the child. Observation of the child getting on and off the examination table can be revealing; children with appendicitis avoid sudden movements (jumping off the table). The abdomen is auscultated for bowel sounds first, then gently palpated for the area of maximal tenderness and rigidity. Gentle finger percussion assesses for peritoneal irritation ("rebound tenderness"). If performed, a rectal examination should occur last.

Although not a specific finding, **leukocytosis with a predominance of polymorphonuclear cells (a "left shift") on a CBC supports an inflammatory process.** Hematuria and pyuria raise the possibility of a genitourinary etiology, but they can occur with acute appendicitis if it also causes irritation of the bladder or ureteral wall. Plain abdominal radiographs are frequently obtained but infrequently helpful: psoas shadow obliteration, right lower quadrant intestinal dilatation, scoliosis toward the affected region, and an appendicolith (seen in 10%-20% of cases) support appendicitis. Chest radiographs eliminate pneumonia as an alternate diagnosis. **Ultrasonography is more sensitive than plain films for appendicitis and is particularly useful in female adolescents,** in whom the differential diagnosis includes ovarian cysts and pregnancy. **Computerized tomography** has become the diagnostic test of choice in most centers. CT is particularly helpful for patients who are **neurologically impaired, immunologically suppressed, or obese,** and when **perforation** is suspected. CT images are used as a guide for periappendiceal abscess drainage.

**Definitive treatment is surgical removal of the appendix,** accomplished as soon as the diagnosis is strongly suspected to prevent perforation (if it has not already occurred). For perforated appendicitis, recovery requires intravenous antibiotics and fluid replacement, and may be complicated by sepsis, abscess formation, or prolonged (4 to 5 days) paralytic ileus.

**Table 36–1** PARTIAL DIFFERENTIAL DIAGNOSIS OF ACUTE ABDOMINAL PAIN IN CHILDREN BEYOND INFANCY

| CONDITION | SIGNS AND SYMPTOMS |
|---|---|
| Appendicitis | Right lower quadrant pain, abdominal guarding, and rebound tenderness |
| Bacterial enterocolitis | Diarrhea (may be bloody), fever, vomiting |
| Cholecystitis | Right upper quadrant pain, often radiating to subcapsular region of the back |
| Constipation | Infrequent, hard stools, and recurrent abdominal pain; sometimes enuresis |
| Diabetic ketoacidosis | History of polydipsia, polyuria, and weight loss |
| Ectopic pregnancy | Lower abdominal pain, vaginal bleeding, and an abnormal menstrual history |
| Gastroenteritis | Fever, vomiting, and hyperactive bowel sounds |
| Hemolytic-uremic syndrome | Irritability, petechiae, and edema |
| Henoch-Schönlein purpura | Purpuric lesions, especially of lower extremities and joint pain |
| Hepatitis | Right upper quadrant pain and jaundice |
| Inflammatory bowel disease | Weight loss, diarrhea, and malaise |
| Mittelschmerz | Sudden onset of right or left lower quadrant pain with ovulation, copious mucoid vaginal discharge |
| Nephrolithiasis | Hematuria, colicky abdominal pain |
| Ovarian cyst | White blood cell count less than 11,000/mm$^3$; vomiting rare |
| Pancreatitis | (Severe) epigastric abdominal pain, fever, and persistent vomiting |
| Pelvic inflammatory disease | Cervical motion tenderness; white blood cells in the vaginal secretions |
| Pneumonia | Fever, cough, and crackles on auscultation of the chest |
| Sickle cell crisis | Anemia, and extremity pain |
| Streptococcal pharyngitis | Fever, sore throat, and headache |
| Urinary tract infection | Dysuria, fever, vomiting, and back pain |

## Comprehension Questions

36.1 A 7-year-old has right-sided abdominal pain and fever to 102°F (38.9°C). His mother says that he has had 2 days of poor appetite and cough; he had two loose stools earlier in the day. On examination, his temperature is 101.7°F (38.7°C), his heart rate is 120 bpm, and his respiratory rate is 50 breaths/min. Breath sounds are diminished, and the abdomen is diffusely tense with hypoactive bowel sounds. Which of the following would likely lead to the diagnosis?

A. Abdominal computerized tomography
B. Chest radiograph
C. Liver function tests
D. Stool leukocytes
E. Stool for culture, ova, and parasites

36.2 A 14-year-old adolescent female with a 3-day history of abdominal pain, anorexia, and vomiting and a 1-day history of fever underwent laparoscopic surgery for suspected appendicitis, which was perforated at the time of surgery. Intravenous ampicillin, gentamicin, and clindamycin were initiated prior to surgery and continued postoperatively. On the seventh postoperative day, she continues to have fevers to 102°F (38.9°C). Which of the following is the next most appropriate step in management?

A. Add metronidazole to the antibiotic regimen.
B. Change the antibiotics to amikacin and a cephalosporin.
C. Order a computerized tomography scan *stat.*
D. Send a urinalysis and urine culture.
E. Perform a pelvic examination.

36.3 A previously healthy 8-year-old boy presents to your office with abdominal pain, anorexia, and vomiting that have worsened over the previous 24 hours. The pain is located in the umbilical region. Despite the emesis, he appears well hydrated. A CBC reveals a white blood count of 17,000 cells/$mm^3$ with 50% polymorphonuclear cells. A urine dipstick on a clean-catch specimen shows 2+ leukocytes and 1+ protein but no nitrites. Which of the following is the most appropriate management at this point?

A. Obtain a complete chemistry panel and continue to observe him in the office.
B. Send the patient immediately to the hospital for an abdominal ultrasound.
C. Give him a prescription for trimethoprim-sulfamethoxazole; schedule a follow-up visit in 2 days to reevaluate the urine.
D. Admit him to the hospital for intravenous antibiotics to treat presumed pyelonephritis.
E. Schedule a computerized tomography scan of the abdomen for the next morning.

36.4 A 4-year-old girl has a fever of 102.4°F (39.1°C), difficulty swallowing, vomiting, and abdominal pain. Which of the following diagnostic tests is most likely to yield the appropriate diagnosis?

A. Streptococcal antigen test ("rapid strep test")
B. Antigen test for Epstein-Barr virus ("Monospot")
C. Lateral neck radiograph
D. Abdominal ultrasound
E. Complete blood count

## ANSWERS

36.1 **B.** Lower lobe pneumonias can cause abdominal pain, which may be the most distressing symptom in a young patient. Inflammation of the diaphragm can result in an abnormal abdominal examination, which may be mistaken for the source of the child's illness. This child has cough, fever, tachypnea, and diminished breath sounds, which together make pneumonia the most likely diagnosis.

36.2 **C.** This adolescent female is at risk for an intra-abdominal abscess despite her appendectomy and intravenous antibiotics. It would be unusual for a urinary tract infection or pelvic inflammatory disease to cause persistent fever despite broad-spectrum intravenous antibiotics.

36.3 **B.** This boy's symptoms and signs are most consistent with a diagnosis of acute appendicitis. A urinary tract infection in an otherwise healthy boy would be unusual. His pyuria is most likely the result of bladder wall or ureter irritation caused by an inflamed appendix.

36.4 **A.** Her symptoms are most consistent with streptococcal pharyngitis. In addition to throat pain and fever, group A *Streptococcus* infections commonly cause abdominal pain and emesis.

### Clinical Pearls

- Acute appendicitis typically causes periumbilical abdominal pain that eventually migrates to the right lower quadrant. Emesis usually follows, rather than precedes, the onset of pain.
- Surgical management of appendicitis occurs as soon as the diagnosis is suspected in order to minimize the potential risks of perforation and intra-abdominal abscess formation.
- Appendicitis often is not confirmed until surgery. A history and physical examination, urinalysis, CBC, and abdominal ultrasound or computerized tomography scan are the most useful tools for eliminating other preoperative considerations.

## REFERENCES

Aiken JJ, Oldham KT. Acute appendicitis. In: Kliegman RM, Behrman RE, Jenson HB, Stanton BF, eds. *Nelson Textbook of Pediatrics*. 18th ed. Philadelphia, PA: WB Saunders; 2007:1628-1635.

Pegoli W. Appendicitis. In: McMillan JA, Feigin RD, DeAngelis CD , Jones MD, eds. *Oski's Pediatrics: Principles and Practice*. 4th ed. Philadelphia, PA: Lippincott Williams & Wilkins; 2006:2000-2002.

Stevenson RJ. Appendicitis. In: Rudolph CD, Rudolph AM, Hostetter MK, Lister G, Siegel NJ, eds. *Rudolph's Pediatrics*. 21st ed. New York, NY: McGraw-Hill; 2003:1450-1452.

# Case 37

A 19-year-old student presents to the university health center with several days of fever, sore throat, malaise, and a rash that developed today. She first started feeling ill 10 days ago with general malaise, headache, and nausea. Four days ago she developed a temperature of 103°F (39.4°C) that has persisted. She has worsening sore throat and difficulty swallowing solid foods; she is drinking well. She denies emesis, diarrhea, or sick contacts. She takes an oral contraceptive daily and took two doses of ampicillin yesterday (left over from a prior illness). On examination, she is well developed with a diffuse morbilliform rash. She appears tired but in no distress. Her temperature is 102.2°F (39°C). She has mild supraorbital edema; bilaterally enlarged tonsils that are coated with a shaggy gray exudate; a few petechiae on the palate and uvula; bilateral posterior cervical lymphadenopathy; and a spleen that is palpable 3 cm below the costal margin. Laboratory data include a white blood cell (WBC) count of 17,000 cells/mm$^3$ with 50% lymphocytes, 15% atypical lymphocytes, and platelet count of 100,000/mm$^3$.

- ➤ What is the most likely diagnosis?
- ➤ What is the best tool to quickly confirm this diagnosis?
- ➤ What is the best management for this condition?
- ➤ What is the expected course of this condition?

# ANSWERS TO CASE 37:

# Acute Epstein-Barr Viral Infection (Infectious Mononucleosis)

*Summary:* A female college student has 10 days of malaise, headache, and nausea. She now has a fever, sore throat, and morbilliform rash after taking ampicillin. Her examination reveals a fever, rash, tonsillar hypertrophy with exudate, posterior cervical lymphadenopathy, and splenomegaly. She has an elevated WBC count with a lymphocytic predominance, and a mild thrombocytopenia.

- **Most likely diagnosis:** Epstein-Barr virus (EBV) infection (infectious mononucleosis).
- **Best tool:** Assay for heterophil antibodies (Monospot).
- **Best management:** Symptomatic care, avoidance of contact sports while the spleen is enlarged (usually 1-3 months).
- **Expected course:** Acute illness lasts 2 to 4 weeks, with gradual recovery; splenic rupture is a rare but potentially fatal complication. Rarely, some patients have persistent fatigue.

## ANALYSIS

### Objectives

1. Describe the presenting signs and symptoms of acute EBV infection.
2. Contrast EBV infection symptoms in young children with those in adolescents and adults.
3. List potential complications of acute EBV infection.

### Considerations

This case is typical for adolescents with primary EBV infection, although supraorbital edema occurs in only 10% to 20% of patients. Differential diagnosis includes group A β-hemolytic streptococcal pharyngitis; it typically does not have a prodrome similar to this case nor cause splenomegaly. Acute cytomegalovirus (CMV) infection is another possibility; similarities include splenomegaly, fever, and atypical lymphocytosis, but exudative sore throat and posterior cervical lymphadenopathy occur less frequently. Although the patient denied recent ill contacts, EBV infection has a 30- to 50-day incubation; further questioning revealed that her boyfriend had similar symptoms 6 weeks ago. Rash is seen less commonly in adolescents with EBV, but many patients develop a morbilliform rash in response to ampicillin, amoxicillin, or penicillin.

# APPROACH TO Epstein-Barr Infection

## DEFINITIONS

**EPSTEIN-BARR VIRUS (EBV):** A double-stranded DNA herpes virus that infects human oropharyngeal and salivary tissues and B lymphocytes. It can cause persistent viral shedding, is associated with oral hairy leukoplakia in HIV-infected individuals, and causes several malignancies.

**INFECTIOUS MONONUCLEOSIS:** The typical EBV presentation in older children and adolescents. Fever, posterior cervical adenopathy, and sore throat are seen in more than 80% of cases.

## CLINICAL APPROACH

**EBV is ubiquitous in humans.** In developing nations, infection occurs in almost all children by 6 years of age. In the industrialized world, about half of adolescents have serologic evidence of previous EBV infection; 10% to 15% of previously uninfected college students seroconvert each year. The virus is excreted in saliva; infection results from mucosal contact with an infected individual or from contact with a contaminated fomite. Shedding of Epstein-Barr virus in the saliva after an acute infection can continue for more than 6 months, and occurs intermittently thereafter for life.

**After an infection occurs, EBV replicates in the oropharyngeal epithelium and later in the B lymphocytes.** A prodromal period may last for 1 to 2 weeks, with vague findings of fever, nausea, malaise, headache, sore throat, and abdominal pain. The sore throat and fever gradually worsen and frequently cause a patient to seek medical help. **Physical findings during an acute infection may include generalized lymphadenopathy, splenomegaly, and tonsillar enlargement with exudate.** Less common findings include a rash and hepatomegaly.

Primary EBV infection presents as typical infectious mononucleosis in older children and adults, but this presentation is less common in young children and infants. In small children, many infections are asymptomatic. In others, fever may be the only presenting sign. Additional acute findings in small children include otitis media, abdominal pain, and diarrhea. Hepatomegaly and rash are seen more often in small children than in older individuals.

The **Monospot is a useful diagnostic test in children older than approximately 5 years**; the results are unreliable in younger children. Early in the illness the Monospot may be falsely negative. **More definitive testing includes assays of EBV viral capsid antigen (EBV-VCA), early antigen (EA), and Epstein-Barr nuclear antigen (EBNA).** Typically, immunoglobulin (Ig) G and IgM antibodies to EBV-VCA appear first. Anti-EBNA antibodies appear

1 to 2 months following infection and persist for years. Anti-EA antibodies are seen in most children during acute infection and persist for years in approximately one-third of patients. VCA-IgG and EBNA-IgG antibodies indicate past infection. Other laboratory findings include a **lymphocytic leukocytosis**, with approximately **20% to 40% atypical lymphocytes**. Mild **thrombocytopenia** is common, rarely precipitating bleeding or purpura. More than half of patients with EBV infection develop **mildly elevated liver function tests**; jaundice is uncommon.

Infection complications are rare but can be life-threatening. Neurologic sequelae include Bell palsy, seizures, aseptic meningitis or encephalitis, Guillain-Barré syndrome, optic neuritis, and transverse myelitis. Parotitis, orchitis, or pancreatitis may develop. Airway compromise may result from tonsillar hypertrophy; treatment may include steroids. **Splenomegaly** is seen in approximately half of those with infectious mononucleosis; **rupture is rare, but the blood loss is life-threatening.**

Typical infectious mononucleosis requires only rest. Strict bed rest is not useful except for patients with debilitating fatigue. Children with splenomegaly should avoid contact sports to prevent splenic rupture until the enlargement resolves. Acyclovir, which is effective in slowing viral replication, does not affect disease severity nor outcome.

Epstein-Barr virus initially was identified from Burkitt lymphoma tumor cells and was the first virus associated with human malignancy. Other associated malignancies include Hodgkin disease, nasopharyngeal carcinoma, and lymphoproliferative disorders. Epstein-Barr virus can stimulate hemophagocytic syndrome. HIV-infected patients may develop oral hairy leukoplakia, smooth muscle tumors, and lymphoid interstitial pneumonitis with EBV infection.

## Comprehension Questions

37.1 A 17-year-old adolescent male has left shoulder and left upper quadrant abdominal tenderness and vomiting. He reports having "mono" last month but says he is completely recovered. He was playing flag football with friends when the pain started an hour ago. On examination, his heart rate is 150 bpm and his blood pressure is 80/50 mm Hg. He is pale, weak, and seems disoriented. He has diffuse rebound abdominal tenderness. Emergent management includes which of the following?

A. Laparoscopic appendectomy
B. Fluid resuscitation and blood transfusion
C. Intravenous antibiotics
D. Hospital admission for observation
E. Synchronized cardioversion for supraventricular tachycardia

37.2 You are asked to see a 2-year-old boy in consultation. His general practice doctor admitted him to the hospital 2 days ago because of 3 days of fever. He has generalized lymphadenopathy but is otherwise well. Results of Monospot, HIV testing, and CMV antigen tests are negative; his liver function test values are mildly elevated. His physician diagnosed the boy's 7-year-old sibling with "mono" the month prior. You should suggest which of the following?

A. Start intravenous immunoglobulin and obtain an echocardiogram; the patient likely has Kawasaki disease.
B. Send an EBV culture for confirmation of the physician's suspicions.
C. Acyclovir treatment because he has an exposure history positive for EBV.
D. Obtain EBV-VCA IgG and IgM, EBV-EA, and EBV-NA tests.
E. Liver imaging with ultrasonography or computerized tomography.

37.3 The mother of a 15-year-old adolescent female recently diagnosed with infectious mononucleosis calls for more information. She reports that her daughter, although tired, seems comfortable and is recovering nicely. She remembers that her 20-year-old son had "mono" when he was 10 years old, and he received an oral medicine. She requests the same medication for her daughter. Which of the following is the most appropriate course of action?

A. Explain that medications are not routinely used in EBV infection.
B. Call the pharmacy and order oral prednisone, 50 mg daily for 5 days (1 mg/kg/d).
C. Call the pharmacy and order oral acyclovir 250 mg four times per day (20 mg/kg/d).
D. Have her come to the office for a single dose of 50 mg intravenous methylprednisolone (1 mg/kg).
E. Call the pharmacy and order oral amoxicillin 250 mg three times per day for 7 days.

37.4 A teenage boy arrives for a check-up. His friend recently was diagnosed with mononucleosis. He is worried he will contract it. Which of the following is true regarding transmission of EBV?

A. It is common among casual friends.
B. It occurs only in immunodeficient individuals.
C. It requires close contact with saliva (ie, kissing or drinking from the same cup).
D. It is passed only through sexual contact with an infected individual.
E. It does not occur after the infected person recovers from the initial infection.

## ANSWERS

37.1 **B.** The patient described is in hypovolemic shock and likely has splenic rupture with intraperitoneal bleeding. He will die shortly if not aggressively resuscitated with fluids and blood. Evaluation by a surgeon for potential removal of the ruptured spleen should follow quickly.

37.2 **D.** The Monospot heterophil antibody test, useful in older children, is not so reliable in younger children. Antibodies against specific EBV antigens are more helpful in younger children. No imaging study is diagnostic for EBV; acyclovir is not indicated for EBV exposure; EBV culture is not readily available; and while Kawasaki disease must be considered in patients with persistent fever, the exposure history makes EBV more likely.

37.3 **A.** Supportive care alone usually is required for a patient with acute EBV infection. Steroids have been used historically; current literature suggests their use only in impending airway compromise due to tonsillar hypertrophy or other life-threatening complications. Acyclovir suppresses viral shedding acutely but has no long-term benefit and is not routinely recommended. Amoxicillin and ampicillin are ineffective antiviral medications and induce a rash in some EBV-infected patients.

37.4 **C.** EBV is excreted in saliva and is transmitted through mucosal contact with an infected individual (as in kissing) or through a contaminated object. Virus is shed for a prolonged period after symptoms resolve and is intermittently reactivated and shed for years asymptomatically.

### Clinical Pearls

- Most adults show evidence of past Epstein-Barr virus infection; it is a common infection worldwide.
- Children in industrialized nations usually are infected with EBV infection later in life than are children in developing countries.
- Diagnosis of Epstein-Barr virus infection in young children is best achieved by specific antibody assays.
- Infectious mononucleosis is self-limited and usually does not require treatment. Occasional complications of Epstein-Barr virus infection may require steroid administration.

## REFERENCES

Brady MT. Epstein-Barr virus infections (infectious mononucleosis). In: Rudolph CD, Rudolph AM, Hostetter MK, Lister G, Siegel NJ, eds. *Rudolph's Pediatrics*. 21st ed. New York, NY: McGraw-Hill; 2003:1035-1039.

Jenson HB. Epstein-Barr virus. In: Kliegman RM, Behrman RE, Jenson HB, Stanton BF, eds. *Nelson Textbook of Pediatrics*. 18th ed. Philadelphia, PA: Saunders Elsevier; 2007:1372-1376.

Luzuriaga K, Sullivan JL. Epstein-Barr virus infections in children. In: McMillan JA, Feigin RD, DeAngelis CD, Jones MD, eds. *Oski's Pediatrics: Principles and Practice*. 4th ed. Philadelphia, PA: Lippincott Williams & Wilkins; 2006:1241-1246.

# Case 38

A mother says her 2-year-old daughter has had 1 to 2 weeks of perineal and perianal itching. She notes that the itching occurs mostly at night, but she denies fevers, diarrhea, or emesis. The girl spends time in a "Mother's Day Out" program 3 days per week but otherwise is always with her mother. On examination, the perianal area is red and irritated; the anal sphincter tone is normal, and you find no evidence of penetrating trauma. The perineal area is similarly red and excoriated. Other than a slight whitish vaginal discharge, the child's diaper area is clean.

- ➤ What is the most likely diagnosis?
- ➤ How can you confirm the diagnosis?
- ➤ What is the best management for this condition?

# ANSWERS TO CASE 38: Pinworms

*Summary:* A 2-year-old healthy girl with several weeks of nocturnal perianal and perineal pruritus.

- **Most likely diagnosis:** Infection with *Enterobius vermicularis* (pinworms).
- **Confirm the diagnosis:** Cellophane tape test with microscopy to identify pinworm eggs (Figure 38–1).
- **Best management:** Mebendazole, pyrantel pamoate, or albendazole in a single dose, treating the entire family.

## ANALYSIS

### Objectives

1. Describe the presentation of *E vermicularis* infection in the pediatric population.
2. Explain the methods of treatment and prevention of reinfection.

### Considerations

This patient has the typical history for pinworm infection. Although sexual abuse is possible, it is unlikely given the history and examination. Poor personal hygiene is another common problem in 2-year-olds who are toilet training and

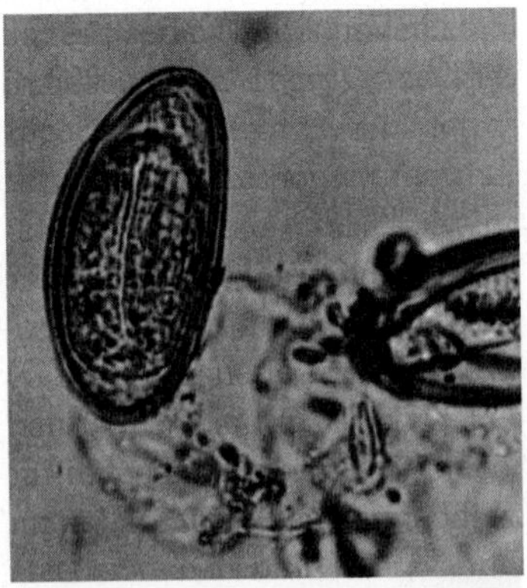

**Figure 38–1.** Pinworm (Enterobius vermicularis) ova on microscopy. *(Reproduced, with permission, from Rudolph CD, Rudolph AM, Hostetter MK, Lister G, Siegel NJ, eds.* Rudolph's Pediatrics. *21st ed. New York, NY: McGraw-Hill; 2003:1106.)*

not cleaning themselves adequately. This results in perianal itching and irritation, yet the genital examination is essentially normal. Occasionally, overzealous cleaning results in similar symptoms.

## APPROACH TO Enterobius Vermicularis Infection

### DEFINITION

**NEMATODE (ROUNDWORMS):** Cylindrical organisms, with thousands of different species, only a few of which are parasitic (Table 38–1). Nematode infection is one of the most common types of infection in humans.

### CLINICAL APPROACH

A patient with perianal itching, especially at night, should be evaluated for *E vermicularis* infection. Unlike many other parasites, feces examination for ova is not useful because the eggs are small and few. Some parents may see a worm in the stool, but *E vermicularis* is difficult to identify positively with the naked eye. Instead, **cellophane tape is applied to the perianal region in the early morning**; from this tape ***E vermicularis* eggs** may be identified. These eggs are infectious; proper infection control practices are indicated.

***Enterobius vermicularis* infection** is the **most common nematode infection in North America**, and humans are the only natural host. Risk factors include exposure to other children in a day care environment or in the home. The adult worm is approximately 1 cm long and lives in the human GI tract, rarely migrating to the appendix, spleen, liver, bladder, and vagina. The pinworm life cycle begins when female worms migrate to the perianal region to deposit their eggs. Within 6 hours a larva is present in each ovum; the larvae are viable for up to 20 days. These eggs are subsequently transferred to clothes, fingers (from itching), and bed sheets. An infection results upon egg ingestion. The larvae "hatch" in the duodenum and grow to adult worms in 4 to 6 weeks.

Many infected patients are asymptomatic. The symptom described most frequently is **nocturnal perianal itching**, a result of worm and ova hypersensitivity. The gravid worms occasionally migrate to the perineal area, resulting in vaginal itching and discharge. Although bruxism historically has been related to pinworm infection, perianal itching is the only consistently reported symptom.

Some experts recommend treating the entire family; others suggest global treatment only in recurrent cases. **Treatment can be with mebendazole, albendazole, or pyrantel pamoate** in a single dose. Often a second dose is given 2 weeks after the first dose to eliminate any new worms released from ova ingested proximate to the treatment time.

**Table 38–1 COMMON NEMATODE INFECTIONS IN HUMANS**

| COMMON NAME | PARASITE NAME(S) | SOURCE OF INFECTION | SIGNS AND SYMPTOMS | DIAGNOSIS | TREATMENT |
|---|---|---|---|---|---|
| Ascariasis | *Ascaris lumbricoides* | Egg ingestion, usually from soil contaminated with human feces | Most asymptomatic; hemoptysis, pulmonary infiltrates, abdominal pain, distention; occasional intestinal obstruction | Embryonate and non-embryonate eggs in stool; occasionally see adult worms in stool or coughed up | Albendazole single dose, mebendazole for 3 d or a single dose of pyrantel pamoate; obstruction may be cleared with piperazine salts (causes worm paralysis and expulsion) |
| Hookworms | *Ancylostoma duodenale; Necator americanus* | Larvae in soil penetrate exposed skin | Pruritus and rash at site of entry; epigastric pain and diarrhea; anemia from blood loss; respiratory symptoms | Characteristic ovoid eggs in stool | Mebendazole for 3 d, or albendazole single dose, or pyrantel pamoate; include iron supplement |
| Pinworms | *Enterobius vermicularis* | Egg ingestion | Many asymptomatic; nocturnal perianal itching most common | Microscopy of cellophane tape applied to anus reveals eggs; routine stool ova and parasites not useful | Pyrantel pamoate, or mebendazole, or albendazole single dose with a second dose 2-3 wk later |

| | | | | | |
|---|---|---|---|---|---|
| Strongyloids | *Strongyloides stercoralis* | Larvae penetrate skin and move to lungs and then intestines; also auto-infectious, larvae can move from intestines into blood stream, to lungs, and back to intestines | Can be asymptomatic; can cause epigastric pain, emesis, diarrhea, malabsorption, weight loss<br>if immunocompromised, can develop 'hyperinfection' (GNR sepsis) | Larvae in feces, or sample of duodenal fluid by a string test | Ivermectin for 1-2 d, or thiabendazole for 2 d; may require up to 2 wk of therapy, based on subsequent stool examinations |
| Visceral and ocular larva migrans | *Toxocara canis; Toxocara cati; Toxocara leonina; Baylisascaris procyonis* | Egg ingestion, usually from soil contaminated with dog or cat feces | Fever, cough, occasional abdominal pain; hepatomegaly, rhonchi, and skin lesions on examination | Clinical presentation and serologic testing; microscopy of affected tissue occasionally reveals larvae | Visceral: none, self-limited disease<br>Ocular; diethylcarbamazine, albendazole for 3-5 d, or mebendazole for 5 d; use with caution, as death of organisms may precipitate inflammatory reaction |
| Whipworms | *Trichuris trichiura* | Egg ingestion | Most asymptomatic; can cause proctitis, bloody diarrhea, abdominal pain, rectal prolapse | Lemon-shaped eggs in the stool | Mebendazole or albendazole for 3 d (single dose for light infections) |

## Comprehension Questions

38.1 A mother states her 4-year-old son has had 2 days of "buttocks pain." She reports several blood-streaked stools and frequent scratching of the area. He is afebrile, but his perianal region is bright red with a clearly demarcated erythematous border. The area is diffusely tender, but no nodularity, fluctuance, or trauma is found. Appropriate diagnostic testing and therapy includes which of the following?

A. Stool sample for ova and parasites; treatment with albendazole
B. Cellophane tape test for ova; treatment with albendazole
C. Rapid streptococcal test of the anal area; oral antibiotics
D. Blood culture; parenteral antibiotics
E. Administration of diaper rash ointment

38.2 A 6-year-old boy who recently moved from the southeastern United States complains of "something coming out" of his buttocks while straining during defecation; it seems to resolve when he relaxes. He also complains of abdominal pain and bloody stools for the last week. Examination reveals a normal external anus without evidence of trauma. When straining, he produces a pink mucosal mass from his anus; it returns when he relaxes. Initial diagnostic evaluation should include which of the following studies?

A. Cellophane tape test upon morning awakening
B. Stool for ova and parasites
C. Rectal culture
D. Abdominal ultrasonography
E. Herpes culture

38.3 A mother brings a stool sample for your review. In the stool are several 15- to 20-cm long, round, whitish worms. You initiate treatment with which of the following?

A. Amoxicillin
B. Mebendazole
C. Praziquantel
D. Niclosamide
E. Paromomycin

38.4 A 14-year-old adolescent male with HIV and AIDS presents for a physical examination prior to traveling to Southeast Asia. In counseling him on health risks in the area, you mention that he must always wear shoes to help prevent *Strongyloides* infection, which is particularly dangerous to him for which of the following reasons?

A. His antiretroviral medications make him more susceptible.
B. His immunodeficiency will make eradication impossible.
C. Antiparasitic agents are not available in Southeast Asia.
D. Teenagers typically have severe disease when infected.
E. *Strongyloides* can develop a "hyperinfection" in immunocompromised hosts.

## ANSWERS

38.1 **C.** Although diagnostic considerations should include pinworm infestation (as well as sexual abuse, contact diaper rash, and candidal diaper rash), the presentation is more consistent with perianal cellulitis. Pinworm infection usually does not cause blood-streaked stool, and any erythema associated with it is not well demarcated. Perianal cellulitis is commonly caused by *Streptococcus* and usually responds to oral or topical (mupirocin [Bactroban]) antibiotics.

38.2 **B.** Pinworms are not known to cause rectal prolapse, whipworms (*Trichuris trichiura*) are. The whipworm nematode lives in warm and humid areas and is commonly found in the southeastern United States. Routine microscopy for ova is sufficient for the diagnosis (whipworms produce many more ova than do pinworms). Treatment is albendazole or mebendazole. Cystic fibrosis should be a consideration in a child with rectal prolapse, although the history might include frequent pneumonias, failure to thrive, or foul-smelling stools.

38.3 **B.** Worms of this size and description typically are *ascaris*; treatment is mebendazole or albendazole. Amoxicillin is an antibacterial agent. Praziquantel, niclosamide, and paromomycin are effective against cestodes (tapeworms) and are not recommended for nematodes.

38.4 **E.** The life cycle of *Strongyloides* does not require a period outside the host. Therefore, the organism can "autoinfect" the host (larvae in the intestines move through the intestinal wall, into the circulation, through the lungs, and back into the intestines). This autoinfection can lead to disseminated strongyloidiasis in immunocompromised hosts with massive invasion of organs with tissue destruction; sepsis with gram-negative intestinal organisms can result.

## Clinical Pearls

- Patients with nocturnal perianal itching are evaluated for *Enterobius vermicularis* infection.
- Typical stool ova and parasites studies may not identify *Enterobius vermicularis* ova (the count is low). A cellophane tape test is more useful to confirm the diagnosis.

## REFERENCES

Cherian T. The nematodes. In: McMillan JA, Feigin RD, DeAngelis CD, Jones MD, eds. *Oski's Pediatrics: Principles and Practice*. 4th ed. Philadelphia, PA: Lippincott Williams & Wilkins; 2006:1361-1369.

Dent AE, Kazura JW. Enterobiasis (Enterobius vermicularis). In: Kliegman RM, Behrman RE, Jenson HB, Stanton BF, eds. *Nelson Textbook of Pediatrics*. 18th ed. Philadelphia, PA: Saunders Elsevier; 2007:1500-1501.

Oberhelman RA. Enterobiasis (pinworm). In: Rudolph CD, Rudolph AM, Hostetter MK, Lister G, Siegel NJ, eds. *Rudolph's Pediatrics*. 21st ed. New York, NY: McGraw-Hill; 2003:1105-1106.

Sanfilippo JS. Vulvovaginitis. In: Kliegman RM, Behrman RE, Jenson HB, Stanton BF, eds. *Nelson Textbook of Pediatrics*. 18th ed. Philadelphia, PA: Saunders Elsevier; 2007:2277.

# Case 39

A 5-month-old infant arrives at the emergency center strapped to a backboard with a cervical collar in place. The father was holding him in his lap in the front passenger seat of their sedan when the driver lost control and crashed. The child was ejected from the car through the windshield. The paramedics report his modified Glasgow coma scale score is 6 (opens eyes to pain, moans to pain, and demonstrates abnormal extension); they intubated him at the scene. He had a self-limited, 2-minute generalized tonic-clonic seizure en route to the hospital.

Your assessment reveals a child with altered mental status. His endotracheal tube is in the correct position, and his arterial blood gas reflects effective oxygenation and ventilation. He is euthermic and tachycardic. He has no evidence of fractures, and his abdominal examination is benign. He has several facial and scalp lacerations. His anterior fontanelle is bulging, his sutures are slightly separated, and his funduscopic examination reveals bilateral retinal hemorrhages.

- ➤ What is the most likely etiology for this child's altered mental status?
- ➤ What is the most appropriate study to confirm this etiology?

# ANSWERS TO CASE 39: Subdural Hematoma

*Summary:* An unrestrained infant is ejected through the windshield. He has altered mental status, he has experienced seizure activity, and his examination is consistent with increased intracranial pressure (ICP).

- **Most likely diagnosis:** Subdural hematoma.
- **Best study:** Urgent computerized tomography (CT) of the head.

## ANALYSIS

### Objectives

1. Describe the typical clinical findings in head trauma.
2. Compare the typical findings of subdural hematoma with those of epidural hematoma.
3. Discuss the possible treatment options for intracranial hemorrhage.

### Considerations

This child is younger than 1 year, and subdural hematomas are more common in this age group; epidural hematomas are more common in older children. Seizures are more common with subdural hematomas, occurring in 75% of affected patients; seizures occur in less than 25% of epidural hematoma patients. His altered mental status could be caused by a simple cerebral concussion, but the CT scan would be normal or show nonspecific changes. The infant's ejection at the crash provides an appropriate mechanism of injury, making other considerations (such as shaken baby syndrome, more recently referred to as abusive head trauma) less likely. This child's lack of a car seat must also be addressed.

# APPROACH TO Subdural Hematoma

## DEFINITIONS

CONCUSSION: Altered mental state immediately after blunt head trauma; no consistent brain abnormality is seen; can cause retrograde and anterograde memory loss.

**EPIDURAL HEMORRHAGE:** Bleeding between the dura and the skull; commonly occurs with skull fracture and middle meningeal artery laceration but can result from disruption of dural sinuses or middle meningeal veins (Figure 39–1).

**GLASGOW COMA SCALE (GCS):** A clinical tool developed to assist in head injury severity prediction. For infants and toddlers, several "modified" scales exist that attempt to adapt the verbal portion to reflect language development and modify the motor component to reflect the lack of purposeful movement in early infancy (Table 39–1).

**SUBDURAL HEMORRHAGE:** Bleeding between the dura and the arachnoid space; occurs with disruption of bridging veins connecting cerebral cortex and dural sinuses (Figure 39–1).

## CLINICAL APPROACH

The child in the case is seriously ill, with increased ICP and retinal hemorrhages. Some form of cerebral hemorrhage is likely. Initial management follows the **ABC**s of resuscitation: evaluate the patient's **A**irway first, followed by his **B**reathing, and then his **C**irculatory status. Care can then be directed at his injuries.

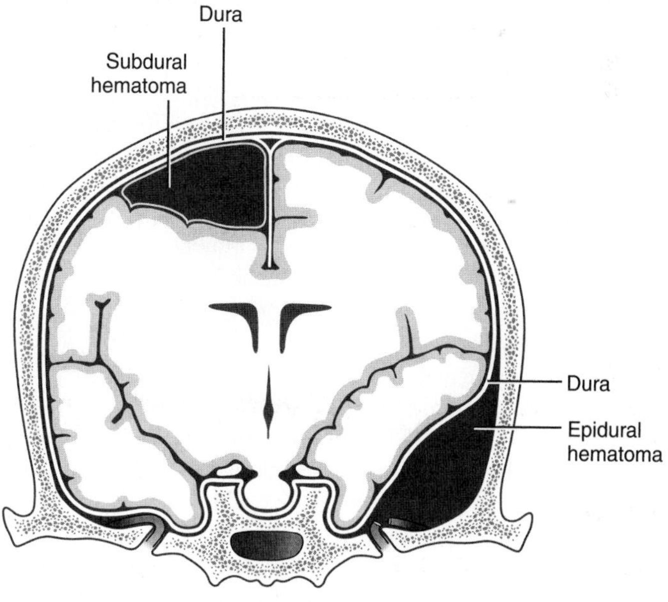


**Figure 39–1.** Anatomy of subdural and epidural hematomas.

**Table 39–1 MODIFIED GLASGOW COMA SCORE FOR CHILDREN YOUNGER THAN 3 YEARS OF AGE**

| | |
|---|---|
| Eye opening: | |
| 1 | None |
| 2 | To pain |
| 3 | To speech |
| 4 | Spontaneous |
| Verbal communication: | |
| 1 | No response |
| 2 | Incomprehensible sounds |
| 3 | Inappropriate words |
| 4 | Confused conversation, cries |
| 5 | Oriented, cries to indicate needs |
| Motor response: | |
| 1 | None |
| 2 | Abnormal extension |
| 3 | Abnormal flexion |
| 4 | Withdraws from pain |
| 5 | Localizes pain |
| 6 | Spontaneous movement in infants <6 mo and goal-directed movements in children 6-36 mo |

**Subdural hemorrhage is more common in children younger than 1 year and is far more common than a supratentorial epidural hemorrhage. Approximately one-third of CT-identified subdural hemorrhages have an associated skull fracture**; almost all are venous in origin, and approximately **three-fourths are bilateral**. The CT images typically show a crescentic hematoma. **Seizures occur in 60% to 90% of afflicted patients**, and retinal hemorrhages are frequently associated. Increased ICP is typical. Subdural hemorrhage is generally associated with less mortality than that seen with epidural hemorrhage, but long-term morbidity is more significant because the brain parenchyma is more often involved.

Subdural hematomas may be acute, subacute, or chronic. In acute hematomas, symptoms occur in the first 48 hours after injury. Patients with subacute subdural hematoma display symptoms between 3 and 21 days after injury, whereas chronic hematomas cause symptoms after 21 days. **Chronic subdural hematomas are more common in older children** than in infants; symptoms may include chronic emesis, seizures, hypertonicity, irritability, personality changes, inattention, poor weight gain, fever, and anemia. Magnetic resonance imaging is more useful than CT for evaluating subacute and chronic hematomas because the hematoma age can be estimated by signal intensity.

**Epidural hemorrhages occur more commonly in older children and adults** and are seen more typically in the infratentorial space. **Two-thirds of epidural hemorrhages are associated with skull fracture.** Although most adult epidural hemorrhages are arterial in origin; in children approximately half originate from venous injuries. **Most epidural hemorrhages are unilateral,** are located in the temporoparietal region, and present on CT scan as a lens-like, or biconvex, hematoma. **Fewer than 25% of epidural hematoma patients have seizures,** and retinal hemorrhages are uncommon. **Mortality is greater with epidural hemorrhage than with subdural hemorrhage,** but in survivors long-term morbidity is low.

Increased ICP, which can be caused by both hemorrhage forms, is important to recognize and treat. Epidural hematomas are frequently rapidly progressive and may require urgent surgical evacuation with identification of the bleeding source. Subdural hemorrhage usually does not require urgent evacuation but may require evacuation at a later date.

## Comprehension Questions

39.1 You are the team physician for a high-school football team. During the first quarter of the latest game, you watch as your star quarterback is sacked with a helmet-to-helmet tackle. He does not get up from the initial impact. You sprint onto the field and assess the injured player. He is breathing and has a steady pulse, but he is unconscious. As you begin your evaluation, he wakes up. He remembers his name but cannot remember the day, his position on the team, or how he got to the game. He has no sensory or motor deficit suggestive of a cervical spine injury, and you assist him off the field. After 10 minutes he is fully oriented (although he still cannot remember what he had for breakfast) and wants to go back in. The coach tells him he is sitting out for the rest of the game. The player appeals to you. Which of the following is the most appropriate management?

A. Affirm the coach's decision. Tell the player that he will need sequential evaluations before he can come back to practice.
B. Affirm the coach's decision. Tell the player he can come back and practice tomorrow.
C. Refute the coach's decision. Tell the player he can resume playing now.
D. Refute the coach's decision. Tell the player he can resume playing after half-time.
E. Strap the player to a backboard and take him to the hospital.

39.2 A 17-year-old adolescent female is brought to the hospital after a motor vehicle crash. She and her boyfriend had been drinking beer and were on their way home when she lost control of the car and hit the side wall of the local police station. She reportedly had a brief loss of consciousness but currently is oriented to name, place, and time. She responds appropriately to your questions. While waiting for her cervical spine series, she vomits and lapses into unconsciousness. She becomes bradycardic and develops irregular respirations. Which of the following brain injuries is most likely in this case?

A. Subdural hemorrhage
B. Epidural hemorrhage
C. Intraventricular hemorrhage
D. Posttraumatic epilepsy
E. Concussion

39.3 Several days after emergent management, the adolescent in question 39.2 is transferred to your general inpatient ward service from the intensive care unit. She is concerned about her prognosis. Which of the following statements is correct?

A. She will need extensive neuropsychiatric evaluation before she can return to school.
B. She will likely have headaches, fatigue, nausea, and sleep disturbances.
C. She will likely develop seizures and needs 2 years of prophylactic seizure medicine.
D. She can no longer be legally permitted to drive because she has had brain surgery.
E. She should have few long-term problems.

39.4 A 7-month-old child presents to the emergency room after reportedly falling from his high chair. The parents report no loss of consciousness, other trauma, or medical problems. Your examination reveals a few old bruises but no evidence of acute trauma or fracture. He is irritable, so you request a CT scan of the brain without contrast. The pediatric radiologist reports bilateral frontal subdural hematomas and notes two healing skull fractures that she estimates to be approximately 2 weeks old. Which of the following is the best next step in this child's management?

A. Observe him for 6 hours in the emergency center.
B. Assess bleeding time and prothrombin time.
C. Order magnetic resonance imaging of the head.
D. Discharge him from the emergency center with head injury precautions.
E. Order an electroencephalography and a neurology consultation.

## ANSWERS

39.1 **A.** Although controversial, the correct answer is for a player who sustains a concussion resulting in loss of consciousness to refrain from play for the remainder of the day. The most recent clinical report from the American Academy of Pediatrics concerning conditions affecting sports participation references the 2nd International Conference on Concussion in Sports from 2004. This report suggests that individualized and frequent reassessment over time, and a stepwise return to play, is more useful than a predetermined length of time to refrain from additional sports.

39.2 **B.** This teen displays the typical adult course of epidural hemorrhage (an initial period of altered mental status [initial concussion], a period of lucidity, and then redevelopment of altered mental status and symptoms of increased ICP [hematoma effect]). Younger children typically do not display this pattern. Immediate neurosurgical evaluation is required.

39.3 **E.** The acute epidural hemorrhage mortality rate is higher than that of acute subdural hemorrhage, but long-term morbidity is less. The complaints in answer B are common after a subdural hemorrhage. A seizure disorder may preclude driving; a cranial surgery history does not.

39.4 **C.** This child has evidence of old skull fractures with subdural hematomas. Head magnetic resonance imaging would help to determine the hematoma age. If the hematoma blood age correlates with the estimated skull fracture age, child abuse is considered. Neurology may be helpful later, but an immediate consultation would be of limited benefit before additional data were gathered. Discharge with the information presented in the case is dangerous; the child likely requires hospital admission and the involvement of social services. Bleeding studies are unlikely to be helpful; the child has no history consistent with a bleeding disorder, nor would a bleeding disorder explain the old fractures.

### Clinical Pearls

- Subdural hemorrhage is more common in children younger than 1 year and in the supratentorial space; seizures and retinal hemorrhages are frequently associated findings, and increased ICP is typical.
- Epidural hemorrhages are more commonly seen in older children and adults and in the infratentorial space. Fewer than 25% of patients have seizures; retinal hemorrhages are uncommon.
- Mortality with subdural hemorrhage is generally less than that seen with epidural hemorrhage, but long-term morbidity is more significant with subdural injury because the brain parenchyma is more often involved.

## REFERENCES

Chiriboga CA. Trauma to the nervous system. In: Rudolph CD, Rudolph AM, Hostetter MK, Lister G, Siegel NJ, eds. *Rudolph's Pediatrics*. 21st ed. New York, NY: McGraw-Hill; 2003:2241-2252.

Landry GL. Head and neck injuries. In: Kliegman RM, Behrman RE, Jenson HB, Stanton BF, eds. *Nelson Textbook of Pediatrics*. 18th ed. Philadelphia, PA: Saunders Elsevier; 2007:2862-2863.

McCrory P, Johnston K, Meeuwisse W, et al. Summary and agreement statement of the 2nd International Conference on Concussion in Sport, Prague 2004. *Clin J Sport Med*. 2005;15(2):48-55.

Prasad MR, Ewing-Cobbs L, Swank PR, Kramer L. Predictors of outcome following traumatic brain injury in young children. *Pediatr Neurosurg*. 2002;36:64-74.

Rice SG; and the Council on Sports Medicine and Fitness. Medical conditions affecting sports participation. *Pediatrics*. 2008;121:841-848.

Rosman NP. Acute head trauma. In: McMillan JA, Feigin RD, DeAngelis CD, Jones MD, eds. *Oski's Pediatrics: Principles and Practice*. 4th ed. Philadelphia, PA: Lippincott Williams & Wilkins; 2006:730-746.

Teasdale G, Jennett B. Assessment of coma and impaired consciousness: a practical scale. *Lancet*. 1974;2:81-84.

Wojtys EM, Hovda D, Landry G, et al. Concussions in sports. *Am J Sports Med*. 1999;27:676-687.

# Case 40

A 16-year-old adolescent female presents to your office complaining of very heavy menstrual bleeding for the last 6 months. She notes that her cycles are regular, occuring every 29 days, but they last for 10 days and she goes through 10 to12 pads per day. Her last period ended a week ago, and she now complains of dizziness when she stands up. She denies concurrent vaginal discharge or abdominal pain. Her past medical and family histories are negative for bleeding problems. Her menarche was at 12 years of age, and she started having regular menstrual cycles at 14 years of age. She denies all forms of sexual activity. Her examination is significant for mild resting tachycardia and orthostatic hypotension. Her nail beds and conjunctiva are pale. A urine pregnancy test is negative, and her hemoglobin is 10 g/dL.

- What is the most likely diagnosis?
- How would you manage this patient?

# ANSWERS TO CASE 40:
# Dysfunctional Uterine Bleeding

*Summary:* An adolescent female complains of heavy but regular menstrual bleeding that has resulted in anemia and orthostatic hypotension.

- ➤ **Most likely diagnosis:** Dysfunctional uterine bleeding (DUB).
- ➤ **Management:** Iron supplement and monophasic low-dose oral contraceptive pills (OCPs) for 3 to 6 months with a follow-up hemoglobin in 6 weeks.

## ANALYSIS

### Objectives

1. List the diagnostic possibilities for abnormal uterine bleeding.
2. Describe the appropriate evaluation of abnormal uterine bleeding.
3. Differentiate between the different managements of DUB based on symptoms and type of bleeding.

### Considerations

Menstrual bleeding that leads to anemia and orthostatic hypotension is not typical, and requires further investigation. Excessive bleeding may be caused by pregnancy; although she denies sexual activity, a urine pregnancy test should be part of the evaluation. Sexually transmitted diseases, malignancy, and trauma should also be considered.

# APPROACH TO
# Dysfunctional Uterine Bleeding

## DEFINITIONS

**MENORRHAGIA:** Excessive and/or prolonged uterine bleeding with a regular menstrual cycle.

**METRORRHAGIA:** Irregular uterine bleeding between menstrual cycles.

**MENOMETRORRHAGIA:** Irregular uterine bleeding with excessive and/or prolonged flow.

## CLINICAL APPROACH

Dysfunctional uterine bleeding is excessive flow that occurs either in a regular cycle (menorrhagia) or irregularly and not related to the normal menstrual flow (metrorrhagia). Dysfunctional uterine bleeding is a diagnosis of exclusion; other diagnoses must be considered first. Of young women presenting with abnormal vaginal bleeding, about 9% will have an organic cause such as ectopic pregnancy or threatened abortion; other potential causes include infections (cervicitis, human papillomavirus [HPV], trichomonas), trauma, hormonal contraceptives and other medications, foreign body, or malignancy. The remainder of women will have no demonstrable cause for their bleeding and are diagnosed with dysfunctional, or abnormal, uterine bleeding.

The typical presentation is that of a teen with regular menstrual cycles that then develops prolonged or heavy menstrual bleeding, or irregular bleeding. The bleeding is usually painless. Important aspects of the history include prior episodes of bleeding, the length of the woman's cycle, the number of days of bleeding, and the severity of the bleeding (can be established by asking about the number of pads or tampons used per day). Family history should include others with bleeding problems such as excessive hemorrhage after surgery and women requiring hysterectomy after childbirth.

After verifying the patient is not pregnant, the next most important laboratory evaluation is the hemoglobin. The degree of anemia helps categorize the severity of bleeding and helps guide management (Figure 40–1). Women with a hemoglobin more than 12 g/dL are considered to have mild bleeding, and may be managed with iron supplements alone and with careful follow up. A hemoglobin of 9 to12 g/dL is considered a result of moderately severe bleeding; treatment includes iron and monophasic OCP. Women with a hemoglobin less than 9 g/dL are considered to have severe bleeding, and may need hospitalization and transfusion. Intravenous estrogen (Premarin) and high-dose oral contraceptives are used until the bleeding stops; further bleeding despite these measures may require dilatation and curettage. Although these high doses of estrogen raise theoretical concerns about thrombotic events, none have been reported with the short-term use required in this diagnosis.

Patients with dysfunctional uterine bleeding continue oral contraceptives for 3 to 6 months. After the menstrual cycle is regular and irregular bleeding has ceased, careful withdrawal of the OCP may be attempted with close follow-up. Iron supplementation should be continued for 2 months after the anemia is resolved.

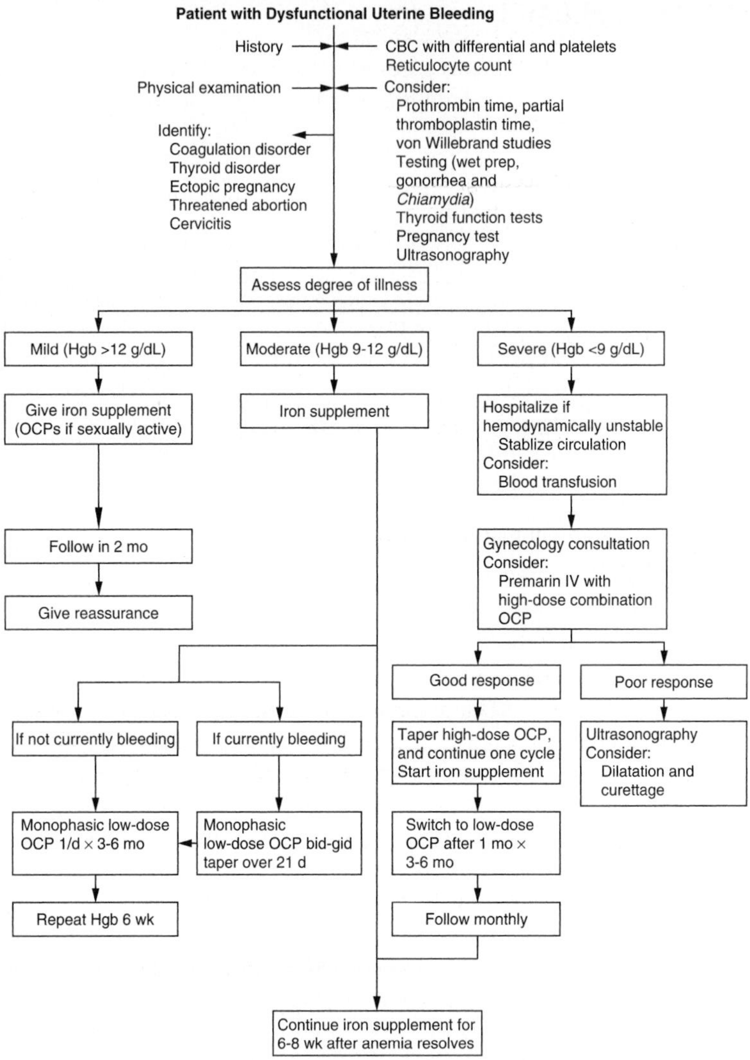


**Figure 40–1.** Evaluation of dysfunctional uterine bleeding. CBC, complete blood count; Hgb, hemoglobin; OCP, oral contraceptive pills. (*Reproduced, with permission, from Kaplan DW, Love-Osborne L. Adolescence. In: Hay WW, Levin MJ, Sondheimer JM, Deterding RR, eds.* Current Diagnosis and Treatment in Pediatrics. *19th ed. New York, NY: McGraw-Hill; 2009:128.*)

## Comprehension Questions

40.1 A 15-year-old adolescent female presents to the local hospital emergency center complaining of several days of left sided abdominal pain, mild vaginal bleeding, and dizziness. Upon further questioning you learn that she has had near-syncopal episodes the last few times she has tried to stand up. She denies fever, sexual activity, previous episodes of mid-cycle vaginal bleeding, and abdominal or genitourinary trauma. On examination, she is pale and tachycardic. She has abdominal pain with rebound and guarding in the upper and lower left quadrants that radiates to the back. Her hemoglobin is 5 g/dL, her white count is 12,000/$mm^3$, and her platelet count is 210,000/$mm^3$. Her serum ß-HCG is 1800 IU/mL. Which of the following is the most likely diagnosis?

A. Metrorrhagia with subsequent anemia
B. Pelvic inflammatory disease
C. Salicylate overdose
D. Ruptured ectopic pregnancy
E. Uterine malignancy

40.2 A 13-year-old adolescent female comes to the office for a preparticipation sports physical before the start of the basketball season. She has no complaints, but wants to discuss the human papillomavirus (HPV) vaccine some of her friends have received. Which of the following is an accurate statement about human papillomavirus and the vaccine?

A. The HPV vaccine is indicated only once a woman becomes sexually active.
B. HPV types 6 and 11 are high cancer risk serotypes and are included in the vaccine.
C. HPV vaccine helps prevent cervical cancer but not genital warts.
D. HPV types 16 and 18 are associated with the majority of cervical cancers.
E. Syncope after injection has been reported and is a unique adverse reaction to HPV vaccine.

40.3 A 16-year-old presents to your office with a complaint of persistent vaginal bleeding. She had been seen 3 months ago when you noted a mild anemia of 13 g/dL, diagnosed her with dysfunctional uterine bleeding and started her on iron supplements. Today she is listless and pale. Her hemoglobin in your office is 6 g/dL, her platelet count is normal, and her urine pregnancy test remains negative. You admit her to your local hospital and order a transfusion of packed red blood cells. In addition to stabilizing her circulatory system, which of the following is the most appropriate next step in the acute management of her condition?

A. Monophasic low-dose oral contraceptive (OCP)
B. Intravenous conjugated estrogens (Premarin) and high-dose combination OCP
C. Hysterectomy
D. Discharge after transfusion with iron supplementation
E. Triphasic low-dose OCP

40.4 A 19-year-old adolescent female presents with a temperature of 101.2°F (38.4°C), lower abdominal pain, bloody vaginal discharge, and dyspareunia. She has no nausea or vomiting, and is tolerating fluids well. She has cervical motion tenderness on examination. Her urine pregnancy test is negative, and an ultrasound of her right lower quadrant is negative for appendicitis. Appropriate outpatient management for her likely condition is which of the following?

A. Levofloxacin, 500 mg orally once a day for 14 days as monotherapy
B. Ofloxacin, 400 mg orally twice a day for 14 days as monotherapy
C. Ceftriaxone, 250 mg IM in a single dose as monotherapy
D. Levofloxacin, 500 mg orally once a day, *and* doxycycline, 100 mg orally twice a day, both for 14 days
E. Ceftriaxone, 250 mg IM as a single dose *and* doxycycline, 100 mg orally twice a day for 14 days

## ANSWERS

40.1 **D.** The classic triad of abdominal pain, vaginal bleeding, and amenorrhea only occurs in about 50% of cases of ectopic pregnancy. As ectopic pregnancy is the leading cause of pregnancy-related death in the first trimester; a physician must consider the diagnosis for any woman of childbearing age with abdominal pain. Risk factors for an ectopic pregnancy include pelvic inflammatory disease (PID), intrauterine device (IUD), previous ectopic pregnancy, previous tubal surgery, increasing age, use of fertility drugs, and smoking. Since this patient is hemodynamically unstable, admission and surgery is indicated; however, hemodynamically stable patients may be managed expectantly or treated with methotrexate.

40.2 **D.** Quadrivalent human papillomavirus vaccine (Gardasil) was licensed in 2006, and is indicated for the prevention of HPV types 6, 11, 16, and 18. Types 6 and 11 cause about 90% of all genital warts, but carry a low risk of malignancy. Types 16 and 18 cause about two-thirds of all cervical cancer cases. Immunization before sexual debut is ideal, but even women who are sexually active may benefit from the vaccine; as there is no commercially available screening test to determine the serotypes to which a woman has been exposed, the vaccine may still provide some protection. The vaccine is a three-dose series. Common side effects include headache and pain at the injection site. Anaphylaxis to yeast is a contraindication. Syncope has been reported in the adolescent population with all vaccines; current recommendations suggest observing adolescents for 15 minutes after immunization.

40.3 **B.** Based on her anemia, this adolescent's dysfunctional uterine bleeding is classified as severe, and warrants hospitalization. Stabilization of her circulatory system is the first priority, and then steps must be taken to stop the bleeding. Intravenous premarin in conjunction with a high-dose OCP is the next step. If this treatment is successful in decreasing the bleeding, she can be continued on high-dose OCP for a month and then moved to a low-dose OCP. If she continued to have bleeding after IV Premarin and a high-dose OCP, dilatation and curettage may be necessary.

40.4 **E.** More than one million women develop pelvic inflammatory disease (PID) in the United States each year, and more than a quarter of these require hospitalization. PID is most common in the teen population, with decreasing incidence with increasing age. As presenting signs and symptoms are variable, diagnosis can be difficult. The CDC recommends that empiric treatment should be started if a young woman at risk for PID presents with lower abdominal or pelvic pain, no other cause for the pain can be identified, and the woman has: (1) cervical motion tenderness, (2) uterine tenderness, or (3) adnexal tenderness. Treatment is aimed at both gonorrhea and chlamydia. Recent surveillance by the CDC has shown fluoroquinolone resistant gonorrhea is widespread in the United States, so fluoroquinolones are no longer recommended in the treatment of PID.

## Clinical Pearls

- Pregnancy and STDs must be considered in any adolescent with abnormal vaginal bleeding.
- Dysfunctional uterine bleeding can be excessive flow with normal intervals (menorrhagia), or flow with irregular intervals (metrorrhagia).
- Cessation of bleeding can usually be achieved through the use of oral contraceptives; occasionally, intravenous estrogen is required.

## REFERENCES

Buzzini SR, Gold MA. Menstrual disorders. In: McMillan JA, Feigin RD, DeAngelis CD, Jones MD, eds. *Oski's Pediatrics: Principles and Practice*. 4th ed. Philadelphia, PA: Lippincott Williams & Wilkins; 2006:561-566.

Centers for Disease Control and Prevention et al. Sexually transmitted diseases treatment guidelines, 2006. *MMWR Recomm Rep./CDC*. 2006;55(RR-11):56-61.

Centers for Disease Control and Prevention (CDC). Update to CDC's sexually transmitted diseases treatment guidelines, 2006: fluoroquinolones no longer recommended for treatment of gonococcal infections. *MMWR Morb Mortal Wkly Rep*. 2007;56(14):332-336.

Cunningham FG, Leveno KL, Bloom SL, Hauth JC, Gilstrap LC III, Wenstrom KD. Ectopic pregnancy. In: Cunningham FG, Leveno KL, Bloom SL, Hauth JC, Gilstrap LC III, Wenstrom KD, eds. *Williams Obstetrics*. 22nd ed. Available at http://www.accessmedicine.com/content.aspx?aID=721129.

Daley Matthew F, Simoes Eric A, Nyquist Ann-Christine. Immunization. In: Hay WW, Jr., Levin MJ, Sondheimer JM, Deterding RR, eds. *Current Diagnosis and Treatment: Pediatrics*. 19th ed. New York, NY: McGraw-Hill; 2009:262-263.

Jenkins RR. Menstrual problems. In: Kliegman RM, Behrman RE, Jenson HB, Stanton BF, eds. *Nelson Textbook of Pediatrics*. 18th ed. Philadelphia, PA: Saunders Elsevier; 2007:836-842.

Kaplan DW, Love-Osborne L. Gynecological disorders in adolescence. In: Hay WW, Levin MJ, Sondheimer JM, Deterding RR, eds. *Current Diagnosis and Treatment in Pediatrics*. 19th ed. New York, NY: McGraw-Hill; 2009:120-130.

# Case 41

The emergency department (ED) notifies you that one of your patients is being evaluated for new-onset seizures. The 2-year-old boy was in his normal state of good health until this morning, when he complained of a headache and then fell to the floor. While waiting for the ED physician to come to the phone, you review the patient's chart and find that he has had normal development. His family history is significant for a single seizure of unknown etiology that his father had at age 4 years. According to the ED physician, the boy's mother saw jerking of both arms and legs. When the ambulance arrived 5 minutes later, the child had stopped jerking but was not arousable; his heart rate was 108 bpm, respiratory rate 16 breaths/min, blood pressure 90/60 mm Hg, and temperature 104°F (40°C). His blood sugar level was 135 mg/dL. By the time the child arrived to the ED, he was awake and he recognized his parents. His physical examination in the ED is normal, as are his complete blood count and urinalysis.

- ➤ What is the most likely diagnosis?
- ➤ What is the best management for this condition?
- ➤ What is the expected course of this condition?

# ANSWERS TO CASE 41:
# Simple Febrile Seizure

*Summary:* An otherwise normal 2-year-old boy, with a family history of seizure in his father, has a brief, generalized, self-limited seizure associated with an elevated temperature. His examination is nonfocal. He has completely recovered within 1 to 2 hours of the seizure.

- **Most likely diagnosis:** Simple febrile seizure.
- **Best management:** Parental education, injury prevention during seizures, and fever control.
- **Expected course:** More seizures with fever may occur, but he is likely to "grow out" the condition by 5 to 6 years of age. He is likely to have no sequelae and is expected to have normal development.

## ANALYSIS

### Objectives

1. Describe a typical febrile seizure.
2. Explain the typical course of febrile seizures.
3. List factors that increase the risk of further seizure activity.

### Considerations

This patient likely had a simple febrile seizure. The seizure was short, self-limited, and generalized without focal findings. The child had an elevated temperature and is between the ages of 6 months and 6 years. He had a short postictal state and then quickly returned to normal. He is old enough to have reliable neck examination findings and has no evidence of meningeal irritation. The father might have had a febrile seizure; data are insufficient to make that conclusion.

# APPROACH TO
# Febrile Seizure

## DEFINITIONS

**EPILEPSY:** Recurrent seizure activity; may or may not have identifiable cause.

**FEBRILE SEIZURE:** A seizure occurring in the absence of central nervous system (CNS) infection with an elevated temperature in a child between the ages of 6 months and 6 years.

**SEIZURE:** Abnormal electrical activity of the brain resulting in altered mental status and/or involuntary neuromuscular activity.

## CLINICAL APPROACH

A diagnosis of febrile seizure must be made only after considering CNS infection as the cause. **Two classic physical findings** suggest **meningeal** irritation: **Kernig sign** (patient is supine, leg flexed at the hip and knee at 90° angle, pain is induced with leg extension) and **Brudzinski sign** (while supine, passive neck flexion results in involuntary knee and hip flexion). If the **neurologic examination is abnormal** after the seizure, the **seizure occurred several days into the illness,** or if the **child is unable to provide adequate feedback** during a neck examination, a **lumbar puncture (LP) may be necessary.** The **meningeal signs** described above usually are **not reliable in children younger than 1 year;** therefore, an **LP is recommended for such patients with fever and seizure. Contrast-enhanced brain imaging should occur before LP when a space-occupying lesion, such as a brain abscess, is a possibility.**

**Febrile seizures** are a uniquely pediatric entity. **Typically occurring between 6 months and 6 years of age,** these convulsions are distressing to the parent but only occasionally pose a threat to the child. Febrile seizures are common, occurring in 2% to 4% of all children; they seem to have a **genetic basis** (many children have a family history of febrile seizure). Febrile seizure risk is increased (10% to 20%) when a **first-degree relative** has been diagnosed with the same.

**Febrile seizures frequently are classified as simple or complex;** the distinction helps to clarify the recurrence risk and prognosis. **Simple febrile seizures last less than 15 minutes without focal or lateralizing signs or sequelae.** If more than one seizure occurs in a brief period, the total episode lasts less than 30 minutes. A complex febrile seizure lasts for more than 15 minutes and may have lateralizing signs. If several seizures occur in a brief period, the entire episode may last for more than 30 minutes.

The timing of the febrile seizure in relation to the temperature elevation is variable. Whereas many children will have a febrile seizure during the initial temperature upswing (many parents are unaware that the child is ill until the seizure and the subsequent temperature recording), some children will have seizures at other points during the febrile illness.

A febrile seizure usually is self-limited. If it lasts longer than 5 minutes, lorazepam or diazepam can be used to interrupt the seizure. Airway management is a priority, as benzodiazepines occasionally cause respiratory depression. Ongoing seizures unresponsive to lorazepam or diazepam can be interrupted with fosphenytoin.

The evaluation of a simple febrile seizure need not be extensive (Figure 41–1). Electroencephalography (EEG) is not recommended unless focal findings were present during or after the seizure, or if the seizure was prolonged. EEG is not predictive of future febrile or afebrile seizures. Laboratory studies (except

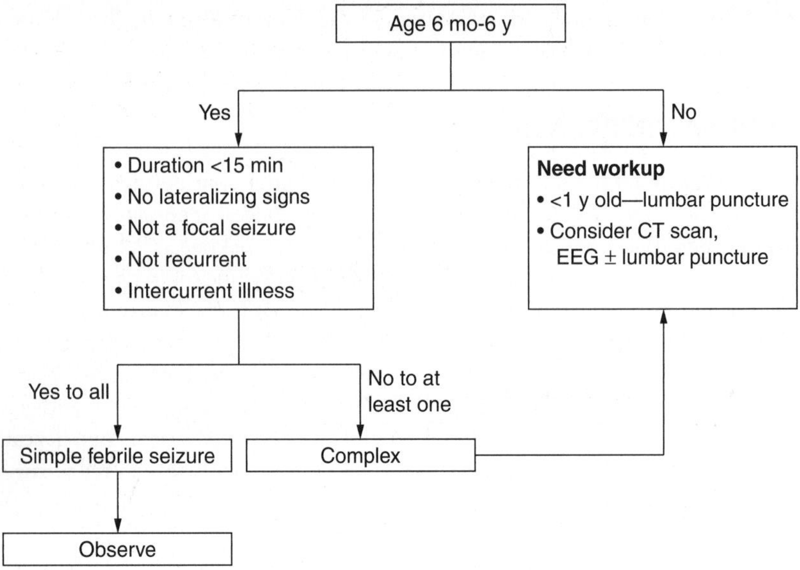


**Figure 41–1.** Algorithm for managing febrile seizures.

as needed to determine the cause of fever) and brain imaging usually are not helpful. Imaging may be indicated for a complex febrile seizure or in patients with evidence of increased intracranial pressure. An LP is not routinely indicated, except as outlined above.

Prophylactic medications usually are not necessary. In the practice parameter published in 2008, the American Academy of Pediatrics emphasized that prophylactic medications for the usually benign condition of febrile seizures were not routinely useful.

**Prognosis is generally good;** most children who develop febrile seizures will not develop neurologic or developmental consequences. **Children younger than 12 months at the time of their first seizure have a 50% to 65% chance of having another febrile seizure; older children have a 20% to 30% chance of recurrence.** The chance of developing epilepsy increases from 0.5% in the general population to 1% in the child with a febrile seizure history. Children at highest risk for developing epilepsy following a febrile seizure often have preexisting neurologic problems and have complex febrile seizures; these children have 30 to 50 times the baseline risk of developing epilepsy.

## Comprehension Questions

41.1 Paramedics bring to the ED a 7-month-old infant with seizure activity. The father reports the infant was in a normal state of health until approximately 3 days ago when she developed a febrile illness, diagnosed by her physician as a viral upper respiratory tract infection. Approximately 30 minutes ago she began having left arm jerking, which progressed to whole-body jerking. The episode spontaneously ceased on the way to the hospital. Vital signs include heart rate 90 bpm, respiratory rate 25 breaths/min, and temperature 100.4°F (38°C). Your examination reveals a sleeping infant in no respiratory distress. The child's anterior fontanelle is full. The oropharynx is clear, and crusted mucous is found in the nares. The tympanic membranes are dark and without normal landmarks. The lungs are clear, and the heart and abdominal examinations are normal. She has a bruise over the occiput and several parallel bruises along the spine. Which of the following is the best next step in management?

A. Computerized tomography (CT) of the head
B. Electroencephalogram
C. Lumbar puncture
D. Observation
E. Phenobarbital

41.2 A 2-year-old boy who had a simple brief febrile seizure comes to your office 1 day after his ED visit. He is currently afebrile, is happily pulling the sphygmomanometer off the wall, and is taking antibiotics for an ear infection diagnosed the previous day. His mother wants to know what to expect in the future regarding his neurologic status. You correctly tell her which of the following?

A. He has no risk of further seizures because he was age 2 years at the time of his first febrile seizure.
B. He will need to take anticonvulsant medications for 6 to 12 months to prevent further seizure activity.
C. You want to schedule an EEG and a magnetic resonance scan of his head.
D. Although he does have a risk of future febrile convulsions, seizures of his type are generally benign and he is likely to outgrow them.
E. This is an isolated disorder, and his children will not have seizures.

41.3 A 10-month-old boy presents to the ED with a 1-day history of fever to 104°F (40°C), increased irritability, decreased breast-feeding, and refusal of solid foods. The parents brought him in after two 30-second episodes of generalized jerking that occurred over a 20-minute span. Your examination reveals an awake but lethargic infant. The anterior fontanelle is flat, the tympanic membranes and oropharynx are moist and not erythematous, the lungs are clear, and the heart and abdominal examinations are normal. He has no focal neurologic findings. Which of the following is the best next step in management?

A. Intravenous ceftriaxone
B. Admission overnight for observation
C. Computerized tomography of the head
D. Discharge from ED to follow up with his primary care provider in 24 hours
E. Lumbar puncture

41.4 The father of a 4-year-old girl calls your office to report her second febrile seizure. He states that this seizure was identical to the first one that happened 4 months ago: she developed an elevated temperature and within a short time had a generalized convulsion lasting 90 seconds. She was sleepy for approximately 2 minutes afterward. Upon awaking, she was given ibuprofen. She is now running around the house, chasing her younger brother and the family's chihuahua. The parents wonder if she needs to take anticonvulsants now that she has had another seizure. You should tell the father which of the following?

A. Febrile seizures frequently are recurrent but usually have no significant long-term effect.
B. You will prescribe an anticonvulsant because it will reduce the risk of future epilepsy.
C. You will order an EEG and CT scan of her head to be done on an outpatient basis.
D. He needs to take his daughter to the hospital for inpatient admission.
E. He should stop the ibuprofen and observe the fever curve.

## ANSWERS

41.1 **A.** This child's history is worrisome for trauma. The fontanelle is full, bruises are found along the spine and on the occiput, and she has hemotympanum. A CT scan is of paramount importance; this child likely had a seizure from acute intracranial hemorrhage associated with physical abuse. Although this child is febrile and within the proper febrile seizure age range, the history and physical findings are more consistent with a diagnosis other than febrile seizure. Performing an

LP in a patient who may have increased intracranial pressure is not advisable, an EEG would probably not reveal the diagnosis, and phenobarbital is not immediately necessary in a patient who is not actively seizing.

41.2 **D.** Part of the anticipatory guidance for parents of children with febrile seizures is to impress upon them that the child may have another seizure; it is similarly important to emphasize the usual benign nature of this condition. In a simple febrile seizure, imaging and EEG generally are not recommended, nor are prophylactic anticonvulsants. Because febrile seizures seem to have a genetic basis, it is possible that your patient's children will also have febrile seizures.

41.3 **E.** Although this child ultimately may be diagnosed as having had a simple febrile seizure, the patient's age (<1 year) precludes a reliable neck examination. An LP is required to evaluate the child for meningitis. Administering antibiotics before the LP (or other cultures are obtained) is inadvisable unless the patient's condition is such that he would not tolerate the procedure.

41.4 **A.** Some children will develop recurrent febrile seizures. Anticonvulsants will decrease the risk of further febrile seizures, but they do not decrease the risk of developing epilepsy. The possible adverse reactions with antiepileptic medications are numerous, including severe allergic reactions and interference with school performance; often the benefit is not worth the risk. Fever reduction with medications is generally encouraged in children with a febrile seizure history. Hospital admission and diagnostic studies are not necessary in simple febrile seizures.

## Clinical Pearls

- Febrile seizures usually are benign and self-limited. They do not require an extensive diagnostic evaluation unless they are prolonged or focal.
- A diagnosis of febrile seizure must be made only after considering the possibility of central nervous system infection as the seizure cause.
- Febrile seizures rarely lead to epilepsy; risk factors for nonfebrile seizures include preexisting developmental abnormalities and complex febrile seizures.

## REFERENCES

American Academy of Pediatrics. Febrile seizures: clinical practice guideline for the long-term management of the child with simple febrile seizures. *Pediatrics*. 2008; 121:1281-1286.

Feigin RD. Bacterial meningitis beyond the newborn period. In: McMillan JA, Feigin RD, DeAngelis CD, Jones MD, eds. *Oski's Pediatrics: Principles and Practice*. 4th ed. Philadelphia, PA: Lippincott Williams & Wilkins; 2006:924-933.

Fishman MA. Febrile seizures. In: McMillan JA, Feigin RD, DeAngelis CD, Jones MD, eds. *Oski's Pediatrics: Principles and Practice*. 4th ed. Philadelphia, PA: Lippincott Williams & Wilkins; 2006:2297-2299.

Johnston MV. Febrile seizures. In: Kliegman RM, Behrman RE, Jenson HB, Stanton BF, eds. *Nelson Textbook of Pediatrics*. 18th ed. Philadelphia, PA: Saunders Elsevier; 2007:2457-2458.

Prober CG. Acute bacterial meningitis beyond the neonatal period. In: Kliegman RM, Behrman RE, Jenson HB, Stanton BF, eds. *Nelson Textbook of Pediatrics*. 18th ed. Philadelphia, PA: Saunders Elsevier; 2007:2513-2521.

Ryan SG. Febrile seizures. In: Rudolph CD, Rudolph AM, Hostetter MK, Lister G, Siegel NJ, eds. *Rudolph's Pediatrics*. 21st ed. New York, NY: McGraw-Hill; 2003: 2270-2271.

Tureen J. Meningitis. In: Rudolph CD, Rudolph AM, Hostetter MK, Lister G, Siegel NJ, eds. *Rudolph's Pediatrics*. 21st ed. New York, NY: McGraw-Hill; 2003:901-904.

# Case 42

Parents worry about their 4-year-old son's ability to walk. He began walking at 16 months, but he was clumsy and fell frequently; they were reassured by another pediatrician that he would "outgrow it." He remains clumsier than his peers, falls during simple tasks, and has developed a "waddling" gait. Within the last month he has experienced increasing difficulty arising from a sitting position on the floor.

- What is the most likely diagnosis?
- What is the diagnostic test of choice?
- What is the mechanism of disease?

# ANSWER TO CASE 42:
# Muscular Dystrophy

*Summary:* A 4-year-old boy has delayed walking, a waddling gait, clumsiness, and proximal muscle weakness.

- **Most likely diagnosis:** Muscular dystrophy (MD), probably Duchenne type.
- **Diagnostic test:** DNA peripheral blood analysis or immunohistochemical detection of abnormal dystrophin on a muscle biopsy tissue section.
- **Mechanism of disease:** Duchenne MD is an **X-linked recessive** trait. The abnormal gene is at the Xp21.2 locus and encodes for an aberrant form of the protein dystrophin.

## ANALYSIS

### Objectives

1. Know the presentation of children with inherited MD.
2. Understand the inheritance pattern of the common MDs.
3. Understand the progression of the MD.

### Considerations

This 4-year-old boy exhibits classic Duchenne muscular dystrophy (DMD) signs: **waddling gait** and **progressive proximal muscle weakness**. Initial testing includes serum creatine kinase (CK) assessment and DNA analysis of peripheral blood for diagnosis. After the diagnosis of DMD, the family is introduced to support organizations and is offered genetic counseling. Ongoing cardiac evaluation for the development of cardiomyopathy is routine. Medical therapy is supportive.

# APPROACH TO
# Muscular Dystrophy

## DEFINITIONS

**GOWER SIGN:** A description of patients with proximal muscle weakness arising to a standing position. The legs are brought under the torso and weight is shifted to the hands and feet. The hands are walked toward the feet and up the thighs as the patient attempts to rise.

**TRENDELENBURG GAIT:** A pelvic waddling gait from proximal muscle weakness.

## CLINICAL APPROACH

**DMD is the most common hereditary neuromuscular degenerative disease,** with an incidence **of 1 in 3600 male births**; 30% of cases are new mutations. It is the most severe progressive primary myopathy of childhood.

DMD usually is asymptomatic during infancy, with normal or mildly delayed developmental milestones, but by 3 to 5 years of age patients have increasing lumbar lordosis (gluteal weakness), **frequent falling, difficulty climbing stairs, hip waddle, and proximal muscle weakness (Gower sign). Muscular enlargement, caused by hypertrophy of muscle fibers and infiltration of fat and collagen proliferation**, causes calf, gluteal, and deltoid muscle **pseudohypertrophy**. Contractures of hip flexors, heel chords, and iliotibial bands develop, limiting joint range of motion. **Cardiomyopathy** with ECG findings on the precordial leads of tall R waves on the right and deep Q waves on the left can be seen. Nonprogressive intellectual impairment is common (mean IQ 80); brain atrophy can be seen on brain CT.

**Patients generally become wheelchair dependent by 10 and 12 years of age** and have rapid progression of scoliosis after the loss of ambulation. Distal muscles remain functional, permitting adequate manual dexterity. Respiratory muscle involvement and the scoliosis result in diminished pulmonary function and recurrent pulmonary infections. Oropharyngeal dysfunction can lead to aspiration, further compromising respiratory capacity.

**DNA blood analysis is diagnostic in two-thirds of cases. Muscle biopsy tissue testing** for abnormal dystrophin can be performed when blood samples are not diagnostic. Muscle biopsy findings include endomysial connective tissue proliferation, inflammatory cell infiltrates, areas of regeneration interspersed with areas of degeneration, and areas of necrosis. Other laboratory findings include elevated CK levels. This enzyme is elevated before clinical signs (helpful in diagnosing familial cases); **in 80% of cases, female carriers have elevated CK levels.** Electromyogram findings reveal myopathy, but patients with Becker MD also have a genetic defect at the Xp21.2 locus, resulting in similar, but less severe, disease.

Treatment consists of medical therapies to slow disease progression. Orthopedic intervention, including bracing and tendon lengthening, can prolong the duration of ambulation and slow the progression of scoliosis. Caution must be exercised with surgical interventions, as these patients are prone to hyperthermia with anesthesia. Physiotherapy may delay the onset of contractures but is not intended for muscle strengthening because significant exercise can hasten muscle degeneration. The Collaborative Investigation of Duchenne Dystrophy (CIDD) group has performed clinical trials of steroid use to slow the progression of muscle weakness with promising results. **All DMD patients have some degree of cardiomyopathy**; it does not correlate with the degree of skeletal involvement. Thus, routine cardiac evaluation is required. Early cardiac dysfunction may be responsive to digoxin.

**Respiratory failure is often the cause of death.** Pulmonary infections are treated early and aggressively; exposure to respiratory illnesses should be limited when possible. Routine immunizations are supplemented with yearly influenza vaccine.

The nutritional status of patients is monitored to ensure appropriate caloric intake. Caloric needs are lower for wheelchair-bound patients because of their decreased activity, but calcium supplementation may be required to minimize osteoporosis. Patients are at risk for depression, often resulting in overeating, weight gain, and added burden to their already limited muscle function.

Another common form of MD is myotonic muscular dystrophy, the second most common type of MD in the United States. It is inherited as an autosomal dominate trait. Infants born with this condition may have an inverted V-shaped upper lip, thin cheeks, and wasting of the temporalis muscles. The head is abnormally narrow and the palate is high and arched. In the ensuing years weakness of the distal muscles leads to progressive challenges in walking. A variety of other findings arise including speech difficulties, gastrointestinal tract problems, endocrinopathies, immunologic deficiencies, cataracts, intellectual impairment, and cardiac involvement.

## Comprehension Questions

42.1 The parents of a 3-year-old child are worried about the child's apparent clumsiness with frequent falls and a waddling gait. The child had normal development of motor skills during the first year of life and has normal language development. Which of the following is consistent with Duchenne muscular dystrophy?

A. Female sex
B. Hypertrophy of the quadriceps
C. 22-year-old sister with Becker muscular dystrophy
D. Gower sign
E. Positive antinuclear antibodies in the blood

42.2 Which of the following is the best *screening* test for the child discussed in Question 42.1?

A. Muscle biopsy
B. Measurement of serum creatinine
C. Electromyogram
D. Blood analysis for antinuclear antibodies
E. Measurement of serum creatine kinase level

42.3 A 12-year-old healthy boy has noticed some muscle weakness. He has experienced increasing difficulty lifting his backpack and walking long distances. He has no trouble with schoolwork, and he continues to play the piano and video games without tiring. His 38-year-old maternal uncle recently became wheelchair-bound for unclear reasons. Which of the following is the most likely diagnosis?

A. Cerebral palsy
B. Duchenne muscular dystrophy
C. Myasthenia gravis
D. Becker muscular dystrophy
E. Guillain-Barré syndrome

42.4 A 16-year-old has just delivered a newborn via cesarean section; the delivery paperwork states the indication for the cesarean section as "ineffectual uterine contractions." The newborn has contractures of multiple joints, facial wasting, generalized hypotonia, and weakness. The infant is transferred via helicopter to your facility. In your neonatal intensive care unit the infant's suck is noted to be weak suggesting that gavage feeds will be required, but the child's respiratory status worsens resulting in his requiring intubation and ventilator support. Little prenatal history is known until the great grandmother arrives. She reports the mother of the child attends special education classes and walks with braces; she knows little else since the infant's mother only recently began to live with her. Which of the following is the likely explanation for this child's condition?

A. Infantile botulism
B. Congenital myotonic dystrophy
C. Duchenne muscular dystrophy
D. Congenital Guillain-Barré syndrome
E. Becker muscular dystrophy

## ANSWERS

42.1 **D.** Duchenne muscular dystrophy is an X-linked recessive disease and is clinically evident only in males. Affected boys may have calf hypertrophy that occurs as a compensation for **proximal muscle weakness**. They will generally develop a Gower sign.

42.2 **E.** A definitive diagnosis can be made only using muscle biopsy tissue, but serum creatine kinase measurement is preferred because it is less invasive and results can be obtained rapidly. Electromyography will reveal nonspecific myopathy.

42.3 **D.** This patient does not have muscle weakness that precludes extended use of distal muscles (hands) or limits his manual dexterity. The child's presentation at age 12 years and a 38-year-old, wheelchair-bound maternal uncle suggest a diagnosis of Becker MD.

42.4 **B.** A severe, congenital form of myotonic dystrophy can be seen in infants born to mothers with myotonic dystrophy. Those that require ventilation longer than about 30 days have a poorer outcome. For none of the other entities listed would *in utero* findings be expected.

## Clinical Pearls

- Duchenne muscular dystrophy (DMD) is an X-linked recessive disorder.
- A Gower sign reflects proximal muscle weakness and is a classic feature of DMD.
- Creatine kinase level is elevated in patients with DMD and in many female carriers of the gene.

## REFERENCES

DeVivo DC, DiMauro S. Hereditary and acquired types of myopathy. In: McMillan JA, Feigin RD, DeAngelis CD, Jones MD, eds. *Oski's Pediatrics: Principles and Practice*. 4th ed. Philadelphia, PA: Lippincott Williams & Wilkins; 2006:2322-2324.

DiMauro S, Hays AP, Bonilla E. Myopathies. In: Rudolph CD, Rudolph AM, Hostetter MK, Lister G, Siegel NJ, eds. *Rudolph's Pediatrics*. 21st ed. New York, NY: McGraw-Hill; 2003:2289-2293.

Sarnat HB. Muscular dystrophies. In: Kliegman RM, Behrman RE, Jenson HB, Stanton BF, eds. *Nelson Textbook of Pediatrics*. 18th ed. Philadelphia, PA: WB Saunders; 2007:2540-2544.

# Case 43

A 10-day-old infant has a 12-hour history of fever, irritability, and decreased oral intake. She was delivered vaginally at 39-week gestation to a gravida 2, para 1 woman after an uncomplicated pregnancy with routine prenatal care. The infant went home on day 2 of life. She has surpassed her birth weight of 3.7 kg and had been well until today. On examination, she has a temperature of 101.5°F (38.6°C), and she is fussy. Her only finding on physical examination is a small cluster of 2 mm, fluid-filled lesions on her parietal scalp. The infant has an episode in the emergency department of right-sided body shaking that then generalizes. The episode lasts approximately 2 minutes, and subsequently she is somnolent. Initial lumbar puncture results show 850 white blood cells with 90% lymphocytes, red cells, and a protein of 200 mg/dL; a blood count reveals a platelet count of $57{,}000/mm^3$.

- ➤ What is the most likely diagnosis?
- ➤ What are the potential complications of this condition?

# ANSWERS TO CASE 43:
# Congenital Herpes

*Summary*: A 10-day-old previously healthy infant with fever, irritability, decreased oral intake, and vesicles on her scalp has an episode of seizure-like activity. Laboratory studies reveal lymphocytic meningitis and thrombocytopenia.

- **Most likely diagnosis:** Congenital herpes.
- **Potential complications of this condition:** Left untreated, the majority of infants with disseminated or central nervous system (CNS) infection die. The use of high-dose, long-duration antiviral therapy has reduced mortality and improved long-term outcomes among survivors.

## ANALYSIS

### Objectives

1. Recognize the importance of early recognition of congenital herpes infection.
2. Know how to diagnose congenital herpes infection.
3. Know the appropriate management of congenital herpes infection.

### Considerations

A **young infant with fever and irritability is presumed to have a serious bacterial or viral infection.** Bacterial causes in this age include group B *Streptococcus*, *Listeria*, and gram-negative pathogens. The history in this case of a **focal seizure**, the finding of **vesicles on the infant's scalp**, and the **laboratory findings make herpes simplex virus (HSV) the most likely pathogen**. The absence of a maternal history of herpes is not unusual; only 15% to 20% of mothers of HSV-infected infants have a history of herpes and only approximately 25% have relevant symptoms at delivery. The risk of maternal passage of HSV to the neonate is higher in cases of primary herpes outbreaks because the viral inoculum in the genital tract is high and protective antibody is not present.

Blood, urine, and cerebrospinal fluid (CSF) specimens are obtained for routine bacterial cultures; HSV cultures are obtained from the blood, nasopharynx, eyes, urine, stool or rectum, and CSF. Cerebrospinal fluid is tested by polymerase chain reaction (PCR) for HSV. A complete blood count and liver function and coagulation studies may reveal abnormalities. Pending test results, this infant is placed on intravenous antibiotics and antiviral therapy.

# APPROACH TO Suspected Congenital Herpes Infection

## DEFINITIONS

**GENITAL HERPES:** Infection of the genital tract with HSV type 1 or 2, the majority caused by HSV-2.

**PRIMARY HERPES INFECTION:** HSV infection in a previously seronegative host. Most primary infections are subclinical, but they can cause localized lesions or severe systemic symptoms.

**RECURRENT INFECTION:** Reactivation of a latent infection in an immune host. Lesions tend to be localized and are not associated with systemic symptoms.

## CLINICAL APPROACH

Approximately **20% to 30%** of American women of childbearing age have antibodies to HSV-2, with a higher rate in women of lower socioeconomic groups and those in crowded living conditions. Approximately 75% of congenital herpes cases are caused by HSV-2. Usually HSV-2 is transmitted via sexual contact, and most genital diseases are the result of type 2 infection; HSV-1 can be transmitted sexually and occasionally is found in the genital tract. HSV-2 is associated with greater morbidity among congenital infection survivors than HSV-1.

**Cesarean delivery is generally indicated in delivering women with an outbreak of genital herpes or symptoms of HSV infection.** The infant's risk of HSV infection is increased significantly if the maternal outbreak represents **primary infection**. As many as 50% of such infants will become infected if delivered vaginally, whereas fewer than 5% will acquire the disease if the outbreak is recurrent disease. HSV surveillance cultures are not recommended in pregnant women; women at greatest risk for infecting their infants are those without prior infection history.

**Neonatal HSV disease** can result in premature delivery and can manifest in the neonate as **localized skin, eye, and mouth involvement (SEM); CNS disease; disseminated disease**; or a combination of these. Asymptomatic infection can occur but is uncommon. Nonspecific presenting clinical signs and symptoms often occur in the absence of lesions and can include fever, lethargy, irritability, anorexia, vomiting, respiratory distress, apnea, jaundice, a bulging fontanelle, seizures (focal or generalized), decerebrate posturing, and coma. Shock and disseminated intravascular coagulation (DIC) can occur in severe cases. Organomegaly, pneumonitis, and pleural effusion may occur. The risk of death is highest among infants with disseminated or CNS disease, particularly if pneumonitis and DIC occur. Among survivors, morbidity is associated with disseminated disease, CNS involvement, HSV-2 infection, seizures, and frequent cutaneous recurrences.

**Cell culture of samples taken from various body sites and PCR of CSF** are the most useful diagnostic tests. Serologic tests for herpes virus are not helpful in the acute setting (titers rise late in the infection's course). **Tzanck preparation** of lesions and antigen detection methods applied to the specimens can aid in **rapid diagnosis, but the sensitivity is low.** Infected individuals often have moderate peripheral leukocytosis, elevated serum liver transaminase levels, hyperbilirubinemia, and thrombocytopenia. When the CNS is involved, the CSF frequently contains an elevated number of red cells, lymphocytes, and protein; CSF glucose usually is normal but may be reduced. Electroencephalography (EEG) shows characteristic patterns in acutely affected infants, and brain computerized tomography (CT) will become abnormal as the disease progresses. HSV encephalitis in the neonatal period tends to be global, but electroencephalography (EEG) and magnetic resonance imaging (MRI) obtained in patients beyond the neonatal period may show temporal lobe abnormalities.

**Parenteral acyclovir is the preferred treatment.** Children with isolated skin, eye, and mouth disease generally have the best outcomes. The use of long-duration, high-dose acyclovir has reduced mortality among children with localized central nervous system disease to 4%, and to about 30% in children with disseminated disease. Most survivors of central nervous system disease have neurologic sequelae, but as many as 80% of survivors of disseminated infection have normal development at 12 months of age.

## Comprehension Questions

43.1 A 10-day-old infant has a painful, red vesicular rash in the diaper area. He is mildly fussy but afebrile, and he has good oral intake. Which of the following is the most appropriate management of this infant?

A. Hospitalize the patient, obtain HSV cultures, and initiate parenteral acyclovir.
B. Order an EEG and brain MRI *stat*.
C. Perform a Tzanck smear and send the patient home if it is negative.
D. Prescribe an antifungal cream and follow up by telephone in 24 hours.
E. Schedule an appointment with a pediatric dermatologist.

43.2 A woman presents for her first prenatal visit at 9-week gestation. She reports that she is generally healthy, except that she has an outbreak of genital herpes approximately once per year. To prevent transmission of the virus to her infant, her physician should do which of following?

A. Anticipate a cesarean section delivery.
B. Order titers to determine if the infection is HSV-1 or HSV-2.
C. Perform weekly genital viral cultures starting at 36-week gestation.
D. Perform a cesarean delivery if herpetic lesions or prodromal symptoms are present when labor has begun.
E. No change in management is indicated; the risk of infant transmission is low even if she has an outbreak at delivery.

43.3 A 5-year-old with dysuria is found on examination to have herpetic genital lesions. Which of the following is the best next step in management?

A. Ask the parent to leave the room and then ask the girl in an open-ended fashion whether she has ever been inappropriately touched in her private area.
B. Prescribe oral acyclovir and ask her to follow up in 2 days.
C. Admit her to the hospital for parenteral antiviral therapy.
D. Ask how often the mother has outbreaks of genital herpes.
E. Send a urine culture and have the mother apply petroleum jelly until the lesions heal.

43.4 The results of PCR of CSF from a 15-year-old adolescent male with encephalitis demonstrate an HSV infection. His parents ask about his prognosis. Which of the following is likely to be true?

A. He will most likely die.
B. He will likely survive, but will certainly have serious neurologic impairment.
C. Most children with HSV encephalitis survive; many (but not all) are left with some permanent neurologic deficits.
D. They should consider placing him in a long-term care facility upon discharge.

## ANSWERS

43.1 **A.** In contrast to older children and adults, infants with suspected herpes skin lesions require parenteral antiviral therapy to prevent more serious sequelae.

43.2 **D.** Even though the viral transmission risk in the setting of a recurrent HSV outbreak is low, cesarean section is indicated if lesions are present at the time of delivery. Surveillance cultures are not recommended; negative results a few days prior to delivery do not preclude a later outbreak, and results of analysis of a more recently obtained specimen may not be available.

43.3 **A.** The possibility of sexual abuse is considered in a child who presents with genital herpes beyond the neonatal period. It is important to know who helps to bathe the child, and whether these persons have ever had herpes, as nonsexual transmission is also possible.

43.4 **C.** Although the majority of children with HSV encephalitis suffer permanent neurologic impairment, good outcomes are possible with appropriate medical and rehabilitative therapy.

## Clinical Pearls

- Most infants with congenital herpes simplex virus are born to mothers without a prior history of herpes simplex virus infection.
- The presenting signs and symptoms of congenital herpes simplex virus may be nonspecific, without any visible herpetic lesions.
- Infants with suspected herpes simplex virus infection should be hospitalized for testing and parenteral antiviral therapy pending test results.
- Children with herpes simplex virus skin, eye, and mouth (SEM) disease generally have the best outcomes, whereas the majority of infants with central nervous system disease develop neurologic sequelae. Approximately 30% of infants with systemic infection die despite aggressive antiviral therapy.

## REFERENCES

American Academy of Pediatrics. Herpes simplex. In: Pickering LK, ed. *2006 Red Book: Report of the Committee on Infectious Diseases*. 27th ed. Elk Grove Village, IL: American Academy of Pediatrics; 2006:361-371.

Prober CG. Herpes simplex virus infections. In: Rudolph CD, Rudolph AM, Hostetter MK, Lister G, Siegel NJ, eds. *Rudolph's Pediatrics*. 21st ed. New York, NY: McGraw-Hill; 2003:1029-1031.

Sánchez PJ, Siegel JD. Herpes simplex virus. In: McMillan JA, Feigin RD, DeAngelis CD, Jones MD, eds. *Oski's Pediatrics: Principles and Practice*. 4th ed. Philadelphia, PA: Lippincott Williams & Wilkins; 2006:516-520.

Stanberry LR. Herpes simplex virus. In: Kliegman RM, Behrman RE, Jenson HB, Stanton BF, eds. *Nelson Textbook of Pediatrics*. 18th ed. Philadelphia, PA: WB Saunders; 2007:1360-1366.

# Case 44

A mother brings her 11-month-old daughter to the clinic because of a persistent facial rash. The child is restless at night and scratches in her sleep. She is otherwise healthy. Physical examination reveals a well-nourished, healthy-appearing white female with dry, red, scaly areas on the cheeks, chin, and around the mouth. The areas on the cheeks have a plaque-like, weepy appearance. The diaper area is spared. The remainder of the child's examination is normal.

- ➤ What is the most likely diagnosis?
- ➤ What is the most appropriate next step in the evaluation?

# ANSWERS TO CASE 44:
# Atopic Dermatitis

*Summary:* An 11-month-old female infant has dry, red, scaly areas on the cheeks, chin, and around the mouth, with sparing of the diaper area.

- **Most likely diagnosis:** Atopic dermatitis.
- **Next step in evaluation:** Further history to determine rash duration and exacerbating factors, and family history for atopic dermatitis, allergic rhinitis, and asthma.

## ANALYSIS

### Objectives

1. Describe incidence, etiology, and risk factors for atopic dermatitis.
2. Discuss diagnostic criteria and differential diagnoses for atopic dermatitis.
3. Describe treatment and follow-up of atopic dermatitis.
4. Be familiar with other conditions associated with atopic dermatitis.

### Considerations

This child's history and examination are consistent with atopic dermatitis. Further history may reveal additional risk factors for allergic disease. Treatment involves avoiding aggravating factors and ensuring intensive skin hydration.

# APPROACH TO
# Atopic Dermatitis

## DEFINITIONS

**EMOLLIENT:** Cream or lotion that restores water and lipids to the epidermis; those containing urea or lactic acid are more lubricating and may be more effective; creams lubricate better than lotions.

**FLEXURAL AREAS:** Areas of repeated flexion and extension, which often perspire on exertion (antecubital fossae, neck, wrists, ankles).

**LICHENIFICATION:** Epidermal thickening, with normal skin lines resembling a washboard.

## CLINICAL APPROACH

**Atopic dermatitis (eczema) typically is pruritic, recurrent, and flexural in older children and symmetrical in adults.** The term *atopy* was coined to describe a group of patients who had a personal or family history of hay fever, asthma, dry skin, and eczema. More than 15 million American adults and children have atopic dermatitis. The highest incidence is seen among children, and the lifetime prevalence of atopic dermatitis is 20% in children aged 3 to 11 years. Sixty-five percent of patients develop symptoms in the first year of life and 90% before age 5 years. The etiology is unknown, but is thought to be related to immune factors. Seventy percent of atopic patients have a family history of asthma, hay fever, or eczema.

**Atopic dermatitis occurs in three phases: infant** (birth to 2 years), **childhood** (2 to 12 years), and **adult** (>12 years). Infants are rarely born with atopic dermatitis, but typically develop the first signs of inflammation during the third month of life. A common scenario is a baby who, during winter months, develops dry, red, scaling cheeks without perioral and paranasal involvement. The chin is often involved; the diaper area is usually spared. The infant is uncomfortable because of pruritus and is often restless during sleep. Atopic dermatitis resolves in approximately 50% of infants by age 18 months. The most common finding in the childhood phase is inflammation in flexural areas. Perspiration stimulates burning and itching, initiating an itch–scratch cycle. Initial papules rapidly coalesce into plaques that ultimately become lichenified when scratched. The exudative lesions typical of the infant phase are not common in the childhood phase. The adult phase begins near the onset of puberty. The reason for the resurgence of inflammation may be related to hormonal changes. Flexural inflammation ensues, often accompanied by hand dermatitis, inflammation around the eyes, and lichenification of the anogenital area.

Two misconceptions about atopic dermatitis are common. The first is that eczema is an emotional disorder. Patients with skin inflammation lasting for months or years are often irritable, a normal response to a frustrating disorder. The second misconception is that atopic skin disease is precipitated by an allergic reaction. Atopic individuals frequently have respiratory allergies and, when skin tested, are informed that they are "allergic to everything." Individuals with atopy may react with a wheal when challenged with a needle during skin testing, but this is a characteristic of atopic skin and is not necessarily an allergic response. Evidence to date indicates that most cases of atopic dermatitis are precipitated by environmental stress on genetically compromised skin and not by interaction with allergens.

### Patient Evaluation

Evaluation of the child with atopic dermatitis involves ruling out other potential causes of the child's rash through a complete personal history (Table 44–1), family history, and physical examination to obtain a proper diagnosis and initiate treatment. Physical examination includes temperature measurement to identify possible infection. Skin is evaluated for locations and nature of affected areas (patches, weepiness, lichenification), extent of skin dryness, and warmth or tenderness (possible secondary infection). Eyes, nose, throat, and chest are examined for evidence of allergic rhinitis or asthma (rhinnorhea, watery eyes, dark circles under eyes, wheezing).

**Laboratory studies are not particularly helpful** in diagnosing atopic dermatitis. **A serum immunoglobulin E (IgE) level is often elevated.** Culture of the skin is performed if superinfection is suspected.

The differential diagnosis includes seborrheic dermatitis (cradle cap), which usually begins on the scalp in the first few months of life and may involve the ears, nose, eyebrows, and eyelids. The greasy brown scales of seborrheic dermatitis are in contrast to the erythematous, weeping, crusted lesions of infantile atopic dermatitis. Other considerations include scabies, irritant dermatitis (perioral fruit juice dermatitis), allergic contact dermatitis (poison ivy), and eczematoid dermatitis (infectious lesion near a draining ear).

## Treatment

Treatment goals include preserving and restoring the skin barrier by using emollients, eliminating inflammation and infection with medications, reducing scratching through antipruritic use, and controlling exacerbating factors. Some recommend limiting bathing to brief baths or showers of moderate temperature with mild and preferably nonsoap cleansers (Cetaphil). Drying soaps (Ivory) are avoided. Lubricants (Eucerin) are applied immediately after bathing and air- or pat-drying. Some products contain urea (Nutraplus) or lactic acid (Lac-Hydrin); they have special hydrating qualities and may be more effective than other moisturizers. Lotions and creams may sting shortly after application due to bases or specific ingredients, such as lactic acid. If itching and stinging continue with each application, another product should be selected.

Topical corticosteroids used to control inflammation vary in potency; percentage is not an indication of potency. Lower-potency preparations (glucocorticoid groups VI and VII) can be used for longer periods to treat chronic symptoms involving the trunk and extremities. Lower-potency steroids are

**Table 44–1 QUESTIONS TO ASK WHEN INVESTIGATING RASHES**

| |
|---|
| How long have the symptoms been present? Were there previous episodes of similar outbreaks? |
| How itchy are the affected areas? Is the child becoming irritable or awakening at night because of itching and scratching? |
| Do symptoms appear to get worse with exposure to cold weather, wool, perspiration, or stress? |
| Do other family members have eczema, asthma, or allergic diseases? |
| Has the child had fever or other signs of infection? |

generally used for infants and can be added to moisturizers to cover large areas of affected skin. Fluticasone propionate (Cutivate) is the only Food and Drug Administration (FDA)-approved topical corticosteroid cream for infants as young as 3 months. **Fluorinated corticosteroids are generally avoided on the face, genitalia, and the intertriginous area because they may depigment and thin the skin.** Higher-potency steroids (glucocorticoid groups I and II) are used only for short periods and on lichenified areas; the face and skin folds are avoided. Ointment preparations are generally preferable because they result in better penetration of the corticosteroid, thus reducing the incidence of irritant and hypersensitivity reactions. Administration of agents is usually twice daily unless the chosen agent requires only once-daily application. Lubrication is continued after corticosteroids are discontinued.

Tacrolimus (Protopic) and pimecrolimus (Elidel) are nonsteroidal, immunomodulator topicals for treatment of atopic dermatitis. Tacrolimus 0.03% and pimecrolimus 1% are approved for use in children 2 years and older. These agents are recommended for short-term and long-term intermittent therapy, on a twice-daily basis, in patients not adequately responsive to, or intolerant of, conventional therapy. Because of a possible link with lymphoma, their exact role for use in children is under investigation; consultation with a pediatric dermatologist may be indicated.

Oral antihistamines are used to reduce itching. Because symptoms of atopic dermatitis are often worse at night, sedating oral antihistamines (hydroxyzine, diphenhydramine) may offer an advantage over non-sedating agents. Less-sedating agents include loratadine and cetirizine. Doxepin has tricyclic antidepressant and antihistamine effects and may be useful in some cases. Topical antihistamines (Caladryl) are avoided because of the potential for skin irritation or toxicity due to absorption. Fingernails should be cut short to prevent further skin damage via scratching.

Patients with secondary bacterial infections (*Staphylococcus or Streptococcus* sp) often require antibiotic therapy. Topical antibiotic therapy with mupirocin (Bactroban) may be used for limited areas of infection or in the nose to reduce chronic *Staphylococcus aureus* carriage. Oral antibiotics are indicated for more extensive areas of infection. First-generation cephalosporins, erythromycin, penicillinase-resistant penicillins, or clindamycin are chosen based on local susceptibility patterns. Patients with evidence of superinfection with herpes simplex virus may require oral or intravenous acyclovir.

The role of food allergies in the management of atopic dermatitis is controversial. Dietary manipulation in a child with a strong history of exacerbation of symptoms upon exposure to a particular food may be helpful. A 4- to 6-week trial excluding eggs and milk in children, followed by a rechallenge, may be justified, especially in a child who does not respond to first-line treatment.

Consultation with a pediatric dermatologist may be warranted for patients with an unclear diagnosis, who fail to respond to treatment, or who have extensive exfoliation. Consultation also may be appropriate for patients with ocular or serious infectious complications and for patients requiring oral steroid therapy.

## Comprehension Questions

44.1 A mother brings her 2-week-old son to the clinic for a well-baby visit. Her only concern is a rash on his face and scalp that began 1 week earlier. Examination reveals a healthy white male with normal vital signs and a normal examination except for yellowish, waxy-appearing, adherent plaques on the scalp, forehead, cheeks, and nasolabial folds. Which of the following therapies is appropriate for this condition?

A. High potency topical steroids
B. Topical mupirocin
C. Phototherapy
D. Ketoconazole-containing shampoo
E. Topical antifungals

44.2 An 8-year-old girl arrives at your clinic complaining about a minimally itchy rash on her chest, abdomen, and arms. It started with one small, scaly, red area on her chest and then spread. She is taking no medications. Physical examination reveals salmon-colored, flat, finely scaly, oval eruptions on her chest, abdomen, back, and upper arms. Which of the following is the most likely explanation for these findings?

A. Topical mupirocin
B. High-dose topical steroids
C. Supportive therapy
D. Three sequential weekly penicillin injections
E. Topical antifungals

44.3 A father brings his 8-month-old daughter to an emergency room for worsening skin rash and fever. He reports that his daughter usually has weepy, red lesions on her face that is relatively well controlled with bathing her with gentle soaps, using topical emollients and steroids, and giving oral antihistamines. Over the previous few days, however, the rash has gotten progressively worse and the child has become "sicker." Your physical examination reveals a lethargic child with an oral temperature of 103°F (39.4°C). The child's cheeks are red and contain numerous red, punched-out, and umbilicated vesicles; some lesions are pustular. Which of the following is the best therapy at this point?

A. Prescribe intravenous acyclovir.
B. Prescribe prednisolone.
C. Prescribe topical bacitracin.
D. Prescribe cephalexin.
E. Prescribe topical acyclovir.

44.4 An 8-month-old child has refractory eczema that was first noticed at 2 months of age. His past medical history reveals multiple episodes of otitis media and pneumonia, and he has now developed severe nosebleeds. His CBC shows a white blood count of 8500/mm$^3$, his hemoglobin is 11.1 mg/dL, his hematocrit is 33.4%, and his platelet count is 15,000/mm$^3$. Which of the following is the most likely diagnosis?

A. Bruton agammaglobulinemia
B. DiGeorge anomaly
C. Job syndrome
D. Severe combined immunodeficiency
E. Wiskott-Aldrich syndrome

## ANSWERS

44.1 **D.** Seborrheic dermatitis presents in infancy and adolescence. The chronic, symmetrical eruption, characterized by overproduction of sebum, affects the scalp, forehead, retroauricular region, auditory meatus, eyebrows, cheeks, and nasolabial folds. Treatment includes softening the scales with mineral oil, avoiding scrubbing, and daily shampooing with a mild shampoo. Low to medium potency topical corticosteroids or ketoconazole (Nizoral) shampoo may be helpful.

44.2 **C.** Pityriasis rosea is preceded by a "herald patch," an annular, scaly, erythematous lesion. The lesions are salmon-colored and in a Christmas-tree formation, following the lines of the skin. The cause is unknown. Treatment may include antihistamines, topical antipruritic lotions and creams, low-dose topical corticosteroids, and phototherapy. The rash usually lasts up to 6 weeks and then resolves. It can be confused with nummular eczema and tinea versicolor. In the sexually active adolescent, syphilis should also be considered.

44.3 **A.** Atopic infants may develop rapid onset of diffuse cutaneous herpes simplex. The disease is most common in areas of active or recently healed atopic dermatitis, particularly the face. High fever and adenopathy occur 2 to 3 days after the onset of vesiculation. Viral septicemia can be fatal. Eczema herpeticum of the young infant is a medical emergency. The child should be admitted immediately for intravenous acyclovir.

44.4 **E.** Wiskott-Aldrich syndrome is an X-linked condition with recurrent infections, thrombocytopenia, and eczema. Infections and bleeding usually are noted in the first 6 months of life. Potential infections include otitis media and pneumonia caused by poor antibody response to capsular polysaccharides, and fungal and viral septicemias caused by T-cell dysfunction. Thrombocytopenia usually is in the 15,000 to 30,000/mm$^3$ range, and platelets are typically small. In addition to eczema, these children have autoimmune disorders and a high incidence of lymphoma and other malignancies.

## Clinical Pearls

- Atopic dermatitis is a chronic, itchy disease that often begins in childhood. In infancy, the itchy eruption is found on the face and cheeks; by childhood, the rash is noted in flexural areas.
- Baseline therapy for atopic dermatitis is avoidance of drying soaps and replenishment of skin hydration with emollients; topical steroids may be required.

## REFERENCES


Buckley RH. Immunodeficiency with thrombocytopenia (Wiskott-Aldrich syndrome). In: McMillan JA, Feigin RD, DeAngelis CD, Jones MD, eds. *Oski's Pediatrics: Principles and Practice*. 4th ed. Philadelphia, PA: Lippincott Williams & Wilkins; 2006:2467-2468.

Chatila TA. Wiskott-Aldrich syndrome. In: Rudolph CD, Rudolph AM, Hostetter MK, Lister G, Siegel NJ, eds. *Rudolph's Pediatrics*. 21st ed. New York, NY: McGraw-Hill; 2003:799.

Leung DYM. Atopic dermatitis (atopic eczema). In: Kliegman RM, Behrman RE, Jenson HB, Stanton BF, eds. *Nelson Textbook of Pediatrics*. 18th ed. Philadelphia, PA: WB Saunders; 2007:970-975.

Prose NS. Atopic dermatitis. In: Rudolph CD, Rudolph AM, Hostetter MK, Lister G, Siegel NJ, eds. *Rudolph's Pediatrics*. 21st ed. New York, NY: McGraw-Hill; 2003:1177-1180.

Sampson HA. Atopic dermatitis. In: McMillan JA, Feigin RD, DeAngelis CD, Jones MD, eds. *Oski's Pediatrics: Principles and Practice*. 4th ed. Philadelphia, PA: Lippincott Williams & Wilkins; 2006:2423-2427.

# Case 45

A father reports his 3-year-old daughter has decreased energy, loss of appetite, and an enlarging abdomen over the past few weeks. Intermittent emesis began yesterday. Physical examination reveals pallor, proptosis, periorbital discoloration, and a large, irregular abdominal mass along her left flank that crosses the midline. Her vital signs and the remainder of her examination are normal.

➤ What is the most likely diagnosis?

➤ What is the next step in evaluation?

# ANSWERS TO CASE 45: Neuroblastoma

*Summary:* A toddler with fatigue, decreased appetite, periorbital discoloration, and a multiquadrant abdominal mass.

- **Most likely diagnosis:** Neuroblastoma.
- **Next step in evaluation:** Select laboratory testing and imaging to ascertain tumor genetic characteristics, location and extent, and impact on surrounding structures. Resultant staging and risk stratification help guide decision-making regarding perisurgical chemotherapy and/or irradiation.

## ANALYSIS

### Objectives

1. Recognize the signs and symptoms of neuroblastoma.
2. Describe the diagnosis and treatment of neuroblastoma.

### Considerations

Since neuroblastoma origin and progression varies from patient to patient and a mass may not always be readily apparent on examination, clinicians must perform thorough histories and comprehensive examinations to ensure timely and accurate diagnosis and diminish the potential for metastatic disease at discovery. Within the diagnostic evaluation includes questioning and examining for syndromes associated with neuroblastoma.

# APPROACH TO Suspected Neuroblastoma

## DEFINITIONS

**HORNER SYNDROME:** Characterized by eyelid ptosis and sluggish pupillary reflex; related to sympathetic nervous system dysfunction.

**PARANEOPLASTIC SYNDROME:** Characterized by hypertension and secretory diarrhea; related to tumor production of catecholamines and vasoactive intestinal peptide.

**OPSOCLONUS-MYOCLONUS SYNDROME:** Characterized by chaotic eye movements and myoclonic jerks; described as "dancing eyes, dancing feet"; related to autoantibodies produced against neuronal elements.

## CLINICAL APPROACH

Neuroblastoma is comprised of primitive neuroendocrine tissue. Its etiology is poorly understood, but believed to be multifactorial. It is the most prevalent solid, extracranial tumor in children and accounts for more than half of all cancers in infancy. Most arise in the abdomen from the adrenal gland, with other origins including intrathoracic and paraspinal neuronal ganglia.

Signs and symptoms related to neuroblastoma depend on tumor location; cervical ganglia tumors may cause Horner syndrome, intrathoracic tumors (most commonly seen in infancy) may be associated with wheezing and respiratory distress, and paraspinal tumors may cause compressive neuralgias, back pain, and urinary or stool retention. Abdominal masses are typically nontender, irregular, and cross the midline. Dependent on a tumor's location and impact on surrounding structures, intrathoracic or paraspinal decompressive surgery may emergently be required.

Metastatic disease typically involves the skin, lungs, liver, and bone. Bluish skin discoloration (most often seen in infancy) represents subcutaneous infiltration. Pulmonary involvement can promote increased work of breathing, dyspnea, and pneumonia. Bone marrow infiltration may cause bone pain and pancytopenia; petechiae, bruising, pallor, and fatigue may occur. If the orbital bones are involved, proptosis and bluish periorbital discoloration, described as "raccoon eyes," may be noted. Generalized lymphadenopathy also is common. Some patients develop paraneoplastic syndrome related to tumor neuroendocrine mediators, or opsoclonus-myoclonus syndrome (an autoimmune-mediated phenomenon that may be characterized by cerebellar ataxia).

The major differential diagnostic consideration is Wilms tumor. These tumors typically are associated with hematuria, hypertension, and a localized abdominal mass that rarely crosses the midline. In general, patients with neuroblastoma are slightly younger and sicker than patients with Wilms tumor.

Computerized tomography (CAT) or magnetic resonance imaging (MRI) is useful in identifying and assessing the extent of neuroblastoma. Laboratory markers include **elevated urinary vanillylmandelic acid and homovanillic acid levels (catecholamine metabolites), observed in approximately 90% of neuroblastoma patients**; other markers include elevated enolase, ferritin, and lactate dehydrogenase levels.

Treatment involves surgical excision of the tumor, usually after chemotherapy and/or radiotherapy to decrease tumor size. Combined multi-agent chemotherapy and radiotherapy often is used in patients with advanced-stage neuroblastoma. Staging is classically dependent on tumor location and extent, with risk assessment and therapeutic decision-making based on variables such as age at diagnosis and staging (eg, stage 2 disease localized to the abdomen of a 1-year-old requiring only limited post-excision chemotherapy versus stage 4 disease with bony metastases in a toddler mandating multi-agent chemotherapy and bone marrow transplantation). Other therapies under investigation include monoclonal antibody immunotherapy and radionuclide therapy.

Overall cure rates for neuroblastoma can exceed 90%, with infants typically having a better prognosis than older children. Select features, such as skeletal metastases or N-*myc* ongogene amplification at the cellular level, often denote a poor prognosis.

## Comprehension Questions

45.1 A mother recently feels a mass in the abdomen of her 4-year-old son during a bath, and brings him to your clinic for evaluation. He has no history of emesis, abnormal stooling, or abdominal pain. Physical examination reveals a resting blood pressure of 130/88 mm Hg, heart rate of 82 beats/minute, pallor, and a firm left-sided abdominal mass that doesn't cross the midline. Which of the following is the most likely explanation for these findings?

A. Constipation
B. Intussusception
C. Neuroblastoma
D. Wilms tumor
E. Volvulus

45.2 A 1-week-old infant presents with a right midquadrant abdominal mass and decreased urinary output. There has been no temperature lability, irritability, or abnormal stooling or urine appearance. Which of the following is the most likely diagnosis?

A. Intussusception
B. Hydronephrosis
C. Neuroblastoma
D. Sepsis
E. Wilms tumor

45.3 A father presents his otherwise healthy 15-month-old daughter to the emergency center with cough, post-tussive emesis, and subjective fever over the past 3 days. He also thinks her abdomen has been hurting her. Diarrhea started yesterday, with "regular" stooling prior to this illness. She has been drinking well and recently had a wet diaper. Physical examination reveals a temperature of 98.9°F (37.2°C), congested nares, shoddy neck lymphadenopathy, and a mildly distended and apparently tender abdomen without obvious guarding. Which of the following is the most likely etiology for her abdominal pain?

A. Constipation
B. Lymphoma
C. Neuroblastoma
D. Appendicitis
E. Mesenteric lymphadenitis

45.4 During a routine preventive health visit for a 3-year-old boy, you incidentally note an irregular abdominal mass involving both lower quadrants. His mother denies having noted this previously and declares her son to be generally healthy. There has been neither gastrointestinal distress nor apparent abdominal pain. Beyond the abdominal mass and pallorous conjunctivae, his vital signs and physical examination are normal. Which of the following tests would be most helpful in determining the etiology of his abdominal mass?

A. Abdominal radiograph
B. Chest radiograph
C. Urinary catecholamines
D. Complete blood count
E. Urine myoglobin

## ANSWERS

45.1 **D.** The scenario presented is typical for Wilms tumor. Beyond abdominal imaging, checking a urinalysis for hematuria, metabolic panel for renal or hepatic dysfunction, and complete blood count for anemia should be considered in the workup of Wilms tumor.

45.2 **B.** Urinary tract obstruction is often silent. In the newborn, a palpable abdominal mass is commonly a hydronephrotic or multicystic dysplastic kidney.

45.3 **E.** Upper respiratory tract infection symptoms, neck lymphadenopathy, and diarrhea are consistent with viremia; viral-mediated mesenteric lymph node enlargement can occur and cause nonspecific abdominal pain. This otherwise healthy child with classic viremia lacks history or findings consistent with an intra-abdominal tumor, enteritis, or intestinal dysmotility. An abdominal CAT scan may show diffuse, mildly enlarged lymph nodes in mesenteric lymphadenitis, but imaging is rarely warranted unless an etiology for abdominal pain remains elusive. Other nonmalignancy-related causes of abdominal pain include enteritis caused by bacteria (*salmonella*, *E. coli*, *Yersinia* sp., and typical or atypical mycobacteria) or viruses (mononucleosis, coxsachie, and adenovirus).

45.4 **C.** This boy's history and examination are consistent with neuroblastoma. Given the vast majority of neuroblastoma patients have elevated urinary catecholamines, a 24-hour quantitative assessment of these metabolites should be confirmatory.

## Clinical Pearls

- Neuroblastoma may present with an abdominal mass, pallor, proptosis, and "raccoon eyes."
- Masses are often discovered incidentally by a family member or on routine physical examination.
- Patients with neuroblastoma are slightly younger and appear sicker than patients with Wilms tumor.
- Approximately 90% of neuroblastoma patients have elevated levels of the catecholamine metabolites, vanillylmandelic acid, and homovanillic acid.

## REFERENCES

Jaffe N, Huff V. Neoplasms of the kidney. In: Kliegman RM, Behrman RE, Jenson HB, Stanton, BF, eds. *Nelson Textbook of Pediatrics*. 18th ed. Philadelphia, PA: WB Saunders; 2007:2140-2143.

Strother DR, Russell HV. Neuroblastoma. In: McMillan JA, Feigin RD, DeAngelis CD, Warshaw JB, eds. *Oski's Pediatrics: Principles and Practice*. 4th ed. Philadelphia, PA: Lippincott Williams & Wilkins; 2006:1778-1781.

Strother DR. Neuroblastoma. In: Rudolph CD, Rudolph AM, Hostetter MK, Lister G, Siegel NJ, eds. *Rudolph's Pediatrics*. 21st ed. New York, NY: McGraw-Hill; 2003: 1778-1781.

# Case 46

A mother reports that her 4-year-old daughter complains of sore throat and difficulty swallowing for 3 days. She has been irritable and does not want to move her neck. Her appetite and intake have decreased, and she has vomited twice overnight. She exhibits no symptoms of upper respiratory tract infection (URI). She is otherwise healthy with up-to-date immunizations. Her physical examination is remarkable for fever to 102°F (38.9°C), bilateral tonsillar exudates, and an erythematous posterior oropharynx with right posterior pharyngeal wall swelling.

- ➤ What is the most likely diagnosis?
- ➤ What is the most appropriate next step in the evaluation?

# ANSWERS TO CASE 46:
# Retropharyngeal Abscess

*Summary:* An ill-appearing toddler with sore throat, odynophagia, fever, and an abnormal oropharyngeal examination.

- **Most likely diagnosis:** Retropharyngeal abscess.
- **Next step in evaluation:** Laboratory testing might include group A beta-hemolytic *Streptococcus* (GAS) immunoassay and culture. Radiologic evaluation might include lateral cervical x-ray and computed tomography (CT) or magnetic resonance imaging (MRI) to elucidate location and extent of infection.

## ANALYSIS

### Objectives

1. Discuss the diagnosis and treatment of retropharyngeal abscess.
2. Differentiate between various forms of neck abscess.
3. Discuss neck conditions presenting similarly to retropharyngeal abscess.

### Considerations

History and examination for this toddler with odynophagia, fever, and posterior pharyngeal swelling is consistent with retropharyngeal abscess. Because a variety of head and neck lesions can present similarly, the diagnostic challenge lies in determining whether a bacterial infection is present, the extent of infection, the possible need for surgical intervention, and whether the potential exists for spread to surrounding vital structures.

# APPROACH TO
# Retropharyngeal Abscess

## DEFINITIONS

**RETROPHARYNGEAL SPACE:** Bordered by layers of the deep cervical fascia; located posterior to the esophagus; contains lymphatics draining the middle ears, sinuses, and nasopharynx; contiguous with the posterior mediastinum.

**PARAPHARYNGEAL (LATERAL) SPACE:** Comprises anterior and posterior compartments containing lymph nodes, cranial nerves, and carotid sheaths; infections in the lateral space can originate from the oropharynx, middle ears, and teeth.

**PERITONSILLAR SPACE:** Bordered by tonsils and pharyngeal musculature; peritonsillar abscess is typically an extension of acute tonsillitis.

**EPIGLOTTITIS:** Infection of the cartilaginous structure protecting the airway during swallowing; bacterial etiology (classically *Haemophilus influenzae*) requiring intravenous antibiotics; fever, drooling, and toxicity are common; emergent airway obstruction is possible.

**RAPID STREP IMMUNOASSAY:** Detects GAS antigen by latex agglutination or enzyme-linked immunosorbent assay; high specificity and variable sensitivity with false-negative results possible.

**MONOSPOT:** Latex agglutination of heterophile antibodies to erythrocytes in Epstein-Barr virus (EBV) infection; high specificity and sensitivity in patients older than 3 years; infection may be confirmed by EBV immunoglobulin (Ig)M antibody if heterophile negative.

**STRIDOR:** Abnormal, musical breathing as a result of large airway obstruction.

**DYSPHAGIA:** Difficulty swallowing.

**ODYNOPHAGIA:** Pain on swallowing.

**TRISMUS:** Inability to open the mouth secondary to pain or inflammation or mass effect involving facial neuromusculature.

## CLINICAL APPROACH

**Categorization of deep neck infections** is based on a combination of **examination findings** and **neck imaging**. The type and extent of infection ultimately determine whether a patient requires surgery and could be at risk for infection of nearby vital structures, including the mediastinum. Multiple compartments exist within the neck, bordered by musculature and fascia and containing various neurovascular structures (cranial nerves and carotid arteries); infections can easily spread along these fascial planes.

Some age predilections are noted in neck abscess. The typical pediatric patient with **retropharyngeal abscess**, for example, is a **toddler younger than 4 years,** coinciding with the time when the majority of upper respiratory and otitis cases are seen. **Peritonsillar abscess** can be seen at any age, but **prevalence is greater in the adolescent or young adult**. Of all abscess types, **peritonsillar abscess is the most common type in the pediatric population**.

Infections of the retropharyngeal, parapharyngeal, and peritonsillar space may present similarly. Patients usually complain of **sore throat and odynophagia**. Fever, irritability, and toxicity are also common. As in **epiglottitis, drooling and increased work of breathing or frank stridor** can be seen. Patients may present with dysphagia or **trismus,** the latter noted more frequently with

**peritonsillar or parapharyngeal infection.** On examination, neck lymphadenopathy is noted more often in patients with peritonsillar or parapharyngeal abscess. Peritonsillar or soft palatal swelling is more prominent with peritonsillar abscess. A patient who **passively refuses to move the neck secondary to pain is likely to have retropharyngeal infection.**

Imaging in the patient with suspected neck abscess starts with a **lateral cervical x-ray.** Radiographic evidence for retropharyngeal abscess on a lateral film includes widening of the retropharyngeal space. Findings on a lateral film in a patient with sore throat and fever may lead to an alternative diagnosis, as in the patient with epiglottic edema and **classic "thumb sign" in epiglottitis.** Cervical CT imaging is an excellent study for determining whether a patient has only cellulitis and edema surrounding a space or hypodensity and rim enhancement consistent with an abscess. It also delineates whether there has been extension to contiguous structures. An MRI is an alternative when there is a concern for infection involving a compartment with neurovascular elements and more accurate visualization is desired.

Specific neck space infections have specific complications. **Retropharyngeal infection** has the **potential for spread to the mediastinum**, where impact on cardiorespiratory function or mediastinitis could develop; **parapharyngeal infection** can ultimately **impact on neurovascular elements in the lateral space**, either because of erosion or mass effect. An infection in one compartment can always spread to another. Infections involving the teeth, ears, and sinuses may spread to the parapharyngeal space, and lymph chains draining the sinuses and oropharynx can seed the retropharyngeal space. Generally, a neck abscess results when there is contiguous spread of bacteria in a patient with pharyngitis, odontogenic infection, otitis, mastoiditis, sinusitis, or other head and neck infection.

Bacterial etiologies for neck abscess include *Streptococcus pyogenes*, *Staphylococcus* sp, *Hemophilus influenzae*, *Peptostreptococcus*, *Bacteroides*, and *Fusobacterium* sp. Polymicrobial infection is typically seen, often reflective of the organisms most commonly found in infections involving the oropharynx, ear, or sinuses.

Viral etiologies include EBV, cytomegalovirus, adenovirus, and rhinovirus and may present similarly to bacterial infection. Viruses can present with oropharyngeal exudate and swelling or neck masses in the form of lymphadenopathy. A viral process usually can be differentiated from a more concerning bacterial process by ancillary testing previously described and taking into consideration symptomatology more frequently seen in viremia. For example, an exudative pharyngitis with neck findings, rhinorrhea, and cough is more consistent with viral infection.

Standard therapies include intravenous penicillins, third-generation cephalosporins, or carbapenems. Clindamycin or metronidazole is added if anaerobes are suspected and broad coverage is desired. Clindamycin often is a good choice for monotherapy in the patient with penicillin allergy. Broad-spectrum antibiotics are started in the patient with neck abscess, with treatment modification if an organism is identified from oropharyngeal or surgical samples. Ultimately, pediatricians and surgeons determine whether to pursue a "watchful waiting" approach with a patient taking antibiotics or to proceed quickly with needle aspiration or incision and drainage based on infection extent, current impact on surrounding structures, and expectations for progression.

Other abnormalities, unrelated to deep neck infection, also can cause sore throat, odynophagia, or swelling and pain of the oropharynx or neck. They include anatomic variants such as thyroglossal duct cyst or second branchial cleft cyst. Arising from vestigial structures, these cysts can become secondarily infected and develop overlying tenderness and erythema that might be confused with deeper infection. Thyroiditis and sialadenitis also present with fairly localized neck findings. Depending on location, one also should consider thyroid nodule, goiter, or salivary gland tumor, particularly in the case of an initially nontender mass that grows slowly.

## Comprehension Questions

46.1 A mother notices a lump on her 5-year-old son's neck. He complains about pain in the region and difficulty swallowing. Appetite and intake are normal. He had a "chest cold" last week that has since resolved. His past medical history is otherwise unremarkable. On examination, he is afebrile with a 3-cm × 3-cm area of mild erythema, fluctuance, and tenderness of the central anterior neck. The mass moves superiorly when he opens his mouth. His oropharynx is clear. Which of the following is the most likely explanation for these findings?

A. Contact dermatitis
B. Lymphadenopathy
C. Salivary gland tumor
D. Streptococcal pharyngitis
E. Thyroglossal duct cyst

46.2 A 9-year-old girl complains of sore throat and anterior neck pain of 1-day duration, and nasal congestion and cough over the past 3 days. There has been no nausea or change in appetite. She describes "lumps growing in her neck" over the past day. Her past medical history is unremarkable. She is afebrile with a clear posterior oropharynx and a supple neck. She has four firm, fixed, and minimally tender submandibular masses without overlying skin changes; the largest mass is 1 cm in diameter. Which of the following is the most likely explanation for these findings?

A. Lymphadenopathy
B. Peritonsillar abscess
C. Retropharyngeal abscess
D. Sialadenitis
E. Streptococcal pharyngitis

46.3 A father states that his 7-year-old daughter has a 1-week history of mouth and neck pain. She describes pain on chewing and swallowing. Slight swelling around her right, lower jaw was first noted yesterday. She has been afebrile and exhibits no URI symptoms. Her examination reveals a temperature of 100.2°F (37.9°C) with swelling, tenderness, and warmth overlying the right, posterior mandible without fluctuance or skin changes. Scattered, bilateral neck lymphadenopathy is appreciated. Her posterior oropharynx is minimally erythematous, with marked swelling and tenderness of the gum surrounding the posterior molars of the right mandible. Which of the following is the most appropriate next step?

A. Admit her immediately to the hospital for intravenous antibiotics.
B. Commence a broad-spectrum antibiotic and advise her to see a dentist as soon as possible.
C. Obtain an immediate surgery consult.
D. Order a cervical CT and obtain ear, nose, and throat (ENT) consultation today.
E. Perform a rapid strep immunoassay in your office.

46.4 A previously healthy, 4-year-old boy has been febrile for 1 day. He does not want to drink and vomited this morning. There have been no URI symptoms nor diarrhea. On examination, he is sleepy, but arousable, and has a temperature of 102.8°F (39.3°C). His posterior oropharynx is markedly erythematous with enlarged, symmetrical, and cryptic tonsils that are laden with exudate. Shoddy cervical lymphadenopathy is noted. He moves his head vigorously in an effort to thwart your examination. Which of the following is the most likely explanation for these findings?

A. Coxsackie pharyngitis
B. Lymphadenitis
C. Parapharyngeal abscess
D. Retropharyngeal abscess
E. Streptococcal tonsillitis

## ANSWERS

46.1 **E.** Thyroglossal duct cysts, arising from the embryonic thyroglossal tract, are typically midline, often move on tongue protrusion, and often are noted after a URI. Treatment is usually surgical excision, sometimes after neck CT imaging to ascertain cyst and thyroid anatomy. About half can become infected. Contact dermatitis does not present as a mass, lymphadenopathy is rarely associated with fluctuance or movement on tongue protrusion, and the oropharyngeal and neck findings make streptococcal pharyngitis and salivary gland tumor unlikely.

46.2 **A.** This patient has viral URI symptoms, most likely causing reactive lymphadenopathy. Supportive care such as analgesics would be a reasonable treatment recommendation. Rapid streptococcal testing usually is not warranted for classic URI symptoms; streptococcal pharyngitis more commonly presents with sore throat, headache, nausea, and/or fever. Signs of viremia and her neck examination do not suggest sialadenitis or neck abscess.

46.3 **B.** Tooth abscess is her most likely diagnosis, as evidenced by obvious gingival inflammation and other signs of ongoing infection in the area, despite the absence of frank pus from an evident cavity. Potential causative organisms include *Streptococcus mutans* and *Fusobacterium nucleatum*. Therapy includes an antibiotic (amoxicillin or clindamycin) and referral to her dentist within the next 24 hours. Deep neck infection is unlikely; imaging and IV antibiotics are not warranted at this time.

46.4 **E.** This child has a fairly classic examination for streptococcal tonsillitis. Coxsackievirus is possible, but usually an ulcerative, rather than exudative, pharyngitis is noted. The potential for a retropharyngeal or peritonsillar process is diminished by the lack of tonsillar asymmetry, soft palatal changes, and nuchal rigidity. A rapid streptococcal immunoassay would be a good initial test; a swab for culture may be sent as well. Standard therapy would include oral or intramuscular penicillin in the nonallergic patient and an analgesic/antipyretic. If the streptococcal immunoassay is negative, some treat patients whose history and examination are consistent with streptococcal infection while awaiting culture.

## Clinical Pearls

- Infections involving specific compartments of the neck have specific complications, such as the potential for mediastinitis in the patient with retropharyngeal abscess.
- Multiple bacterial and viral etiologies, including GAS and Epstein Barr virus (EBV), are possible in the patient with constitutional symptoms and neck findings. Extension of these infections into cervical compartments may endanger surrounding vital structures and potentially require surgery.
- Various head and neck abnormalities (infected thyroglossal duct cyst or extensive reactive lymphadenopathy) may mimic deep neck infection.

## REFERENCES

Inkelis SH. Disorders of the pharynx. In: Osborn LM, DeWitt TG, First LR, Zenel JA, eds. *Pediatrics*. Philadelphia, PA: Elsevier Mosby; 2005:460-470.

Milczuk H. Disorders of the neck and salivary glands. In: Osborn LM, DeWitt TG, First LA, Zenel JA, eds. *Pediatrics*. Philadelphia, PA: Elsevier Mosby; 2005:471-479.

Pappas DE, Hendley JO. Retropharyngeal abscess, lateral pharyngeal (parapharyngeal) abscess, and peritonsillar cellulitis/abscess. In: Kliegman RM, Behrman RE, Jenson HB, Stanton BF, eds. *Nelson Textbook of Pediatrics*. 18th ed. Philadelphia, PA: WB Saunders; 2007:1754-1758.

Weed HG, Forest LA. Deep neck infection. In: Cummings CW, Flint PW, Haughey BH, Robbins KT, Thomas JR, Harker LA, Richardson MA, Schuller DE, eds. *Otolaryngology: Head and Neck Surgery*. 4th ed. Philadelphia, PA: Elsevier-Mosby; 2005:2515-2524.

# Case 47

A term 3700-g male infant is born vaginally to a 27-year-old gravida 2 mother following an uncomplicated pregnancy. Shortly after birth, he begins to cough, followed by a choking episode, difficulty handling secretions, and cyanosis. During the resuscitation, placement of an orogastric tube meets resistance at 10 cm. He is transferred to the level II nursery for evaluation and management of respiratory distress.

- What is the most likely diagnosis?
- What is the best test for evaluation?

# ANSWERS TO CASE 47: Esophageal Atresia

*Summary*: A newborn with cough, choking, cyanosis, and inability to undergo passage of an orogastric tube.

- **Most likely diagnosis:** Esophageal atresia, probably with a tracheoesophageal fistula (TEF).
- **Best test for diagnosis:** A chest and abdomen radiograph with the orogastric tube in place will demonstrate a coiled tube in the esophageal blind pouch.

## ANALYSIS

### Objectives

1. Become familiar with the presentation TEF.
2. Understand the anatomic variants of TEF.
3. Understand emergency management of newborns with TEF.

### Considerations

In this newborn with choking and coughing, esophageal atresia is suspected when an orogastric tube does not pass. Infants with esophageal atresia cannot handle oral secretions and require constant esophageal pouch drainage to prevent aspiration. They are monitored in the neonatal intensive care unit while awaiting surgical intervention.

# APPROACH TO Esophageal Atresia

## DEFINITIONS

**ASSOCIATION:** Sporadic occurrence of two or more clinical features occurring together more commonly than would be expected, but without an identifiable cause.

**POLYHYDRAMNIOS:** Diagnosis of an increased amount of amniotic fluid.

**SYNDROME:** A constellation of features having a common cause (such as the features of Down syndrome being caused by a trisomy 21).

## CLINICAL APPROACH

**Esophageal atresia** occurs in 1 in 4000 live births, usually accompanied by **TEF**. **Polyhydramnios**, which is also seen in duodenal atresia, is a common pregnancy complication seen with TEF. Five different TEF anatomic variants occur; the most common (87%) includes proximal atresia (esophageal pouch) with a distal fistula (Figure 47–1).

Infants with TEF usually present in the newborn period with excessive oral secretions and coughing, choking, and cyanosis secondary to aspirated

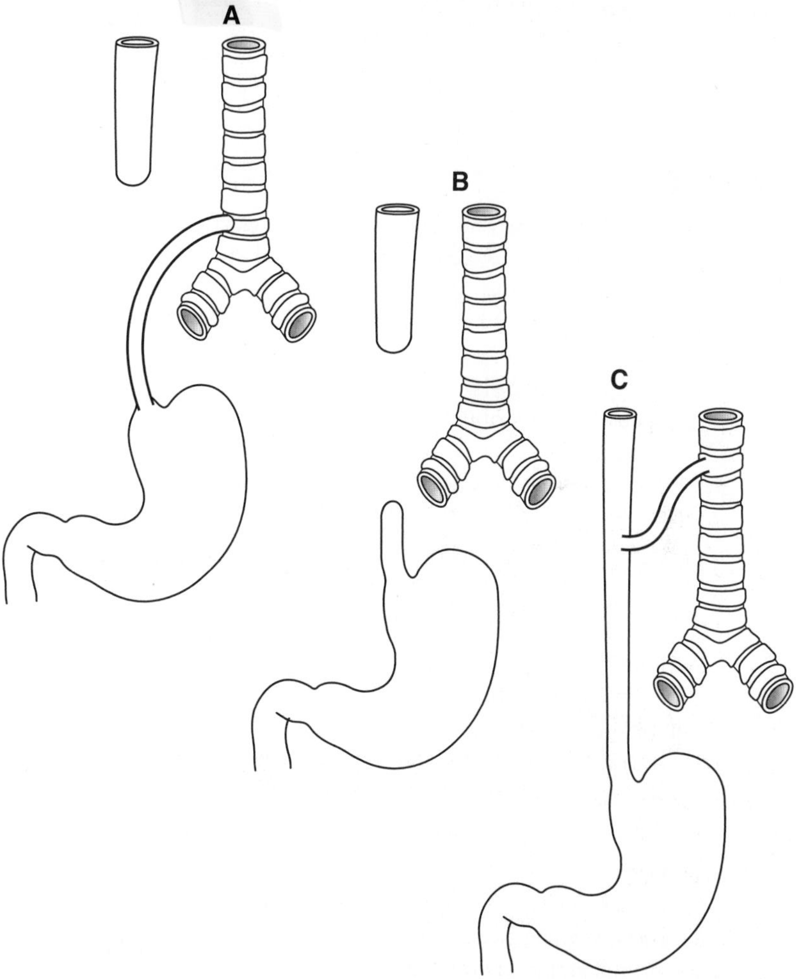


**Figure 47–1.** Types of esophageal atresia/tracheoesophageal fistula. **A.** Proximal esophageal atresia with distal fistula (80-90%). **B.** Esophageal atresia (10%). **C.** H-type tracheoesophageal fistula (3%).

secretions or with initial feeds. Infants with the **"H-type" fistula** (approximately 4% of cases) often present later in life with recurrent aspiration pneumonia or feeding difficulty. Other congenital anomalies occur in approximately 30% to 50% of TEF patients, and a search for them is undertaken. The most common association is the **VATER association** (vertebral abnormality, anal imperforation, tracheoesophageal fistula, radial and renal anomaly).

Neonates with TEF or esophageal atresia are at risk for respiratory compromise due to aspiration. The esophageal pouch requires constant suctioning while awaiting surgery to ligate the fistula and anastomose the esophagus. Staged surgery is required if anatomic conditions preclude primary anastomosis. Postsurgical esophageal dysmotility may persist; chronic gastroesophageal reflux is common.

## Comprehension Questions

47.1 A 2-hour-old term newborn male has coughing, choking, and cyanosis prior to feeding. A nasogastric tube is placed and meets resistance at 10 cm. Prenatal history is significant for polyhydramnios. Which of the following is most likely to be found in this infant?

A. Congenital cataracts
B. Gingival hyperplasia
C. Hepatosplenomegaly
D. Microcephaly
E. Fusion of two lower thoracic vertebral bodies

47.2 An infant with a history of recurrent pneumonia is diagnosed with TEF at 8 months of age. Which of the following statements is correct?

A. The infant most likely has a "H-type" TEF.
B. The infant most likely has proximal esophageal atresia with distal fistula.
C. The infant likely has a previously undetected, associated finding of imperforate anus.
D. The infant is unlikely to have gastroesophageal reflux.
E. The infant is likely to have cystic fibrosis.

47.3 A 2-year-old girl with a history of esophageal atresia and a ventricular septal defect is hospitalized with *Pneumocystis carinii* pneumonia. Her immunodeficiency is likely a result of which of the following?

A. Bruton agammaglobulinemia
B. Chronic granulomatous disease
C. DiGeorge syndrome
D. Hyperimmunoglobulin E syndrome
E. Severe combined immunodeficiency syndrome

47.4 A 2-year-old boy, living with new foster parents for 3 weeks, has become progressively short of breath. When he first arrived at their home, he was active and playful, but now he is too tired to play. They have few details, but they know that he had neonatal surgery for a problem with his "esophagus being connected to his lungs" and that he takes no medications. On examination, he is afebrile, diaphoretic, tachycardic, and tachypneic. His symptoms can most likely be attributed to which of the following?

A. Adjustment disorder
B. Heart failure secondary to ventricular septal defect
C. Kawasaki disease
D. Reactive airway disease
E. Rheumatic heart disease

## ANSWERS

47.1 **E.** The infant probably has esophageal atresia. VATER association, as described in the case, can have vertebral anomalies such as fused or bifid vertebral bodies. None of the other findings listed is commonly associated with VATER.

47.2 **A.** This infant likely has an H-type TEF, found later in infancy with recurrent pneumonias and/or feeding difficulty. Patients with esophageal atresia and distal fistula present in the first hours of life because of their inability to swallow oropharyngeal secretions. Infants with imperforate anus also present as neonates. All patients with TEF are at high risk for gastroesophageal reflux.

47.3 **C.** DiGeorge syndrome (thymic hypoplasia) results from abnormal third and fourth pharyngeal pouch formation during fetal development. Neighboring structures formed during the same fetal growth period are often affected. Associated conditions include anomalies of the great vessels, esophageal atresia, bifid uvula, congenital heart disease, short philtrum, hypertelorism, antimongoloid slant palpebrae, mandibular hypoplasia, and low-set, notched ears. DiGeorge syndrome may present in neonates as hypocalcemic seizures because of parathyroid hypoplasia.

47.4 **B.** This child likely had undergone TEF repair and has associated congenital heart disease with heart failure symptoms.

## Clinical Pearls

- VATER association—vertebral (abnormality), anal (imperforation), tracheoesophageal (fistula), radial and renal (anomaly)—is often seen in patients with tracheoesophageal fistula.
- Esophageal atresia is associated with DiGeorge syndrome.
- The H-type tracheoesophageal fistula often presents later in infancy as recurrent pneumonitis and can be difficult to diagnose.

## REFERENCES

Cox JA, Rudolph CD. Anatomic disorders of the esophagus. In: Rudolph CD, Rudolph AM, Hostetter MK, Lister G, Siegel NJ, eds. *Rudolph's Pediatrics*. 21st ed. New York, NY: McGraw-Hill; 2003:1385-1388.

McEvoy CF. Developmental disorders of gastrointestinal function. In: McMillan JA, Feigin RD, DeAngelis CD, Jones MD, eds. *Oski's Pediatrics: Principles and Practice*. 4th ed. Philadelphia, PA: Lippincott Williams & Wilkins; 2006:369-370.

Orenstein S, Peters J, Khan S, Youssef N, Hussain Z. Congenital anomalies: esophageal atresia and tracheoesophageal fistula In: Kliegman RM, Behrman RE, Jenson HB, Stanton BF, eds. *Nelson Textbook of Pediatrics*. 18th ed. Philadelphia, PA: WB Saunders; 2007:1543-1544.

# Case 48

A term male is born at 38 weeks via a scheduled repeat cesarean section prior to the onset of labor. The infant's mother had good prenatal care including vaginal cultures negative for group B *Streptococcus*. At the delivery, the amniotic fluid was clear and was not foul-smelling. Apgar scores are 8 and 8 at 1 and 5 minutes, respectively. Within the first hour of birth, he has tachypnea, nasal flaring, and mild retractions. Chest auscultation reveals good air movement bilaterally; a few rales are noted.

➤ What is the most likely diagnosis?

➤ What is the best management for this condition?

# ANSWERS TO CASE 48:
# Transient Tachypnea of the Newborn

*Summary:* A term newborn born by cesarean section has respiratory distress.

- **Most likely diagnosis:** Transient tachypnea of the newborn (TTN).
- **Treatment:** Supportive care including supplemental oxygen, if necessary.

## ANALYSIS

### Objectives

1. Know the presentation of TTN.
2. Understand the medical care for TTN.

### Considerations

This infant presents soon after birth with mild respiratory distress following an uneventful pregnancy and delivery. Evaluation of this infant begins with auscultation of the lungs and heart.

# APPROACH TO
# Transient Tachypnea of the Newborn

## DEFINITIONS

**TRANSIENT TACHYPNEA OF THE NEWBORN:** Slow absorption of fetal lung fluid with resultant tachypnea. The condition more commonly is associated with cesarean section deliveries.

**MECONIUM ASPIRATION SYNDROME:** Aspiration of meconium during delivery resulting in respiratory distress. Radiographic findings include hyperinflation with patchy infiltrates. As meconium may plug small airways, areas of air trapping are often present and may lead to the development of pneumothorax.

**RESPIRATORY DISTRESS SYNDROME:** A condition seen in premature infants resulting from surfactant deficiency. Radiographic findings include a characteristic reticulonodular "ground glass" pattern with air bronchograms and decreased aeration.

**CONGENITAL DIAPHRAGMATIC HERNIA (CDH):** The condition of herniation of abdominal contents through the posterolateral foramen of Bochdalek into the thoracic cavity. The incidence is approximately 1 in 5000 live births.

**EXTRACORPOREAL MEMBRANE OXYGENATION (ECMO):** A system using a modified heart-lung machine utilized in severe pulmonary failure. Cannulation of the carotid artery and jugular vein is required to link the neonate to the system.

## CLINICAL APPROACH

Transient tachypnea of the newborn is a self-limited condition usually occurring in a **term infant** after an uneventful cesarean section (more commonly) or vaginal birth. It is felt to be caused by slow absorption of fetal lung fluid. Infants with TTN develop respiratory distress shortly after birth with tachypnea, mild retractions, nasal flaring, and in more severe cases grunting and cyanosis. Chest radiography reveals **perihilar streaking and fluid in the fissures**; lungs are aerated. Most infants with TTN have resolution of their tachypnea in 24 to 48 hours.

For a few infants with TTN, oxygen saturations drop and supplemental oxygen is required; rarely does the oxygen requirement exceed 40%. In the rare, more severe case of TTN consideration for ongoing increased pulmonary vascular resistance leading to persistent pulmonary hypertension must be entertained. Infants with TTN do not require antimicrobial therapy; failure of the infant to follow the expected 24 to 48 hours of mild respiratory distress indicates the need to evaluate the child for more serious pathology.

Infants with **respiratory distress syndrome (RDS)** are usually born prematurely (less than 34 weeks gestational age); these infants have a deficiency of surfactant. Shortly after birth they present with symptoms of respiratory distress including poor oxygenation, grunting, retracting, and poor air movement. Radiographically they have findings including a reticulonodular pattern with air bronchograms and decreased aeration of the lungs. Supportive care includes supplemental oxygen as needed to maintain oxygen saturation of 90% to 95% and intravenous fluids or nasogastric feeding to maintain hydration as the degree of tachypnea usually precludes oral feeding. Exogenous surfactant is available and is administered by the resuscitation team in an effort to ameliorate the effects of surfactant deficiency.

## Comprehension Questions

48.1 A term male is born to a 33-year-old woman who had little prenatal care. Immediately after birth he has cyanosis and respiratory distress. Chest auscultation in the delivery room reveals right-sided heart sounds and absent left-sided breath sounds. Which of the following is the most appropriate next step?

A. Assess the abdomen to evaluate for possible congenital diaphragmatic hernia.
B. Order a computerized tomography of the chest.
C. Order ultrasonography of the chest.
D. Perform a needle thoracostomy for possible pneumothorax.
E. Prepare the infant for ECMO.

48.2 A term female is born via repeat cesarean section to a 30-year-old woman. Immediately after birth she has mild respiratory distress. Chest auscultation in the delivery room reveals clear breath sounds. Which of the following is the most appropriate next step?

A. Endotracheal intubation with direct suction.
B. Begin intravenous antibiotic therapy.
C. Deliver surfactant therapy.
D. Observe and administer supplemental oxygen as needed.
E. Bag-and-mask ventilation.

48.3 A term male is born vaginally to a 22-year-old primigravida woman; the pregnancy was uncomplicated. Just prior to delivery, fetal bradycardia was noted, and at delivery thick meconium is found. The infant has hypotonia and bradycardia. Which of the following is the first step in resuscitation?

A. Administration of epinephrine via endotracheal tube
B. Bag-and-mask ventilation
C. Endotracheal intubation with direct suction
D. Oxygen delivered by cannula in close proximity to the nares
E. Tracheostomy

48.4 After the infant discussed in Question 48.3 is stabilized and admitted to the neonatal intensive care unit, a chest radiograph reveals bilateral patchy infiltrates with coarse streaking and flattening of the diaphragm. He abruptly has an increased oxygen requirement. Physical examination reveals decreased right-sided breath sounds. Which of the following is an accurate statement?

A. High positive end-expiratory pressure (PEEP) is useful in this condition.
B. Needle thoracostomy is contraindicated.
C. Chest radiography is likely to reveal CDH.
D. The infant is likely to have hyperresonance of the chest on the left side.
E. Transillumination of the chest is likely to transmit excessive light on the right side.

## ANSWERS

48.1 **A.** Evaluation of neonates born with respiratory distress and unilateral breath sounds includes an abdominal examination. With asymmetrical breath sounds, pneumothorax and CDH are considered. This infant's scaphoid abdomen suggests CDH; needle thoracostomy is avoided because intestinal perforation may occur. The patient is stabilized and the need for ECMO is ascertained after the infant's initial therapy response is evaluated.

48.2 **D.** As this infant most likely has TTN the next step is to observe and administer supplemental oxygen as needed.

48.3 **C.** Endotracheal intubation with direct suction is performed in a depressed infant with thick meconium noted at delivery. Bag-and-mask ventilation or endotracheal intubation without suction may increase the volume of meconium aspirated.

48.4 **E.** This infant likely has a right-sided pneumothorax; excessive light transmission by transillumination and right-sided hyperresonance with auscultation are expected. Infants with meconium aspiration and respiratory distress are at higher risk for pneumothorax, especially if high PEEP is used for oxygenation. A chest tube for the pneumothorax may be needed. Infants with severe respiratory distress or circulatory involvement may require emergent needle aspiration.

## Clinical Pearls

- Transient tachypnea of the newborn (TTN) is associated with birth by cesarean section.
- TTN is managed with supportive care and does not lead to chronic lung disease.

## REFERENCES

Bland RD. Persistent postnatal pulmonary edema (transient tachypnea of the newborn). In: Rudolph CD, Rudolph AM, Hostetter MK, Lister G, Siegel NJ, eds. *Rudolph's Pediatrics*. 21st ed. New York, NY: McGraw-Hill; 2003:179-181.

Dudell GG, Stol BJ. The respiratory tract. In: Kliegman RM, Behrman RE, Jenson HB, Stanton BF, eds. *Nelson Textbook of Pediatrics*. 18th ed. Philadelphia, PA: WB Saunders; 2007:731-741.

Gross I. Meconium aspiration syndrome. McMillan JA, Feigin RD, DeAngelis CD, Jones MD, eds. *Oski's Pediatrics: Principles and Practice*. 4th ed. Philadelphia, PA: Lippincott Williams & Wilkins; 2006:315.

Gross I. Transient tachypnea of the newborn. McMillan JA, Feigin RD, DeAngelis CD, Jones MD, eds. *Oski's Pediatrics: Principles and Practice*. 4th ed. Philadelphia, PA: Lippincott Williams & Wilkins; 2006:311.

# Case 49

A full-term 1-week-old boy presents with bilious vomiting and lethargy. His mother notes a normal prenatal course and uncomplicated delivery. On physical examination he is noted to have significant abdominal distension and blood in his diaper.

- What is the most likely diagnosis?
- What is the best management for this condition?

# ANSWERS TO CASE 49:
## Malrotation

*Summary:* A full-term 1-week-old boy presents with bilious vomiting and lethargy. He is noted to have significant abdominal distension and blood in his diaper.

- **Most likely diagnosis:** Malrotation with volvulus.
- **Best treatment:** Surgical intervention to remove any necrotic bowel and to ensure adequate blood supply to surviving intestine.

## ANALYSIS

### Objectives

1. Know the presentation of malrotation with volvulus.
2. Understand the treatment of malrotation.
3. Be familiar with the differential diagnosis of acute abdominal pain in children.

### Considerations

In this neonate with bilious emesis, a variety of etiologies are possible (Table 49–1). The clues to the diagnosis are bilious emesis due to intestinal obstruction, abdominal distension, blood per rectum, and lethargy. The most important next step is surgical intervention to prevent death and loss of viable intestine.

**Table 49–1 COMMON ETIOLOGIES OF ACUTE ABDOMINAL PAIN IN INFANTS AND YOUNG CHILDREN**

| CONDITION | SIGNS AND SYMPTOMS |
|---|---|
| Abdominal migraines | Recurrent abdominal pain with emesis |
| Appendicitis | Right lower quadrant pain, abdominal guarding, and rebound tenderness |
| Bacterial enterocolitis | Diarrhea (may be bloody), fever vomiting |
| Cholecystitis | Right upper quadrant pain |
| Diabetes mellitus | History of polydipsia, polyuria, and weight loss |
| Henoch-Schönlein purpura | Purpuric lesions, joint pain, blood in urine, and guaiac positive stools |
| Hepatitis | Right upper quadrant pain and jaundice |
| Incarcerated hernia (inguinal) | Inguinal mass, lower, abdominal or groin pain, emesis |
| Intussusception | Colicky abdominal pain and currant jelly stools |
| Malrotation (with volvulus) | Abdominal distention, bilious vomiting, blood per rectum, usually presents in infancy |
| Nephrolithiasis | Hematuria, colicky abdominal pain |
| Pancreatitis | (Severe) epigastric abdominal pain, fever, and persistent vomiting |
| Pneumonia | Fever, cough, rales on auscultation of the chest |
| Small-bowel obstruction | Emesis, frequent history of prior abdominal surgery |
| Streptococcal pharyngitis | Fever, sore throat, headache |
| Testicular torsion | Testicular pain and edema |
| Urinary tract infection | Fever, vomiting, and diarrhea in infants; back pain in older children |

# APPROACH TO
## Malrotation

### DEFINITIONS

**VOLVULUS:** Twisting of the mesentery of the small intestine leading to decreased vascular perfusion which results in ischemia and ultimately bowel necrosis.

**INTUSSUSCEPTION:** A condition in which a proximal portion of the gastrointestinal tract telescopes into an adjacent distal portion. The most common location is ileocolic portion of the bowel.

### CLINICAL APPROACH

**Malrotation occurs when intestinal rotation is incomplete during fetal development.** During normal fetal development in the first-trimester, the growing intestine exits the abdominal cavity, elongates, and ultimately rotates 270° in a counterclockwise manner before returning into the abdomen. Following normal intestinal rotation, the duodenojejunal junction (ligament of Treitz) is fixed to the posterior body wall to the left of the spine. In cases of malrotation, the ligament of Treitz is located on the right side and the intestine may use the small portion of attached mesentery as axis to turn (volvulus) leading to ischemia and possible necrosis.

Although individuals with intestinal malrotation may present from birth to adulthood, the classic presentation is that of an infant with bilious vomiting due to intestinal obstruction. With prolonged ischemia the bowel becomes necrotic and the patient may have melena or hematemesis, and may develop peritonitis, acidosis, and sepsis. Without surgical intervention, risk of mortality is significant. Patients with malrotation and either partial or intermittent volvulus may present with recurrent abdominal pain or lymphatic congestion leading to failure to thrive because of malabsorption or chylous ascites. Individuals may also have asymptomatic malrotation as an incidental finding.

Abdominal radiographs may be normal or have nonspecific findings in cases of volvulus, thus an upper gastrointestinal contrast series is generally indicated. The characteristic finding in cases of volvulus is a "corkscrew" pattern of the duodenum or "bird's beak" of the second or third portions of the duodenum. In cases of malrotation with or without volvulus, abnormal position (right sided) of the ligament of Trietz or malposition of the colon may be noted with contrast radiography.

Prior to **emergent** surgical intervention, the initial management of patients with malrotation and volvulus includes appropriate evaluation of fluid status as patients may have significant fluid loss with electrolyte abnormalities.

Placement of a nasogastric tube to aid gastrointestinal decompression, and initiation of parenteral antibiotic, in order to address potential sepsis are indicated. Exploratory laporotomy is performed and bowel viability assessed. Areas of necrotic bowel are removed and Ladd procedure of disengaging bowel with anomalous fixation and appendectomy are performed. Complications include short gut syndrome if a significant portion of necrotic bowel is removed and adhesions may develop leading to obstruction. Patients with volvulus have a mortality rate of 5% to 10%. Because of the significant mortality and morbidity associated with volvulus, asymptomatic patients with malrotation require surgical intervention.

## Comprehension Questions

49.1 Malrotation with volvulus is most likely to be present in which of the following patients?

A. A healthy 15-month-old with severe paroxysmal abdominal pain and vomiting
B. A 15-year-old sexually active girl with lower abdominal pain
C. A 3-day-old term infant with bilious emesis, lethargy, and abdominal distension
D. A 4-day-old premature baby (33-week gestation) who has recently started nasogastric feeds; he now has abdominal distention, bloody stools, and thrombocytopenia
E. A 7-year-old girl with abdominal pain, vomiting, fever, and diarrhea

49.2 A 3-day-old boy presents with 12 hours of bilious vomiting, abdominal pain, and abdominal distension. Which of the following is the most appropriate next step in management?

A. Order an abdominal ultrasonography.
B. Order a computerized tomography scan of the abdomen.
C. Order a upper GI contrast series.
D. Order a barium enema.
E. Order a chest radiograph.

49.3 A 9-year-old boy has 24 hours of persistent abdominal pain and vomiting. His physical examination reveals abdominal guarding and right lower quadrant rebound tenderness. Which of the following is the most likely diagnosis?

A. Appendicitis
B. Gastroenteritis
C. Gastroesophageal reflux
D. Intussusception
E. Pyloric stenosis

49.4 A previously healthy 18-month-old child has vomiting and severe, paroxysmal, writhing abdominal pain (he prefers to have his knees flexed to the chest) alternating with periods of relative comfort with a soft, only mildly tender abdomen. On abdominal examination you find a sausagelike mass. He has not stooled, but you find blood upon digital rectal examination. Which of the following is the best next step in management?

A. Administer morphine for pain control.
B. Order a computerized tomography of the abdomen.
C. Obtain an air contrast enema.
D. Obtain serum acetaminophen levels.
E. Begin antibiotics for *Escherichia coli* 0157:H7.

49.5 A 6-week-old male infant has projectile emesis after feeding. He has an olive-shaped abdominal mass on abdominal examination. Which of the following statements is accurate?

A. He likely has hypochloremic metabolic alkalosis.
B. He likely has metabolic acidosis.
C. This condition is more common in female infants.
D. He should be restarted on feeds when the vomiting resolves.
E. He likely will develop diarrhea.

## ANSWERS

49.1 **C.** The 3-day-old term infant with bilious emesis and abdominal distension has classic presenting features of malrotation with volvulus. The 15-month-old child with paroxysmal abdominal pain is most likely to have intussusception. The adolescent female is evaluated for ectopic pregnancy, pelvic inflammatory disease, appendicitis, ovarian torsion, and ruptured ovarian cyst. The premature infant might have necrotizing enterocolitis, whereas the 7-year-old girl more likely has gastroenteritis.

49.2 **C.** Order a upper GI contrast series. Fluid and electrolyte status should also be evaluated.

49.3 **A.** This child most likely has appendicitis.

49.4 **C.** The case describes the typical presentation of intussusception. Although a clinical diagnosis can be made, the diagnostic "gold" standard and often treatment, is contrast enema. Air contrast usually is preferred because the complication risk is lower than with other forms of contrast material. Prior to diagnostic intervention, patients should undergo measurement of serum electrolyte and hemoglobin levels and receive fluid resuscitation. When suspicion for intussusception is high, a pediatric surgeon should be consulted. Classically described "currant jelly stools" are a late finding. Recurrence of intussusception following successful reduction occurs in 5% to 10% of cases.

49.5 **A.** This infant has the features of pyloric stenosis, a condition four times more common in males and more common in first-born children. Affected infants usually present between the third and eighth week of life with increasing projectile emesis. Abdominal examination may reveal an olive-shaped mass and visible peristaltic waves. Serum electrolyte levels usually reveal hypochloremic metabolic alkalosis. Ultrasonography is useful in confirming the diagnosis.

## Clinical Pearls

- Treatment of malrotation with volvulus includes emergent surgical intervention.
- Classic features of intussusception are fever, intermittent colicky abdominal pain, currant jelly stools, and a sausagelike abdominal mass.
- Classic features of pyloric stenosis include projectile vomiting, an olive-shaped abdominal mass, and hypochloremic metabolic alkalosis.

## REFERENCES

Azizkhan RG, Frykman PK. Anomalies of intestinal rotation. In: Rudolph CD, Rudolph AM, Hostetter MK, Lister G, Siegel NJ, eds. *Rudolph's Pediatrics*. 21st ed. New York, NY: McGraw-Hill; 2003:1400-1402.

Brandt ML. Intussusception. In: McMillan JA, Feigin RD, DeAngelis CD, Jones MD, eds. *Oski's Pediatrics: Principles and Practice*. 4th ed. Philadelphia, PA: Lippincott Williams & Wilkins; 2006:1938-1940.

McEvoy CF. Developmental disorders of gastrointestinal function. In: McMillan JA, Feigin RD, DeAngelis CD, Jones MD, eds. *Oski's Pediatrics: Principles and Practice*. 4th ed. Philadelphia, PA: Lippincott Williams & Wilkins; 2006:371-375.

Ryckman FC. Approach to the child with gastrointestinal obstruction. In: Rudolph CD, Rudolph AM, Hostetter MK, Lister G, Siegel NJ, eds. *Rudolph's Pediatrics*. 21st ed. New York, NY: McGraw-Hill; 2003:1376-1379.

Wyllie R. Stomach and intestines. In: Kliegman RM, Behrman RE, Jenson HB, Stanton BF, eds. *Nelson Textbook of Pediatrics*. 18th ed. Philadelphia, PA: WB Saunders; 2007:1554-1564.

# Case 50

A 13-year-old girl complains about "zits" on her face and shoulders. She has tried over-the-counter benzoyl peroxide to no avail, and has stopped eating chocolate and french fries on her mother's advice. She has been invited to an upcoming school dance and wants to look her best. She complains about blackheads, but also lesions that are deep and painful.

- What is the diagnosis?
- What is the best treatment for her condition?

# ANSWERS TO CASE 50: Acne Vulgaris

*Summary:* An adolescent girl presents with acne on her face and shoulders.

- **Most likely diagnosis:** Combination acne.
- **Best therapy:** First-line therapy includes antibacterial soap, keratolytic agent (benzoyl peroxide), comedolytic agent (tretinoin), or topical antibiotic (erythromycin). Oral antibiotics (tetracycline) are a secondary option. Isotretinoin (Accutane) is reserved for severe, resistant nodulocystic acne.

## ANALYSIS

### Objectives

1. Understand the various types of acne vulgaris.
2. Know the treatments for various types of acne.
3. Discuss the potential side effects of isotretinoin (Accutane).

### Considerations

Acne vulgaris has the potential to be as damaging to the psyche as it can be to the skin. Managing acne successfully involves promoting patient understanding of the basics behind its development, creating thoughtful treatment regimens tailored to each patient, and periodically reassessing acne control in an effort to prevent possible emotional and physical scarring.

# APPROACH TO Acne Vulgaris

## DEFINITIONS

**COMEDONES:** Open comedones (blackheads) are composed of compacted melanocytes; closed comedones (whiteheads) contain purulent debris.

**CYST:** Dilated and often tender intradermal follicle.

**INFLAMMATORY PAPULE:** Red "bump" under the skin due to sebum, fatty acids, and bacteria reacting within a follicle.

**PUSTULE:** Inflammation and exudate around comedones occurring in the superficial dermis.

## CLINICAL APPROACH

**Pubertal hormonal surges lead to an increase in sebum production by sebaceous glands.** Proliferation of the bacterium *Propionibacterium acnes* leads to distention of follicular walls, causing obstruction of sebum flow. Follicles reach a maximum capacity and rupture, releasing their inflammatory contents. Neutrophils and liposomal enzymes are released, causing further inflammation. Scarring and pitting often result.

Acne lesions are categorized as inflammatory or noninflammatory. Noninflammatory lesions consist of open and closed comedones. Inflammatory lesions are characterized by the presence of papules, pustules, nodules, or cysts.

Treatment goals are elimination of lesions and diminishment of scarring (Table 50–1). Improvement may not be noticed for at least 1 month after therapy is initiated, with flare-ups possible during treatment. Patients should be discouraged from manipulating skin lesions because doing so will increase inflammation and promote scarring. The affected skin should be gently washed using antibacterial soap and rinsed well to prevent soap buildup on the skin surface. Controversy exists among dermatologists regarding the use of scrubbing agents and alcohol-based drying agents (skin toners), which may stimulate more oil production.

**First-line management should begin with topical benzoyl peroxide or a comedolytic agent such as tretinoin (Retin-A).** The combination of benzoyl peroxide in the morning and tretinoin at night may be effective when either agent alone has failed. Benzoyl peroxide must be washed off prior to application of tretinoin or the retinoid will be rendered ineffective. Benzoyl peroxide is bactericidal and keratolytic, causing follicular desquamation. It is available in over-the-counter preparations with variable uniformity, stability, and efficacy. Although these over-the-counter preparations eliminate bacteria at the skin surface, they do not have a carrier vehicle that allows deep follicular penetration. Therefore, 2.5% to 10% prescription preparations are preferable. A benzoyl peroxide wash is beneficial when lesions are widely distributed or when adherence to a treatment plan is problematic. Washes are applied in the shower and then rinsed off after a few seconds. Benzoyl peroxide can bleach clothing, so thorough drying is recommended.

**Table 50–1 TREATMENT OF VARIOUS TYPES OF ACNE**

| ACNE TYPE | TREATMENT* |
|---|---|
| Pure comedonal acne | Topical tretinoin or adapalene at night |
| Mild papular acne | Benzoyl peroxide in the morning and at night |
| Papulopustular and cystic acne (inflammatory) | Benzoyl peroxide and/or topical antibiotics in the morning and topical tretinoin or adapalene at night |
| Severe pustulocystic acne | Benzoyl peroxide and oral antibiotics |
| Severe cystic acne | Oral retinoid (isotretinoin) |

*Wash all types with antibacterial soap in the morning and at night.

**Topical tretinoin, a vitamin A derivative, inhibits the formation of microcomedones and increases cell turnover.** Therapy should begin conservatively at 0.025%, with 3 to 4 weeks allowed for accommodation. Patients should use a mild soap (Dove) and allow the skin to dry 20 to 30 minutes prior to applying tretinoin. Mild redness and peeling are expected, and patients should avoid sun exposure and use sunscreens. Adapalene 0.1% (Differin) is a retinoid formulation that causes less irritation and photosensitivity, has more activity, and can be used concomitantly with benzoyl peroxide preparations. Tazarotene 0.1% (Tazorac) is a retinoid that is active against psoriasis. This agent is teratogenic and causes irritation, so it should be used with caution. Some believe that azelaic acid applied twice daily for 4 to 6 months may provide acne relief, especially for those sensitive to other agents, and theoretically can reduce scarring.

**Topical, rather than systemic, antibiotics are preferred because of their fewer side effects.** Topical antibiotics (erythromycin, clindamycin) are applied to affected areas twice daily or in combination with benzoyl peroxide or tretinoin. Oral antibiotics are used when inflammatory and pustular acne does not respond to topical treatment. Tetracycline is the most frequently used oral antibiotic because it is inexpensive and has few side effects.

**Isotretinoin (Accutane)** is the **treatment of choice for severe, resistant nodulocystic acne.** A 4-month course often clears a severe case of acne. It is **highly teratogenic** and has many side effects, including **cheilitis, conjunctivitis, hyperlipidemia, blood dyscrasias, elevated liver enzymes, and photosensitivity.** Females should have a negative pregnancy test immediately before isotretinoin is initiated and should maintain effective contraception before, during, and after therapy.

Oral contraceptives (Ortho Tri-Cyclen) are approved for treatment of acne, and intralesional steroid therapy is sometimes used in unresponsive cases.

## Comprehension Questions

50.1 A teenager with severe cystic acne started using isotretinoin 1 month ago. Initially her acne worsened, but is now starting to improve. However, she is "not feeling like herself." She does not want to go to school, cries frequently during the day, and feels hopeless. She also feels "achy" all over. Which of the following is the best course of action?

A. Continue isotretinoin and see her in follow-up in a week.
B. Prescribe an antidepressant.
C. Discontinue isotretinoin and refer her to a psychiatrist.
D. Decrease her isotretinoin dose to determine if the side effects resolve.
E. Counsel her that these symptoms will resolve over time.

50.2 A teenage boy complains of a several-week history of facial "zits" that are painful and itchy. There are no other breakouts. He has inflammatory papules and pustules in the beard and moustache area and has mild cervical lymphadenopathy. He occasionally works weekends on a farm. Which of the following therapies is appropriate?

A. Topical isotretinoin
B. Topical hydrocortisone
C. Oral antifungal
D. Topical mupirocin
E. Oral acyclovir

50.3 A 7-day-old infant is brought to clinic because of "pimples" on his cheeks and forehead. He is breast-feeding well, and the parents have no other concerns. The skin around the pimples and elsewhere is unremarkable, as is the rest of his examination. Which of the following is appropriate advice or therapy?

A. Recommend a different soap.
B. Prescribe topical triamcinolone.
C. Prescribe topical erythromycin.
D. Recommend no treatment.
E. Recommend more frequent bathing.

50.4 A 17-year-old girl is prescribed oral tetracycline, topical tretinoin, and topical benzoyl peroxide. She is sexually active and takes an oral contraceptive. You should counsel her to do which of the following?

A. Take the tetracycline with food or milk.
B. Use a second form of birth control in addition to her oral contraceptive.
C. Get some sun to help dry up her acne.
D. Avoid chocolate and fried foods.
E. Avoid sunscreen because it will irritate her face.

## ANSWERS

50.1 **C.** Depression is a rare side effect of isotretinoin, but it can be severe and suicides have been reported. Myalgias and arthralgias have also occurred. It would be best to stop the drug and have the patient evaluated for depression.

50.2 **C.** Tinea barbae is caused by various dermatophytes and closely resembles tinea capitis. It can be acquired through animal exposure and is more common in farmers. Topical antifungal preparations are ineffective; oral antifungals are required.

50.3 **D.** Approximately 20% of normal neonates develop at least a few comedones within the first month of life. The cause of neonatal acne is unknown, but has been attributed to placental transfer of maternal androgens, hyperactive adrenal glands, and a hypersensitive neonatal end-organ response to androgenic hormones. Such patients may be predisposed to adolescent acne. In most cases a prescription or change in skin care is not warranted.

50.4 **B.** Oral antibiotics may decrease the effectiveness of oral contraceptive pills. Tretinoin can lead to photosensitivity; patients should avoid sun exposure or use sunscreen. Diet has not been found to have an effect on acne. Tetracycline should be taken on an empty stomach; milk products bind tetracycline.

### Clinical Pearls

- Acne is a disorder of the sebaceous follicle in which excess sebum, keratinous debris, and bacteria accumulate, producing microcomedones that may become inflamed.
- Treatment of acne depends on its severity and may include topical benzoyl peroxide, topical retinoic acid, topical antibiotics, oral antibiotics, and/or oral isotretinoin

## REFERENCES

Cuningham BB, Fallon-Friedlander S. Acne. In: Rudolph CD, Rudolph AM, Hostetter MK, Lister G, Siegel NJ, eds. *Rudolph's Pediatrics*. 21st ed. New York, NY: McGraw-Hill; 2003:1208-1210.

Habif TP. *Clinical Dermatology*. 4th ed. St. Louis, MO: Mosby-Year Book; 2003.

Morelli, JG. Acne. In: Kliegman RM, Behrman RE, Jenson HB, Stanton BF, eds. *Nelson Textbook of Pediatrics*. 18th ed. Philadelphia, PA: WB Saunders; 2007:2759-2764.

Tunnessen WW, Krowchuk DP. Acne. In: McMillan JA, Feigin RD, DeAngelis CD, Jones MD, eds. *Oski's Pediatrics: Principles and Practice*. 4th ed. Philadelphia, PA: Lippincott Williams & Wilkins; 2006:875-877.

# Case 51

A 3700-g male infant is born at 38 weeks' gestation after an uncomplicated pregnancy. The infant is noted after birth to have a dribbling urinary stream and a lower abdominal mass. Postnatal ultrasonography reveals bilateral hydronephrosis with bladder wall hypertrophy and an enlarged urethra.

- What is the most likely diagnosis?
- What is the most appropriate next test?

# ANSWERS TO CASE 51: Posterior Urethral Valves

*Summary:* A term newborn male has evidence of severe urinary obstruction.

➤ **Most likely diagnosis:** Posterior urethral valves (PUV).

➤ **Most appropriate next test:** Renal ultrasonography (USG).

## ANALYSIS

### Objectives

1. Know the various presentations of patients with PUV.
2. Know the possible long-term sequelae associated with PUV.
3. Be familiar with common abdominal masses in the newborn period.

### Considerations

Many conditions cause abdominal masses in the newborn (Table 51–1). In this infant's case, the dribbling urinary stream suggests PUV. An abdominal USG is a useful and noninvasive tool to aid in the diagnosis.

**Table 51–1 ABDOMINAL MASSES CAUSING DISTENTION**

| | |
|---|---|
| **Hepatic enlargement**<br>• Cardiac failure, arrhythmias<br>• Hepatic tumors (mesenchymal hamartoma, hemangioma, hemangioendothelioma, metastatic tumors such as neuroblastoma)<br>• Metabolic disorders (storage diseases [lysosomal or carbohydrate], tyrosinemia, galactosemia)<br>• Beckwith-Wiedemann syndrome<br>• Congenital infections (cytomegalic inclusion disease, syphilis, toxoplasmosis, rubella)<br>**Pelvic masses**<br>• Ovarian cyst (follicular, dermoid, teratoma)<br>• Hydrocolpos, hydrometrocolpos<br>• Imperforate hymen<br>• Vaginal atresia/stenosis<br>• Cloaca | **Adrenal masses**<br>• Adrenal hemorrhage<br>• Neuroblastoma<br>**Renal mass**<br>• Multicystic or polycystic kidney<br>• Hydronephrosis (posterior urethral valves, ureterovesical or ureteropelvic junction obstruction)<br>• Renal vein thrombosis<br>**Retroperitoneal masses**<br>• Neuroblastoma<br>• Wilms tumor<br>• Mesoblastic nephroma<br>• Sacrococcygeal teratoma<br>• Lymphangioma<br>**Gastrointestinal masses**<br>• Duplication<br>• Mesenteric cyst |

*(Adapted, with permission, from Seashore JH. Distended abdomen. In: McMillan JA, DeAngelis CD, Feigin RD, Warshaw JB, eds.* Oski's Pediatrics. *3rd ed. Philadelphia, PA: Lippincott Williams & Wilkins; 1999:323.)*

# APPROACH TO
## Posterior Urethral Valves

### DEFINITIONS

**VESICOURETERAL REFLUX (VUR):** Retrograde urine flow from the bladder into the ureter(s) and, if severe, into the kidney. In general this condition is more common in females and may lead to recurrent urinary tract infections (UTI) and diminished renal function. Depending on the degree of reflux, treatment ranges from antibiotic prophylaxis to surgical intervention.

**VOIDING CYSTOURETHROGRAM (VCUG):** A radiographic study in which a catheter is placed in the bladder and contrast is instilled. Upon voiding, the urethra is visualized and, in cases of vesicoureteral reflux, the ureters are outlined.

### CLINICAL APPROACH

**Fetal ultrasonography** assists in the prenatal diagnosis of urinary tract obstruction. Sonographic findings include **bilateral hydronephrosis with bladder distention**. In severe cases oligohydramnios is found and may lead to poor fetal lung development with pulmonary insufficiency and congenital contractures. Boys diagnosed prenatally during the second trimester have a worse prognosis than those diagnosed after birth.

Urethral valves are leaflets of tissue located in the lumen of the distal urethra from the prostate to the external sphincter. **Posterior urethral valves are the most common cause of severe urinary tract obstruction in boys**, occurring in 1 of every 8000 newborn males; 30% ultimately have end-stage renal disease or chronic renal insufficiency. Neonates present with distended bladders, poor or dribbling urinary streams, palpable kidneys, reduced renal function, or UTI. Older infants have failure to thrive, renal dysfunction, or UTI. Older boys may present with voiding difficulty, such as diurnal enuresis or hesitancy. Posterior urethral valve is confirmed with VCUG or postnatal USG. Because of the high incidence of PUV in boys with UTI, evaluation of the boy who has UTI includes VCUG and renal USG.

Immediate relief of PUV obstruction includes bladder catheterization via the urethra with a small feeding tube. If UTI is suspected, antimicrobial therapy is initiated. Serum electrolytes, blood urea nitrogen, and creatinine levels are measured with correction as needed. Hemodynamic status is monitored because sepsis or renal failure can lead to cardiovascular collapse.

After acute obstruction is relieved and the patient has been stabilized, endoscopic transurethral valve ablation may be performed if the serum creatinine level is normal and urethral size permits. If the serum creatinine remains elevated, the urethral lumen is too narrow, or the UTI does not respond to antibiotics, emergent vesicostomy may be necessary. Following ablation, VUR and persistent postobstructive hydronephrosis are common. Antibiotic prophylaxis can be useful in decreasing UTI frequency.

### Follow-Up

After surgery, patients require surveillance of renal function and for possible UTI. Many patients will have polyuria because of diminished ability to concentrate the urine and are at greater risk for dehydration; some develop renal tubular acidosis.

Routine care for boys with a history of PUV includes regular monitoring with urinalysis, renal USG, serum electrolyte levels, blood pressure, and linear growth. They may have prolonged diurnal enuresis and may require urodynamic studies to evaluate their voiding. Renal insufficiency is common, and some may require renal transplantation. Poor prognostic factors for normal renal development include oligohydramnios, hydronephrosis before 24-week gestation, persistently elevated serum creatinine level, bilateral cortical cysts, and diurnal enuresis beyond the age of 5 years.

## Comprehension Questions

51.1 A 3-month-old boy presents with fever without a source. As part of his evaluation a urinalysis is performed; a UTI is suspected. Which of the following is the best next step?

A. If the urine culture reveals UTI, renal USG and VCUG should be performed.
B. VCUG should be performed only after a second UTI is diagnosed
C. Antibiotics should be initiated after urine culture and sensitivities are obtained.
D. Renal biopsy should be performed.
E. Preferred methods of collection for urine culture for this infant include midstream clean-catch and bag urine.

51.2 A 2-month-old girl presents with fever and vomiting. Her serum white blood cell (WBC) count is elevated. Urinalysis reveals 100 WBC per high-power field (unspun); it is positive for nitrates and leukocyte esterase. Urine culture results confirm a UTI; renal USG and VCUG show mild hydronephrosis and grade II VUR on the right. Which of the following is the best next step?

A. She will require surgical reimplantation of her right ureter.
B. Antimicrobial prophylactic therapy should be started when her current course of antibiotics is completed.
C. VCUG should be performed on a monthly basis.
D. Subsequent urine specimen must be obtained only by suprapubic aspiration.
E. Renal arteriography is indicated.

51.3 A 6-month-old infant male presents to your clinic with an abdominal mass, which was discovered by his new foster mother during the child's bath. On physical examination, you also find macroglossia and right-sided hemihypertrophy. This infant is likely to have which of the following?

A. Down syndrome with duodenal atresia
B. Alagille syndrome and biliary atresia
C. Beckwith-Wiedemann syndrome with Wilms tumor
D. Neurofibromatosis and abdominal neurofibromas
E. Zellweger syndrome and hepatomegaly

51.4 An 8-year-old boy presents with bedwetting 3 to 4 times per week for "as long as he can remember." He has a strong urine stream, daytime urine continence, and no UTIs. His physical examination is normal. Which of the following is the most appropriate next course of action?

A. Urodynamic studies.
B. Reassurance; he has secondary nocturnal enuresis.
C. Use of enuresis alarm.
D. Desmopressin acetate can be administered every 6 hours to control enuresis.
E. Behavior modification that includes punishment for wet nights and rewards for dry nights.

## ANSWERS

51.1 **A.** For any infant male with a UTI, evaluation of anatomy and function is necessary. The preferred methods of urine collection include bladder catheterization and suprapubic bladder aspiration. Antimicrobial therapy is started empirically while awaiting urine culture and sensitivity results.

51.2 **B.** Infants and children with VUR receive prophylactic antimicrobial therapy and close monitoring for infection with urinalysis and urine culture at 3- to 4-month intervals. Sulfamethoxazole-trimethoprim, trimethoprim alone, and nitrofurantoin are commonly used for antimicrobial prophylaxis, VUR is graded from I to V based on the degree of reflux. Higher-grade reflux is less likely to resolve spontaneously and is more likely to result in renal damage.

51.3 **C.** This infant with features of Beckwith-Wiedemann syndrome is at high risk for developing Wilms tumor, hepatoblastoma, and gonadoblastoma.

51.4 **C.** Nocturnal enuresis occurs in 15% of 5-year-olds with a resolution rate of 15% per year. Males are more frequently affected, and family history is common. Initial evaluation includes a history of wetting pattern, prior UTI, and developmental, social, and emotional history. Physical examination includes kidney palpation, neurologic examination, and examination of the back looking for sacral dimple or hairy nevus. Some recommend urinalysis and culture to rule out occult infection. The enuresis alarm has a success rate of 70% to 90% and requires parental support. Pharmacologic interventions include night-time doses of imipramine or oral desmopressin acetate. Intransal formulations of desmopressin are no longer approved for the treatment of primary nocturnal emuresis. Following use of desmopressin acetate, fluid intake is restricted to avoid hyponatremia. Pharmacologic treatment usually is reserved for special occasions, such as when the child is sleeping over at a friend's house, summer camp, and so on. Behavior modification does not include punishment.

## Clinical Pearls

- Posterior urethral valve occurs exclusively in males.
- Renal ultrasonography and voiding cystourethrogram are important in the evaluation of infants with urinary tract infection.
- Boys with posterior urethral valve are at risk for end-stage renal disease, even after appropriate therapy.

## REFERENCES

Chintagumpala MM. Wilms tumor. In: McMillan JA, Feigin RD, DeAngelis CD, Jones MD, eds. *Oski's Pediatrics: Principles and Practice*. 4th ed. Philadelphia, PA: Lippincott Williams & Wilkins; 2006:1775-1777.

Colberg JW. Posterior urethral valves. In: Rudolph CD, Rudolph AM, Hostetter MK, Lister G, Siegel NJ, eds. *Rudolph's Pediatrics*. 21st ed. New York, NY: McGraw-Hill; 2003:1737.

Elder JS. Obstructions of the urinary tract, posterior urethral valves. In: Kliegman RM, Behrman RE, Jenson HB, Stanton BF, eds. *Nelson Textbook of Pediatrics*. 18th ed. Philadelphia, PA: WB Saunders; 2007:2241-2242.

Gonzales ET, Roth DR. Urinary tract infection. In: McMillan JA, Feigin RD, DeAngelis CD, Jones MD, eds. *Oski's Pediatrics: Principles and Practice*. 4th ed. Philadelphia, PA: Lippincott Williams & Wilkins; 2006:1836-1840.

Greene DM. Wilms tumor. In: Rudolph CD, Rudolph AM, Hostetter MK, Lister G, Siegel NJ, eds. *Rudolph's Pediatrics*. 21st ed. New York, NY: McGraw-Hill; 2003: 1614-1616.

Kennedy T. Urinary tract infection. In: Rudolph CD, Rudolph AM, Hostetter MK, Lister G, Siegel NJ, eds. *Rudolph's Pediatrics*. 21st ed. New York, NY: McGraw-Hill; 2003:1667-1673.

Norwood VF, Chevalier RL. Obstructive disorders. In: Rudolph CD, Rudolph AM, Hostetter MK, Lister G, Siegel NJ, eds. *Rudolph's Pediatrics*. 21st ed. New York, NY: McGraw-Hill; 2003:1641-1642.

Roth DR, Gonzales ET. Disorders of renal development and anomalies of the collecting system, bladder, penis, and scrotum. In: McMillan JA, Feigin RD, DeAngelis CD, Jones, MD, eds. *Oski's Pediatrics: Principles and Practice*. 4th ed. Philadelphia, PA: Lippincott Williams & Wilkins; 2006:1823-1826.

Sand-Loud N, Rappaport LA. Enuresis. In: McMillan JA, Feigin RD, DeAngelis CD, Jones, MD, eds. *Oski's Pediatrics: Principles and Practice*. 4th ed. Philadelphia, PA: Lippincott Williams & Wilkins; 2006:670-672.

Seashore JH. Distended abdomen. In: McMillan JA, DeAngelis CD, Feigin RD, Warshaw JB, eds. *Oski's Pediatrics: Principles and Practice*. 3rd ed. Philadelphia, PA: Lippincott Williams & Wilkins; 1999:321-325.

Desmopressin Acetate (marketed as DDAVP Nasal Spray, DDAVP Rhinal Tube, DDAVP, DDVP, Minirin, and Stimate Nasal Spray). http://www.fda.gov/cder/drug/Infosheets/HCP/desmopressinHCP.htm. Accessed January 18, 2009.

# Case 52

The mother of a healthy 8-year-old boy is concerned about his school performance. At the last parent–teacher conference, his teacher noted that he is easily distracted and routinely fails to complete both homework assignments and classroom papers. His mother states that at home he also has difficulty in completing tasks and he fidgets constantly. Although the child is very talkative, he does not answer questions clearly. His physical examination is significant only for fidgeting.

➤ What is the most likely diagnosis?

➤ What is the next step in management?

# ANSWERS TO CASE 52: Attention-Deficit/Hyperactivity Disorder

*Summary:* An 8-year-old easily distractible, hyperkinetic boy who cannot complete school work or stay on task at home.

➤ **Most likely diagnosis:** Attention-deficit/hyperactivity disorder (ADHD).

➤ **Next step in management:** An ADHD evaluation, which includes information regarding his behavior obtained from both the caregiver and from the classroom teacher.

## ANALYSIS

### Objectives

1. Understand the basic evaluation of the child with symptoms of ADHD.
2. Know the various treatment options available for this condition.

### Considerations

This boy exhibits ADHD behaviors, including easy distractibility, inability to focus and complete tasks, and excessive fidgeting. The next step is a complete ADHD evaluation as described. If data suggest ADHD, he should undergo developmental and psychological evaluations for coexisting psychiatric conditions or learning disability. Target outcomes then can be identified and a behavioral therapy, classroom modification, and possibly medication treatment plan designed.

# APPROACH TO Attention-Deficit/Hyperactivity Disorder

## DEFINITION

**ATTENTION-DEFICIT/HYPERACTIVITY DISORDER (ADHD):** A condition consisting of developmentally inappropriate inattentiveness, hyperactivity, and impulsivity.

## CLINICAL APPROACH

The *Diagnostic and Statistical Manual of Mental Disorders*, *Fourth Edition (DSM-IV)* describes **criteria** of **inattentiveness** and **hyperactivity/impulsivity** necessary to make an **ADHD diagnosis.** Attention deficit hyperactivity disorder is estimated to affect 3% to 10% of school-aged children; 25% of ADHD patients have an affected primary relative. The pathophysiology of ADHD remains to be elucidated, but decreased activity of certain brain regions in the frontal lobes may be responsible.

**Inattention criteria of ADHD** include careless mistakes, having difficulty paying attention, not listening, not following through on tasks, avoiding sustained mental effort, frequently losing things, easy distractibility, and forgetfulness.

**Hyperactivity criteria of ADHD include** frequent fidgeting, being out of his or her seat frequently, running or climbing excessively, having difficulty playing quietly, and often talking excessively.

**Impulsivity criteria of ADHD include** blurting out answers, having difficulty waiting for his or her turn, and interrupting or intruding frequently.

Attention-deficit/hyperactivity disorder is subdivided into three types: ADHD/I (at least 6 of 9 inattention behaviors), ADHD/HI (at least 6 of 9 hyperactive/impulsive behaviors), and ADHD/C (at least 6 of 9 of both the inattention and hyperactive/impulsive behaviors). Symptoms must be present for **at least 6 months in two or more settings, some symptoms must have been present before age 7, and must result in impaired function.** Caregivers and classroom teacher(s) provide the critical information by filling out checklists, such as the Conners rating, the AHDH index, the Swanson, Nolan, and Pelham checklist (SNAP), or the ADD-H comprehensive teacher rating scale (ACTeRS). Alternatively, information can be surmised via narratives or descriptive interviews.

**Psychological and developmental testing is part of the evaluation of an ADHD child; coexisting psychological and learning disorders occur frequently.** Common coexisting conditions include oppositional-defiant disorder (35.2%), conduct disorder (25.7%), anxiety disorder (25.8%), and depressive disorder (18.2%). Approximately 12% to 60% of ADHD children have concurrent learning disorders and may benefit from special education services.

Management includes the implementation of a long-term treatment program in collaboration with caregivers and teachers. The care plan includes setting specific goals such as increasing independence, decreasing disruptive behavior, improving academic performance, organization, and task completion, and improving relationships with family members, teachers, and peers. **Behavioral modification** can be used alone or in conjunction with **pharmacologic therapy.** Positive reinforcement (providing rewards or privileges) and negative consequences (time-out or withdrawal of privileges) emphasize appropriate behavior. Small class size, structured work, stimulating schoolwork, and appropriate seating arrangements can help **decrease disruptive classroom behaviors. Medications are often used to assist in treatment. Stimulant medications are considered first-line pharmacologic therapy to decrease ADHD behaviors.** Commonly used stimulant medications include **methylphenidate and dextroamphetamine. Atomoxetine (Strattera) is a nonstimulant, selective norepinephrine reuptake inhibitor** approved for use in adults and children.

Tricyclic antidepressants and bupropion, often prescribed under the direction of a psychiatrist or neurologist, are also used.

Long-term sequelae of ADHD include poor peer relationships, poor fine motor control, and increased risk of accidents. Adolescents may develop substance abuse problems as a comorbid condition, but this comorbidity does not seem to be related to treatment of ADHD with stimulants. Approximately 50% of children function well in adulthood; others demonstrate continued inattention and impulsivity symptoms.

## Comprehension Questions

52.1 An 8-year-old boy presents because his mother is concerned that he has ADHD. At home he is always restless, never seems to pay attention, and is always losing things. In the office, the child is cooperative and has a normal examination. Which of the following is the best next step in management?

A. Give the child a 2-week trial of stimulant medication.
B. Obtain further information from the parents and teachers.
C. Reassure the child's mother that this behavior is age appropriate.
D. Send the child for psychological assessment.
E. Send the child for psychiatric evaluation.

52.2 A 7-year-old boy appears distracted. His mother notes that he daydreams "all of the time," and when he is daydreaming he does not respond to her. She describes the episodes as short (lasting several seconds) and occurring many times per day. When he is not daydreaming, he is attentive and can complete tasks. His behavior in class is not disruptive. Which of the following is the best next step in management?

A. Obtain further information from his parents and teachers with the Conners rating scale.
B. Begin a program of behavioral modification.
C. Reassure the child's mother that this behavior is age appropriate.
D. Send the child for an electroencephalogram.
E. Send the child for psychological assessment.

52.3 A 14-year-old adolescent male was recently diagnosed with ADHD. His evaluation for coexisting psychiatric disorders is most likely to identify which of the following?

A. Bipolar disorder
B. Oppositional-defiant disorder
C. Pervasive developmental disorder
D. Posttraumatic stress disorder
E. Schizophrenia

52.4 An 8-year-old boy has completed the initial ADHD evaluation, which demonstrates that he meets 7 of the 9 criteria for inattention and that he also has many impulsive behaviors. Which of the following is the most appropriate next step in management?

A. Give the child a 2-week trial of stimulant medication.
B. Arrange for special education placement.
C. Send the child for a complete psychoeducational assessment.
D. Send the child for an electroencephalogram.
E. Reassure the child's mother that this behavior is age appropriate.

## ANSWERS

52.1 **B.** A physical examination (with emphasis on the neurologic component) is completed to identify any soft signs of neurologic conditions. If none are found, he should undergo an ADHD evaluation with ADHD-specific behavior information obtained from caregivers and teachers. A diagnosis is considered if he has ADHD-specific behaviors in two or more settings. His ability to maintain focus during a brief visit to your office does not preclude the diagnosis of ADHD.

52.2 **D.** This child does not fit the classic ADHD pattern. Episodes of "daydreaming," which last several seconds, may be petit mal or absence seizures; an electroencephalogram is needed.

52.3 **B.** Common coexisting psychiatric conditions include oppositional-defiant disorder (35.2%), conduct disorder (25.7%), anxiety disorder (25.8%), and depressive disorder (18.2%).

52.4 **C.** Prior to developing a management plan, the child is assessed for coexisting psychiatric and learning disorders (psychoeducational testing). Management can include stimulant medication, behavioral modification, and therapy appropriate for coexisting conditions.

### Clinical Pearls

- Attention-deficit/hyperactivity disorder (ADHD) is considered in children who have specific behaviors in two or more settings, such as at home and school or work.
- Children with ADHD frequently have coexisting psychiatric or learning disorders, including oppositional-defiant disorder, conduct disorder, anxiety disorder, and depression.
- Commonly used pharmacologic agents for treatment of ADHD are methylphenidate and dextroamphetamine.

## REFERENCES

American Academy of Pediatrics. Clinical practice guideline: diagnosis and evaluation of the child with attention-deficit/hyperactivity disorder. *Pediatrics*. 2000;105: 1158-1170.

American Academy of Pediatrics. Clinical practice guideline: treatment of the school-aged child with attention-deficit/hyperactivity disorder. *Pediatrics*. 2001;108:1033-1044.

American Psychiatric Association. *Diagnostic and Statistical Manual of Mental Disorders*. 4th ed. (Text Revision). Washington: American Psychiatric Association; 2000:92.

Cutting LE, Mostofsky SH, Denckla MB. School difficulties. In: McMillan JA, Feigin RD, DeAngelis CD, Jones MD, eds. *Oski's Pediatrics: Principles and Practice*. 4th ed. Philadelphia, PA: Lippincott Williams & Wilkins; 2006:674-680.

Dworkin PH. Hyperactivity: overactivity to attention-deficit disorder. In: Rudolph CD, Rudolph AM, Hostetter MK, Lister G, Siegel NJ, eds. *Rudolph's Pediatrics*. 21st ed. New York, NY: McGraw-Hill; 2003:430-434.

Raishevich N, Jensen P. Attention deficit hyperactivity disorder. In: Kliegman RM, Behrman RE, Jenson HB, Stanton BF, eds. *Nelson Textbook of Pediatrics*. 18th ed. Philadelphia, PA: WB Saunders; 2007:146-150.

# Case 53

A previously healthy 12-year-old boy has had right knee pain for 3 weeks. He is athletic, playing basketball and running track, but he denies recent trauma. He describes increased pain when he is running or jumping. He has a normal physical examination except for mild edema and tenderness over his right tibial tubercle.

- What is the most likely diagnosis?
- What is the next step in management?

# ANSWERS TO CASE 53: Osgood-Schlatter Disease

*Summary:* A 12-year-old boy presents with knee pain that increases with activity and tenderness and swelling of his tibial tubercle of the affected knee.

- **Most likely diagnosis:** Osgood-Schlatter disease.
- **Next step in management:** For most patients rest and ice after activity; in severe cases, knee immobilization.

## ANALYSIS

### Objectives

1. Know the presentation and treatment of Osgood-Schlatter disease (OSD).
2. Know differential diagnosis of childhood bone pain and extremity swelling.

### Considerations

A history is critical to determine whether other signs and symptoms are present in this adolescent who has knee pain and swelling. His lack of constitutional signs and symptoms (fever, joint erythema, fatigue, weight loss, night sweats, bruising, and cough) are clues to the relatively benign nature of this condition. If any of these signs or symptoms are present, evaluation for more serious, potentially life-threatening conditions, such as malignancy, is appropriate.

# APPROACH TO Osgood-Schlatter Disease

## DEFINITION

**OSGOOD-SCHLATTER DISEASE (OSD):** A condition of painful inflammation of the tibial tubercle.

## CLINICAL APPROACH

The **knee pain of OSD** is caused by **inflammation of the tibial tubercle, an extension of the tibial epiphysis or growth plate.** Ossification centers begin to form in children between the ages of 9 and 13 years and are completed between the ages of 15 and 17 years. Patients with OSD usually are males who present in late childhood through early adolescence. **Repetitive running and jumping** motions cause traction and microstress fractures to the developing area, resulting in inflammation, edema, tenderness, and bony changes.

The **diagnosis of OSD can be made clinically.** The patient has no history of trauma, but he complains of knee pain that increases with exercise and trauma. Differential diagnosis of knee pain in adolescents includes a number of conditions. Patellofemoral stress syndrome, also common in athletes, causes chronic, dull, nonlocalizing knee pain. Jumper's knee (patellar tendonitis) is caused by microscopic patellar tendon injury; most affected patients have chronic, anterior knee pain and tenderness of the inferior portion of the patella. Iliotibial band friction syndrome causes lateral knee pain in runners. **Slipped capital femoral epiphysis (SCFE)** occurs in **adolescents** during the growth spurt, leading to a limp and groin or thigh pain; however, hip pain may be referred to the knee. Examination of such patients reveals limited hip flexion, internal rotation, and abduction. Radiographs of the hip reveal widening of the femoral epiphysis and osteopenia. Patients with SCFE are at risk for avascular necrosis of the femoral epiphysis and require orthopedic evaluation. Other diagnoses to be considered in the adolescent with knee pain include trauma, tumor, leukemia, and septic joint.

Treatment of OSD consists of decreased activity. Ice after exercise and nonsteroidal anti-inflammatory drugs may provide some relief. In severe cases, knee immobilization and the use of crutches may be required. Symptoms may recur until ossification is complete. Long-term prognosis is excellent.

## Comprehension Questions

53.1 A 12-year-old boy complains of right knee pain that is worse after he runs. His pain started 1 week after he joined the track team. He has tenderness of the tibial tubercle. Which of the following statements is accurate?

A. A left shoe orthotic device will allow him to continue running and will alleviate the pain.
B. Decreasing his activity should alleviate the pain.
C. Initial therapy consists of immobilization.
D. The most likely cause of his pain is a stress fracture.
E. The most likely diagnosis is slipped capital femoral epiphysis.

53.2 A 13-year-old adolescent male has 1 week of limping and right knee pain. On your growth curve you determine that his weight is greater than the 95th percentile for age. His physical examination is remarkable for mild acanthosis and normal knees. His hip examination demonstrates diminished ability to flex and internally rotate his right femur. Which of the following is the best next step in management?

A. Instruct the patient to rest and apply ice to the affected area.
B. Prescribe daily oral nonsteroidal anti-inflammatory drugs until the pain resolves.
C. Order a magnetic resonance imaging of the knee and hip.
D. Arrange for an orthopedic surgery consultation.
E. Prescribe a short course of oral steroids to decrease inflammation.

53.3 A 14-year-old adolescent female arrives for a routine well-child evaluation. The mother reports that her daughter has previously been well, but she wants you to scold the patient since she did not use sunscreen at a recent pool party and returned home 3 weeks ago with a sunburn across her cheeks and nose; the adolescent rolls her eyes at her mother. When the mother leaves the room the patient reports that she did use sunscreen but did not feel like arguing with her mother about the point. She states that she has been well, but also notes that she has had 2 months of intermittent right knee pain that does not appear to be related to exercise. Upon further questioning she reports that she has not been feeling well and is increasingly tired. Your physical examination demonstrates the sunburn across the nose but no knee abnormalities and a normal gait. Which of the following is the most appropriate next step in management?

A. Prescribe ibuprofen and recommend daily sunscreen use.
B. Obtain radiographs of the knee.
C. Obtain further history with regard to fever, weight loss, rashes, and arthritis.
D. Recommend a knee immobilizer.
E. Arrange for an emergent orthopedic consultation for evaluation of possible SCFE.

53.4 A 15-year-old adolescent male presents with right knee pain; he cannot bear weight on the affected joint. The knee is tender, edematous, warm, erythematous, and has significantly diminished range of motion. Which of the following is the best next step in his evaluation?

A. Obtain more history, including sexual history.
B. Prescribe a course of systemic steroids.
C. Administer intra-articular steroids to decrease inflammation.
D. Prescribe anti-inflammatory drugs.
E. Arrange for an outpatient orthopedic surgery consultation.

## ANSWERS

53.1 **B.** This boy's history is consistent with OSD. Initial therapy includes ice after exertion and rest.

53.2 **D.** The most likely diagnosis is SCFE. The patient is put on bed rest, and orthopedic surgery consultation is required.

53.3 **C.** This patient has complaints of joint pain and malaise, and she had a malar facial rash consistent with that of systemic lupus erythematosus (SLE). The next step is to obtain more history of other signs and symptoms of autoimmune disease, medication use (drug-induced SLE), and travel history (tick exposure for Lyme disease).

53.4 **A.** This patient has signs and symptoms of a septic joint. *Neisseria gonorrhoeae* is a major cause of septic arthritis in sexually active adolescents and young adults. If septic arthritis is suspected, immediate orthopedic evaluation and intravenous antibiotics are warranted.

### Clinical Pearls

- Osgood-Schlatter disease is found exclusively in young adolescents prior to closure of the growth plate.
- Edema and tenderness of the tibial tuberosity are classic features of Osgood-Schlatter disease.
- Slipped capital femoral epiphysis can cause limping and is most common in overweight adolescents.

## REFERENCES

Cassidy JT. Rheumatic diseases of childhood. In: McMillan JA, Feigin RD, DeAngelis CD, Jones MD, eds. *Oski's Pediatrics: Principles and Practice*. 4th ed. Philadelphia, PA: Lippincott Williams & Wilkins; 2006:2543-2546.

Crawford AH. Slipped capital femoral epiphysis. In: Rudolph CD, Rudolph AM, Hostetter MK, Lister G, Siegel NJ, eds. *Rudolph's Pediatrics*. 21st ed. New York, NY: McGraw-Hill; 2003:2438-2439.

Eddy AA. Lupus nephritis. In: Rudolph CD, Rudolph AM, Hostetter MK, Lister G, Siegel NJ, eds. *Rudolph's Pediatrics*. 21st ed. New York, NY: McGraw-Hill; 2003: 1687-1688.

Hosalker HS, Wells L. The knee. In: Kliegman RM, Behrman RE, Jenson HB, Stanton BF, eds. *Nelson Textbook of Pediatrics*. 18th ed. Philadelphia, PA: WB Saunders; 2007: 2798-2799.

Landry GL. Sports medicine. In: McMillan JA, Feigin RD, DeAngelis CD, Jones MD, eds. *Oski's Pediatrics: Principles and Practice*. 4th ed. Philadelphia, PA: Lippincott Williams & Wilkins; 2006:897.

Patterson LER. Gonococcal infections. In: McMillan JA, Feigin RD, DeAngelis CD, Jones MD, eds. *Oski's Pediatrics: Principles and Practice*. 4th ed. Philadelphia, PA: Lippincott Williams & Wilkins; 2006:1088-1091.

Sponseller PD. Bone, joint, and muscle problems. In: McMillan JA, Feigin RD, DeAngelis CD, Jones MD, eds. *Oski's Pediatrics: Principles and Practice*. 4th ed. Philadelphia, PA: Lippincott Williams & Wilkins; 2006:2474, 2479.

Staat MA. *Neisseria gonorrhoeae*. In: Rudolph CD, Rudolph AM, Hostetter MK, Lister G, Siegel NJ, eds. *Rudolph's Pediatrics*. 21st ed. New York, NY: McGraw-Hill; 2003: 967-970.

Wall EJ. Osgood-Schlatter disease. In: Rudolph CD, Rudolph AM, Hostetter MK, Lister G, Siegel NJ, eds. *Rudolph's Pediatrics*. 21st ed. New York, NY: McGraw-Hill; 2003:2432.

# Case 54

A 2-week-old male newborn presents with a "twisted neck." He was born at term via a difficult vaginal delivery because of his large size (4550 g). On examination, his head is tilted toward the right side, his chin is rotated toward the left, and he has a palpable, firm, right sternocleidomastoid muscle mass.

- What is the most likely diagnosis?
- What is the best treatment?

# ANSWERS TO CASE 54: Torticollis

*Summary:* A 2-week-old large male born after difficult delivery has torticollis and a palpable sternocleidomastoid muscle mass.

- **Most likely diagnosis:** Muscular torticollis.
- **Best treatment:** Initially, passive stretching of the sternocleidomastoid muscle.

## ANALYSIS

### Objectives

1. Understand the common causes of torticollis.
2. Recognize the differences in treatment of torticollis based on the etiology.

### Considerations

This 2-week-old newborn had a difficult delivery because of his large size. He has torticollis (head tilted toward the right and chin rotated toward the left) as a result of decreased range of movement of the sternocleidomastoid muscle caused by the mass. Such infants are at increased risk for muscular torticollis because of sternocleidomastoid muscle injuries. Breech infants and those with hip dysplasia also are at higher risk for torticollis.

# APPROACH TO Torticollis

## DEFINITIONS

**KLIPPEL-FEIL SYNDROME:** Congenital fusion of portions of the cervical vertebrae, restricted neck movement, short neck, and low hairline. Associated features include Sprengel deformity (see below) and structural urinary tract abnormalities.

**SANDIFER SYNDROME:** Gastroesophageal reflux (GER), hiatal hernia, and posturing of the head.

**SPRENGEL DEFORMITY:** Congenital elevation of the scapula.

## CLINICAL APPROACH

**Torticollis**, identified in a patient with an **obviously twisted neck with the head tilted toward one side and the chin tilted toward the opposite side**, is commonly caused by injury and contracture of the **sternocleidomastoid muscle**. Torticollis presents at or soon after birth; infants may have experienced birth trauma and usually have a palpable, firm mass within the affected muscle. Cervical spine radiography is generally performed to rule out vertebral malformations.

If the spine is normal, therapy by the caregiver (and occasionally a physical therapist) involves **gentle sternocleidomastoid muscle stretching** (moving the head toward a neutral position). If the condition persists beyond the first months of life, an orthopedic consultation is indicated. **Persistent torticollis can lead to facial asymmetry.**

Congenital cervical vertebrae malformations can cause torticollis; gentle stretching does not improve the condition and may result in injury. Radiography demonstrates spinal anomalies such as hemivertebrae or areas of vertebral fusion or subluxation. **Klippel-Feil syndrome** can present as torticollis and includes congenital fusion of portions of the cervical vertebrae, restricted neck movement, short neck and low hairline, Sprengel deformity and urinary tract abnormalities.

**Torticollis presenting beyond infancy requires cautious evaluation** because trauma and inflammation are common. Traumatic torticollis can occur following cervical vertebrae injury with subsequent fracture or atlanto-occipital, atlantoaxial, or C2–3 subluxation or injury to the cervical musculature; radiographic evaluation is essential. Inflammatory torticollis often follows an upper respiratory illness; muscular pain and tenderness and a normal neurologic evaluation are seen. Other inflammatory causes include cervical lymphadenitis, retropharyngeal abscess, cervical vertebral osteomyelitis, rheumatoid arthritis, and upper lobe pneumonia. Children with cervical lymphadenitis are generally febrile and have palpable, tender cervical lymph nodes. Patients with retropharyngeal abscess may present with fever, dysphagia, dyspnea, drooling, or stridor secondary to compression.

A variety of neurologic conditions cause torticollis: visual disturbances, dystonic reactions to medications (phenothiazine, haloperidol, or metoclopramide), spinal cord or posterior fossa tumors, syringomyelia, Wilson disease, dystonia musculorum deformans, and spasmus nutans. A physical examination with particular attention to the neurologic examination may identify findings associated with one of these neurologic causes. Miscellaneous causes include cervical disc calcification, Sandifer syndrome, benign paroxysmal torticollis, bone tumors, soft-tissue tumors, and hysteria.

## Comprehension Questions

54.1 A 3-month-old male infant has intermittent neck contortions and arching. He was term at birth, with an uneventful prenatal course and delivery. He frequently spits up after feeding, and has had one episode of pneumonia. Which of the following is the best next step in management?

A. Begin gentle stretching of the sternocleidomastoid muscle.
B. Evaluate him for gastroesophageal reflux disease (GERD).
C. Refer him for orthopedic evaluation.
D. Obtain cervical spine radiographs.
E. Observe and, if the condition persists, refer him for orthopedic evaluation.

54.2 A 5-month-old female infant presents with sudden onset of torticollis and facial grimacing, but otherwise she appears alert and interactive. She has been doing well and has gained weight for the last month after having been prescribed ranitidine and metoclopramide for GER disease. Which of the following statements is accurate?

A. She is likely having a partial-complex seizure and needs an electroencephalograph.
B. A lumbar puncture for cell count, glucose, and protein is warranted.
C. Measurement of serum electrolyte and glucose levels is unnecessary.
D. She is likely having a dystonic reaction to one of her medications.
E. A cervical spine magnetic resonance image is likely to show a congenital abnormality.

54.3 A 4-year-old boy presents with torticollis, fever, sore throat, and difficulty swallowing but no drooling. He denies headache and dyspnea, and he remains only somewhat playful. Examination reveals posterior pharyngeal edema. Which of the following is the best next step in management?

A. Examine his cerebrospinal fluid.
B. Obtain imaging studies of the airway and soft tissues of the neck.
C. Send a throat culture and begin antibiotic therapy based on the results.
D. Begin oral penicillin.
E. Prescribe ibuprofen and neck stretching exercises.

54.4 A 1-week-old female newborn presents with her new adoptive parents. The family complains that she seems to have a twisted neck. They know only that "delivery was almost a C-section because the baby was lying sideways." She has been feeding well and has had appropriate urine and stool output for the last 24 hours. Physical examination is significant for torticollis. Which of the following statements is most accurate?

A. She is at significant risk for aspiration pneumonia.
B. The parents should immediately begin a regimen of gentle stretching of the neck.
C. Radiographs of the cervical spine should be obtained.
D. Immediate orthopedic consultation should be arranged.
E. Immediate neurologic consultation should be arranged.

## ANSWERS

54.1 **B.** This infant most likely has GER with intermittent torticollis (Sandifer syndrome). He has a history of frequently spitting up and has had pneumonia (possibly aspiration), indicating he has GER. Sandifer syndrome infants have abnormal head posturing associated with reflux. The head movements are thought to occur in response to pain or to protect the airway.

54.2 **D.** This infant has sudden onset of the dystonic features of torticollis and facial grimacing, most likely as a result of the metoclopramide. However, initial evaluation for seizures, including measurement of serum electrolyte, glucose, and calcium levels, is indicated. Diphenhydramine administration may rapidly reverse this drug-induced dystonia. An MRI is unlikely to demonstrate a cervical abnormality because the symptom onset was abrupt. Cerebrospinal fluid analysis as a first step likely will not result in determination of the cause of this type of torticollis.

54.3 **B.** This child has signs and symptoms of retropharyngeal cellulitis or abscess. Such patients may have fever, dysphagia, drooling, stiff neck, dyspnea, or airway stridor. Physical findings include midline or unilateral swelling that may become a fluctuant mass. Management includes antibiotic therapy with possible incision and drainage of the abscess. Computerized tomography may be helpful in early identification of abscess formation.

54.4 **C.** This child appears to have had a difficult delivery, making muscular torticollis likely. If cervical spine radiography is normal, the parents can begin gentle stretching to move the head in a neutral position. If the condition persists, orthopedic referral is necessary.

## Clinical Pearls

- Muscular torticollis is most commonly found in infants as a result of sternocleidomastoid muscle trauma.
- Sandifer syndrome is characterized by gastroesophageal reflux and posturing of the head.
- Drug-induced dystonia is most frequently caused by phenothiazine, metoclopramide, and haloperidol.

## REFERENCES


Crawford AH. Congenital muscular torticollis. In: Rudolph CD, Rudolph AM, Hostetter MK, Lister G, Siegel NJ, eds. *Rudolph's Pediatrics*. 21st ed. New York, NY: McGraw-Hill; 2003:2439-2440.

Goldstein NA, Hammerschlag MR. Peritonsillar, retropharyngeal, and parapharyngeal abscesses. In: McMillan JA, Feigin RD, DeAngelis CD, Jones MD, eds. *Oski's Pediatrics: Principles and Practice*. 4th ed. Philadelphia, PA: Lippincott Williams & Wilkins; 2006:1492-1494.

Hazinski TA. Retropharyngeal and peritonsillar abscess. In: Rudolph CD, Rudolph AM, Hostetter MK, Lister G, Siegel NJ, eds. *Rudolph's Pediatrics*. 21st ed. New York, NY: McGraw-Hill; 2003:1944.

Jankovic J. Dystonia. In: McMillan JA, Feigin RD, DeAngelis CD, Jones MD, eds. *Oski's Pediatrics: Principles and Practice*. 4th ed. Philadelphia, PA: Lippincott Williams & Wilkins; 2006:2371-2373.

Orenstein S, Peters J, Khan S, Youssef N, Hussain SZ. Gastroesophageal reflux disease (GERD). In: Kliegman RM, Behrman RE, Jenson HB, Stanton BF, eds. *Nelson Textbook of Pediatrics*. 18th ed. Philadelphia, PA: WB Saunders; 2007:1547-1550.

Pappas DE, Hendley JO. Retropharyngeal abscess, lateral pharyngeal (parapharyngeal) abscess, and peritonsillar cellulitis/abscess. In: Kliegman RM, Behrman RE, Jenson HB, Stanton BF, eds. *Nelson Textbook of Pediatrics*. 18th ed. Philadelphia, PA: WB Saunders; 2007:1754-1756.

Spiegel DA, Hosalker HS, Dormans JP, Drommond DS. Torticollis. In: Kliegman RM, Behrman RE, Jenson HB, Stanton BF, eds. *Nelson Textbook of Pediatrics*. 18th ed. Philadelphia, PA: WB Saunders; 2007:2822-2823.

# Case 55

A healthy 2-week-old girl has yellow discharge from her left eye. Her mother had early prenatal care, the baby was delivered vaginally, and she was discharged at 48 hours of life. Within the first few days of life, the mother noted that the baby had increased tear production in her left eye, which now has yellow discharge. She has red reflexes bilaterally, her pupils are equal and reactive to light, and she has no scleral injection. She has left-sided mucopurulent ocular discharge.

- What is the most likely diagnosis?
- What is the next step in management?

# ANSWERS TO CASE 55:
# Dacryostenosis

*Summary:* A 2-week-old newborn has excessive unilateral tearing that progresses to mucopurulent eye discharge. The scleral conjunctivae are normal.

- **Most likely diagnosis:** Dacryostenosis (congenital nasolacrimal duct obstruction).
- **Next step in management:** Initial treatment involves nasolacrimal massage and eyelid cleansing. Topical antibiotics are added for purulent discharge.

## ANALYSIS

### Objectives

1. Know about excessive tearing in the newborn period.
2. Know the differential diagnosis of newborn conjunctivitis.

### Considerations

This infant had excessive tear production that later became a mucopurulent discharge but had an otherwise normal ophthalmologic examination. Of note, the conjunctiva is not inflamed and the cornea is not involved. Initial treatment includes topical antibiotic therapy and nasolacrimal duct massage two to three times daily with warm water eyelid cleansing.

# APPROACH TO
# Dacryocystitis

## DEFINITIONS

**CHEMOSIS:** Swelling and fluid collection in the membranes lining the eyelids and conjunctiva.

**DACRYOSTENOSIS:** A condition in neonates and infants caused by tear duct narrowing or blockage.

## CLINICAL APPROACH

The evaluation of a newborn with mucopurulent eye discharge includes examination of the conjunctivae, cornea, and pupils and assessment for a red reflex.

In dacryostenosis, these structures are normal. **Infants with dacryostenosis have unilateral or bilateral increased tearing.**

Dacryostenosis occurs in 2% to 6% of newborns and is caused by a **failure of canalization of the nasolacrimal duct.** Management includes nasolacrimal duct massage twice daily (expulsion of the proximal mucoid contents) and warm water eyelid washes. If mucoid contents become mucopurulent topical, ophthalmic antibiotics are initiated. **In 90% to 96% of cases, dacryostenosis resolves spontaneously, generally by 1 year of age.** For **refractory cases**, an ophthalmologist will **probe the nasolacrimal duct, and nasolacrimal ductal tubes or reconstructive surgery** occasionally is required. If dacryocystitis occurs, systemic antimicrobial therapy is indicated.

**Infantile glaucoma** occurs in 1 in 100,000 births with a **classic triad of tearing, photophobia, and blepharospasm.** It may be isolated or occur with various conditions, including congenital rubella, neurofibromatosis type 1, mucopolysaccharidosis I, Lowe oculocerebrorenal syndrome, Sturge-Weber syndrome, Marfan syndrome, and several chromosomal abnormalities. The increased intraocular pressure can lead to expansion of the globe and corneal damage.

If conjunctivitis is present (Figure 55–1), appropriate evaluation is critical. Ophthalmia neonatorum (conjunctivitis occurring in newborns younger than 4 weeks) is common and has multiple causes with variable prognosis. Physical findings of ophthalmia neonatorum include erythema and chemosis of the conjunctiva, eyelid edema, and discharge that may be purulent or serosanguineous. Timing, quality, and quantity of the discharge aid in diagnosis. Topical erythromycin, tetracycline, or silver nitrate used for gonococcal ocular prophylaxis may cause a mild chemical conjunctivitis that generally begins between 6 and 12 hours of birth and resolves by 48 hours of life. **Common neonatal conjunctivitis pathogens include *Neisseria gonorrhoeae* and *Chlamydia trachomatis*;** gonococcal infections usually present between the second and fifth days of life, whereas chlamydial infections become apparent between 5 and 14 days of life. The discharge of *N gonorrhoeae* begins as serosanguineous and then becomes purulent; corneal and conjunctival inflammation develops with potential complications of corneal ulceration, iridocyclitis, anterior synechiae, and panophthalmitis. Parenteral antimicrobial treatment with ceftriaxone or cefotaxime and frequent saline eye washing are required. Chlamydial conjunctivitis is notable for mild to severe inflammation of the tarsal conjunctivae; a purulent discharge may be present. A 2-week course of oral erythromycin is the preferred therapy for chlamydial infection; because erythromycin given in the neonatal period has been linked to infantile hypertrophic pyloric stenosis, informed consent should be obtained prior to use.

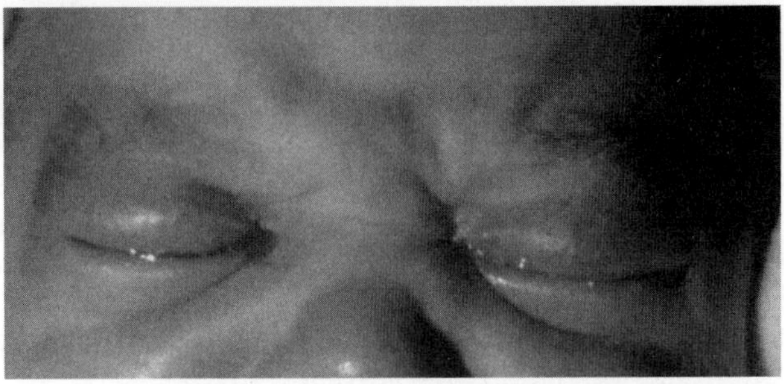

**Figure 55–1.** Infant with conjunctivitis. (*Courtesy of Kathryn H. Musgrove, MD.*)

## Comprehension Questions

55.1 A 6-month-old infant with right-sided dacryostenosis presents with mucopurulent discharge and an indurated, erythematous, tender 1-cm mass on the right side just below his nasal bridge. He has a temperature of 101°F (38.3°C). Which of the following is the best next step in management?

A. Administer intravenous antibiotic therapy.
B. Begin a course of topical antimicrobial treatment.
C. Recommend massage and warm compresses to the affected area.
D. Incise and drain the area.
E. Refer the child for an outpatient ophthalmologic evaluation.

55.2 An 8-hour-old newborn presents with bilateral conjunctivitis following routine newborn care in the nursery. Which of the following is the best next step in management?

A. Administer prophylaxis with topical erythromycin.
B. Send the eye discharge for culture and start antibiotics based on culture results.
C. Start saline eye washes.
D. Begin systemic antibiotic therapy with erythromycin.
E. Begin systemic antibiotic therapy with ceftriaxone.

55.3 A 2-week-old newborn presents with his foster mother because he has bilateral purulent eye discharge. His prenatal history is unknown. The examination demonstrates significant tarsal conjunctivitis and eye discharge. Which of the following statements is most accurate?

A. Initial therapy includes administration of intramuscular ceftriaxone.
B. The organism likely responsible also causes pneumonia in 1- to 3-month-old infants.
C. Immediate referral to a pediatric ophthalmologist is warranted.
D. Warm compresses and gentle massage are first-line therapies.
E. Topical antimicrobial therapy is preferred.

55.4 A 4-month-old infant has excessive right-sided tearing. His mother states he becomes irritable in bright light and calms in a darkened room. On examination, he has eye asymmetry, with the right eye appearing to be larger than the left. Which of the following statements is accurate?

A. Warm compresses and gentle massage are first-line therapy.
B. In most cases, treatment is nonsurgical.
C. The infant has the classic features of Down syndrome.
D. Immediate systemic antibiotic therapy will reduce complications.
E. Immediate referral to a pediatric ophthalmologist is warranted.

## ANSWERS

55.1 **A.** This infant has dacryocystitis and needs immediate systemic (not topical) antibiotics. Surgical treatment may be necessary.

55.2 **B.** Conjunctivitis in the first few hours of life is most likely caused by chemical irritation. Laboratory testing of the discharge is performed; treatment usually can be based upon laboratory results.

55.3 **B.** A chlamydial infection is the most likely cause of this patient's conjunctivitis. *Chlamydia trachomatis* causes infantile pneumonia, generally between 1 and 3 months of age, presenting with cough, tachypnea, and rales but no fever. A complete blood count might show eosinophilia. A 14- to 21-day course of oral erythromycin is given.

55.4 **E.** A history of excessive tearing and photophobia and examination findings of corneal enlargement suggest an immediate evaluation for congenital glaucoma is indicated.

## Clinical Pearls

- Dacryostenosis spontaneously resolves by 1 year of age in 90% to 96% of affected infants.
- Topical erythromycin, tetracycline, and silver nitrate are effective prophylaxis for gonococcal eye infection but not for chlamydial infection.
- Ophthalmologic complications of congenital rubella include glaucoma, cataracts, and retinopathy.
- Prophylactic oral erythromycin for infants of mothers with untreated chlamydial infection generally is not indicated; the efficacy has not been established and its use has been linked to infantile hypertrophic pyloric stenosis.

## REFERENCES

American Academy of Pediatrics. *Chlamydia trachomatis*. In: Pickering LK, ed. *2006 Red Book: Report of the Committee on Infectious Diseases*. 27th ed. Elk Grove Village, IL: American Academy of Pediatrics; 2006:252-257.

American Academy of Pediatrics. Prevention of neonatal ophthalmia. In: Pickering LK, ed. *2006 Red Book: Report of the Committee on Infectious Diseases*. 27th ed. Elk Grove Village, IL: American Academy of Pediatrics; 2006:836-838.

Darville T. *Neisseria gonorrhoeae* (Gonococcus). In: Kliegman RM, Behrman RE, Jenson HB, Stanton BF, eds. *Nelson Textbook of Pediatrics*. 18th ed. Philadelphia, PA: WB Saunders; 2007:1169-1173.

Hammerschlag MR. Chlamydial infections. In: McMillan JA, DeAngelis CD, Feigin RD, Warshaw JB, eds. *Oski's Pediatrics: Principles and Practice*. 3rd ed. Philadelphia, PA: Lippincott Williams & Wilkins; 1999:895-898.

Olitsky SE, Hug D, Smith LP. Disorders of the lacrimal system. In: Kliegman RM, Behrman RE, Jenson HB, Stanton BF, eds. *Nelson Textbook of Pediatrics*. 18th ed. Philadelphia, PA: WB Saunders; 2007:2587.

Patterson LER. Gonococcal infections. In: McMillan JA, Feigin RD, DeAngelis CD, Jones MD, eds. *Oski's Pediatrics: Principles and Practice*. 4th ed. Philadelphia, PA: Lippincott Williams & Wilkins; 2006:1088-1092.

Patterson MJ. Rubella. In: Rudolph CD, Rudolph AM, Hostetter MK, Lister G, Siegel NJ, eds. *Rudolph's Pediatrics*. 21st ed. New York, NY: McGraw-Hill; 2003:1075-1079.

Staat MA. Chlamydial infections. In: Rudolph CD, Rudolph AM, Hostetter MK, Lister G, Siegel NJ, eds. *Rudolph's Pediatrics*. 21st ed. New York, NY: McGraw-Hill; 2003:929-931.

Staat MA. *Neisseria gonorrhoeae*. In: Rudolph CD, Rudolph AM, Hostetter MK, Lister G, Siegel NJ, eds. *Rudolph's Pediatrics*. 21st ed. New York, NY: McGraw-Hill; 2003:967-970.

Tong JT. Lacrimal system. In: Rudolph CD, Rudolph AM, Hostetter MK, Lister G, Siegel NJ, eds. *Rudolph's Pediatrics*. 21st ed. New York, NY: McGraw-Hill; 2003: 2366-2367.

Traboulsi EI. Pediatric ophthalmology. In: McMillan JA, Feigin RD, DeAngelis CD, Jones MD, eds. *Oski's Pediatrics: Principles and Practice*. 4th ed. Philadelphia, PA: Lippincott Williams & Wilkins; 2006:809-812, 819.

# Case 56

A 15-month-old boy presents because his parents are concerned that he does not speak recognizable words, has never made babbling sounds such as "baba" or "dada," does not follow verbal commands, and does not respond to his name. He is appropriately affectionate and makes good eye contact with both of his parents. The child was a full-term baby without hospitalizations or frequent illnesses. He sat without support at 6 months and began walking at 12 months. He is active in the examination room, but he does not respond to his name or to verbal cues from his mother. He is a well-developed, well-nourished normal child otherwise.

- ➤ What is the most likely diagnosis?
- ➤ What is the next step?

# ANSWERS TO CASE 56:
## Severe Hearing Loss

*Summary:* A 15-month-old healthy boy has severe language delay but normal motor development.

➤ **Most likely diagnosis:** Hearing loss.

➤ **Next step:** Audiologic evaluation.

## ANALYSIS

### Objectives

1. Understand the major types of hearing loss.
2. Be aware of common causes of hearing loss.

### Considerations

This 15-month-old boy has never made babbling sounds such as "baba" and "dada," which are the normal precursors to language development and usually are seen by 9 months of age. His history and physical examination do not lead to a specific reason for this speech delay (eg, global developmental delay, syndromic features, or history of prematurity with associated morbidity). The next step is an audiologic evaluation.

# APPROACH TO
## Hearing Loss

## DEFINITIONS

**CONDUCTIVE HEARING LOSS:** Hearing loss caused by disorders of the outer ear (external auditory canal atresia and otitis externa) or middle ear (otitis media and cholesteatoma).

**RETROCOCHLEAR (CENTRAL) HEARING LOSS:** Hearing loss caused by deficits in the auditory nerve or central auditory nervous system.

**SENSORINEURAL HEARING LOSS (SNHL):** Hearing loss caused by cochlea disorders (damage from infection, noise, ototoxic agents, or genetic defects).

## CLINICAL APPROACH

Hearing can be divided into several categories ranging from normal hearing (threshold 0-5 decibels [dB]) to profound hearing loss (>70 dB). With mild hearing loss (25-30 dB), inability to hear some speech sounds is noted; with moderate hearing loss (30-50 dB), most normal speech is indiscernible. One to two newborns per 1000 live births have moderate to profound bilateral SNHL.

**Sensorineural hearing loss can be congenital or acquired.** Approximately half of SNHL cases result from **genetic factors.** The hearing loss may be isolated or occur with other syndromic anomalies. The most **common autosomal dominant syndromes** associated are **Waardenburg syndrome types I and II** (partial albinism [often a white forelock], deafness, lateral displacement of the inner canthi, heterochromic irises, medial eyebrow flare, and a broad nasal bridge and mandible) and **branchio-oto-renal syndrome** (hearing impairment, preauricular pits, branchial fistulas, renal impairment, and external ear abnormalities). Other entities include Alport syndrome (nephritis, progressive renal failure, SNHL, ocular abnormalities), Down syndrome, neurofibromatosis, Jervell and Lange-Nielsen (prolonged QT) syndrome, and Hunter-Hurler syndrome. Ophthalmic or craniofacial abnormalities, external ear malformations, and metabolic, neurologic, or musculoskeletal disorders may be associated with SNHL.

**Prenatal cytomegalovirus (CMV) infection is the most common infectious cause of congenital SNHL;** it can cause hearing loss later in infancy and childhood. Toxoplasmosis, rubella, and syphilis can lead to congenital SNHL; ongoing hearing evaluations are important. Postnatal infections associated with acquired SNHL include group B streptococcal sepsis and *Streptococcus pneumoniae* meningitis. *Haemophilus influenzae* meningitis, mumps, measles, and rubella were common causes prior to current vaccination practices.

Pharmacologic and chemical exposures can cause SNHL. Aminoglycosides, loop diuretics, chemotherapeutic agents (cisplatin), lead, arsenic, and quinine may cause SNHL with *in utero* or postnatal exposure. Other causes include temporal bone fractures, head trauma, extracorporeal membrane oxygenation (ECMO), radiation, and prolonged exposure to loud noise.

Early diagnosis of hearing impairment can impact development of communication skills. Hearing adequacy is evaluated at medical visits by asking parents about their baby's response to sounds and their baby's early language development. Universal newborn hearing screening via otoacoustic emissions (OAE) or auditory brainstem–evoked responses (ABRs) is now recommended and is required by most states; the goal is hearing loss diagnosis prior to age 3 months and intervention before age 6 months. **Early intervention is believed to enhance communication skills and academic performance.**

Various hearing screening methods are used, depending on the child's developmental level and degree of hearing loss. Auditory brainstem–evoked response testing, often used in newborns, measures electrophysiologic response and does not require cooperation. Otoacoustic emissions are absent if the hearing threshold is above 30 to 40 dB. Infants through young preschool children can be assessed via visual reinforcement audiometry, behavioral audiometry, or play audiometry; these methods reveal information specific to each ear. In cooperative children, air conduction audiometry can be performed, using headphones and pure tones between 250 and 8000 Hz. The same sounds are presented via oscillator, usually on the mastoid, thus evaluating bone conduction.

Children with SNHL are evaluated by an audiologist and speech pathologist. Patients with mild to moderate hearing loss can benefit from hearing aids, which can be fitted in infants as young as 2 months. With severe and profound hearing loss, a combination of hearing aids, sign language, lip reading, and attention to appropriate educational surroundings is used. Cochlear implantation is a treatment option for selected children older than 2 years.

## Comprehension Questions

56.1 A 26-month-old boy presents because of maternal concern about his hearing. Over the past few weeks, his mother has had to speak more loudly in order for him to respond. He has a greater than 50-word vocabulary and can put together 2- to 3-word sentences. Three weeks prior he had an upper respiratory infection (URI). Which of the following is the best next step in treatment?

A. Order ABR testing.
B. Perform otoscopy with insufflation.
C. Send him for a complete audiologic evaluation.
D. Perform hearing screening in the office.
E. Explain to the mother that 2-year-old children often do not respond to their parents.

56.2 A 4-month-old boy has a white forelock, a broad mandible, and lateral displacement of his inner canthi. His mother also has a white forelock. Which of the following statements is true?

A. A urinalysis will demonstrate increased protein levels.
B. He is not at risk for hearing loss if his mother has normal hearing.
C. He is at risk for SNHL; order an audiologic evaluation.
D. The inheritance pattern of this disorder is X-linked recessive.
E. He should have ongoing office hearing screening with referral for formal hearing if abnormalities are detected.

56.3 Which of the following groups of children is at especially high risk for hearing loss?

A. A full-term, large-for-gestational-age male born to a mother with gestational diabetes
B. An appropriate-for-gestational age (AGA) infant, the product of a 34-week pregnancy, who had Apgar scores of 7 and 8 at 1 and 5 minutes, respectively
C. A term, 3300-g infant born by cesarean section who had a peak total bilirubin level of 18 mg/dL at 72 hours of life
D. A term AGA baby who received cefotaxime and ampicillin for 48 hours for suspected sepsis
E. A term AGA infant born by cesarean section for placental abruption with Apgar scores of 3 and 5 at 1 and 5 minutes, respectively

56.4 Which of the following would be the expected language development of a normal 24-month-old child?

A. Speech that is 90% understandable
B. A 10-word vocabulary but no combination of words
C. A 50-word vocabulary and 2-word combinations to make a sentence
D. Appropriate use of pronouns
E. A 200-word vocabulary and 4- to 5-word combinations to make a sentence

## ANSWERS

56.1 **B.** This child has normal speech development and was recently noted to have a possible hearing deficit. With the recent URI, he is at risk for otitis media with effusion and conductive hearing loss. Otoscopy with insufflation (gently blowing air into the ear canal to determine tympanic membrane movement) is helpful for qualitative evaluation of middle ear effusion. Tympanometry is a reliable, quantitative tool for assessing middle ear effusion. If he has conductive hearing loss, further evaluation is indicated.

56.2 **C.** This child has features of Waardenburg syndrome (partial albinism, often a white forelock, SNHL, lateral inner canthi displacement, medial eyebrow flaring, and a broad nasal bridge and mandible); inheritance is autosomal dominant. Children with syndromic features strongly associated with hearing loss require hearing evaluation.

56.3 **E.** Infants born with Apgar scores of 4 or less at 1 minute and 6 or less at 5 minutes require audiologic evaluation. Other infants who should undergo testing include those with a family history of childhood SNHL; cytomegalovirus, rubella, syphilis, herpes, or toxoplasmosis infection; craniofacial anomalies; birth weight less than 1500 g; hyperbilirubinemia at a level requiring exchange transfusion; bacterial meningitis; mechanical ventilation for more than 5 days; and stigmata of syndromes associated with hearing loss, especially those with renal abnormalities.

56.4 **C.** At 24 months of age, the average child has a vocabulary of approximately 50 words and forms 2-word sentences. A 12-month-old child has a vocabulary of two to four words in addition to appropriately saying "mama" and "dada." By 36 months, a child should have a vocabulary of 250 words, produce at least 3-word sentences, and use pronouns.

## Clinical Pearls

- Cytomegalovirus infection is the most common infectious cause of congenital sensorineural hearing loss.
- Aminoglycosides and loop diuretics may cause sensorineural hearing loss.
- Syndromes associated with renal abnormalities have a higher incidence of hearing loss.
- Universal hearing screening at birth is recommended.

## REFERENCES


American Academy of Pediatrics. Newborn and infant hearing loss: detection and intervention. *Pediatrics*. 1999;103:527-530.

Haddad J. Hearing loss. In: Kliegman RM, Behrman RE, Jenson HB, Stanton BF, eds. *Nelson Textbook of Pediatrics*. 18th ed. Philadelphia, PA: WB Saunders; 2006:2620-2628.

Joint Committee on Infant Hearing, American Academy of Audiology, American Academy of Pediatrics, American Speech-Language-Hearing Association, and Directors of Speech and Hearing Programs in State Health and Welfare Agencies. Year 2000 position statement: principles and guidelines for early hearing detection and intervention programs. *Pediatrics*. 2000;106;798-817.

Kelly DP. Hearing problems: impairment to deafness. In: Rudolph CD, Rudolph AM, Hostetter MK, Lister G, Siegel NJ, eds. *Rudolph's Pediatrics*. 21st ed. New York, NY: McGraw-Hill; 2003:485-489.

Paller AS. Disorders of pigmentation. In: Rudolph CD, Rudolph AM, Hostetter MK, Lister G, Siegel NJ, eds. *Rudolph's Pediatrics*. 21st ed. New York, NY: McGraw-Hill; 2003:1185-1187.

Robin NH, Jeng LB. The child with hearing loss. In: Rudolph CD, Rudolph AM, Hostetter MK, Lister G, Siegel NJ, eds. *Rudolph's Pediatrics*. 21st ed. New York, NY: McGraw-Hill; 2003:782-784.

# Case 57

A previously healthy 3-year-old boy presents with sudden onset of rash. His mother says he had been playing when she noticed small red spots and a large purple area on his skin. He has had no fever, upper respiratory tract infection (URI) symptoms, or diarrhea, and he is not taking medications. Three weeks previously, he had a mild illness that self-resolved after 48 hours. He is playful on examination, but he has multiple petechiae and purpuric lesions on his upper and lower extremities and on his trunk. He has neither adenopathy nor splenomegaly. His white blood cell (WBC) count is 8500/mm$^3$, hemoglobin level 14 mg/dL, and his platelet count is 20,000/mm$^3$.

- What is the most likely diagnosis?
- What is the next step in management?

# ANSWERS TO CASE 57:
# Idiopathic (Immune) Thrombocytopenic Purpura

*Summary*: A healthy 3-year-old develops thrombocytopenia, petechiae, and purpuric lesions. He is well-appearing but recently had a febrile illness. His WBC count and hemoglobin levels are normal.

- **Most likely diagnosis:** Idiopathic (immune) thrombocytopenic purpura (ITP).
- **Next step in management:** Evaluation of his peripheral blood smear.

## ANALYSIS

### Objectives

1. Know the most common causes of childhood thrombocytopenia.
2. Understand the natural history of ITP.

### Considerations

This 3-year-old has purpuric lesions and petechiae resulting from thrombocytopenia. He lacks the systemic signs of illness expected with disseminated intravascular coagulation or hemolytic-uremic syndrome (HUS). Because his hemoglobin level and WBC count are normal, bone marrow infiltration is less likely the cause of his thrombocytopenia. A peripheral blood smear is examined to identify immature WBCs and red cell morphology. Children with ITP have normal peripheral blood smears without evidence of leukemic or microangiopathic processes. This child has a platelet count of $20{,}000/mm^3$ and lacks evidence of active bleeding; the next step is close observation.

# APPROACH TO
# Thrombocytopenia

## DEFINITIONS

**HEMOLYTIC-UREMIC SYNDROME (HUS):** A syndrome of nephropathy, thrombocytopenia, and microangiopathic hemolytic anemia. It is associated with *Escherichia coli* 0157:H7, *Shigella*, and *Salmonella*. A prodrome of bloody diarrhea is common.

**HENOCH-SCHÖNLEIN PURPURA (HSP):** A syndrome of small-vessel vasculitis in young children. The syndrome may have dermatologic (petechial/purpuric rash), renal (nephritis), gastrointestinal (abdominal pain, gastrointestinal bleeding, intussception), and joint involvement (arthritis).

**IDIOPATHIC (IMMUNE) THROMBOCYTOPENIC PURPURA (ITP):** A condition of increased platelet destruction by circulating antiplatelet antibodies, most frequently antiglycoprotein IIb/IIIa.

## CLINICAL APPROACH

**Acute ITP is the most common cause of thrombocytopenia in a well child usually aged 2 to 5 years.** The evidence suggests an immunologic etiology triggered by a preceding viral illness, but the specific pathophysiologic mechanism is unknown. Acute ITP occurs with an equal gender distribution. Young children usually present with acute onset of petechiae and purpura and a history of a viral illness 1 to 4 weeks previously. Bleeding from the gingivae and other mucous membranes may occur. Examination findings include petechiae and purpura, especially in trauma areas. If significant lymphadenopathy or organomegaly is found, other causes for thrombocytopenia are considered.

Laboratory findings include thrombocytopenia, which can be severe ($<$20,000/mm$^3$), but the platelet size is normal or increased. The WBC count and hemoglobin level are normal (unless excessive bleeding has occurred). Prothrombin time (PT) and activated partial thromboplastin time (aPTT) are normal. The peripheral blood smear may reveal eosinophilia or atypical lymphocytes; immature WBCs and abnormal red cell morphology are absent. Generally, bone marrow aspiration is unnecessary. If the peripheral blood smear is concerning, the WBC count abnormal, or adenopathy or organomegaly is present, **bone marrow evaluation** aids in proper diagnosis, demonstrating an **increased number of megakaryocytes** in ITP. Within 1 month of presentation, more than half of untreated children have complete resolution of their thrombocytopenia and up to another 30% have resolution by 6 months. Persistence beyond 6 months is considered chronic ITP.

The **most serious ITP complication, intracranial hemorrhage**, occurs in less than 1% of affected children. Patients with severe thrombocytopenia ($<$20,000/mm$^3$), extensive mucosal bleeding, severe complications (eg, massive gastrointestinal bleeds), or without a protective environment may require medical intervention. **Treatment is controversial**; data do not demonstrate improved outcomes. Treatment to decrease platelet destruction includes **intravenous immunoglobulin** for 1 to 2 days, **intravenous anti-D therapy,** or a 2- to 3-week course of **systemic corticosteroids.** Platelet transfusion is reserved for life-threatening bleeding. **Splenectomy** may be considered in children with **serious complications not responding to other therapies. After splenectomy, pneumococcal vaccine and penicillin prophylaxis** are required because of risk for sepsis.

**From 10% to 20% of ITP patients have chronic thrombocytopenia lasting for more than 6 months,** occurring more commonly in older children and in females; it may be part of other autoimmune disease or may occur with infection such as human immunodeficiency virus (HIV) or Epstein-Barr virus (EBV). The ITP treatment options listed above are available for chronic ITP patients; the goal remains prevention of serious thrombocytopenia complications.

Many pharmacologic agents may cause immune-mediated thrombocytopenia, including penicillins, trimethoprim-sulfamethoxazole, digoxin, quinine, quinidine, cimetidine, benzodiazepine, and heparin. The measles, mumps, and rubella (MMR) vaccine is associated with thrombocytopenia and is used cautiously in ITP patients.

## Comprehension Questions

57.1 A 2-year-old girl has a rash. She was well until 2 weeks prior when she had fever and URI symptoms that resolved without treatment. On examination, she has petechiae on her upper and lower extremities and trunk. Her platelet count is $25{,}000/mm^3$. Her WBC count is $9000/mm^3$ and hemoglobin level is 11 mg/dL. Which of the following is the best next step in management?

A. Obtain a review of the peripheral blood smear.
B. Administer intravenous immunoglobulin.
C. Send a blood culture and begin empiric antimicrobial therapy.
D. Order a platelet transfusion.
E. Arrange for bone marrow biopsy.

57.2 A 14-year-old adolescent female has a rash on her arms and legs. She was diagnosed with a urinary tract infection 4 days ago, which is being treated with trimethoprim-sulfamethoxazole. She denies fever, vomiting, diarrhea, headache, and dysuria. On examination she has multiple upper- and lower-extremity petechiae. Her WBC count is $7000/mm^3$ and hemoglobin level 13 mg/dL; her platelet count is $35{,}000/mm^3$. Which of the following is the best next step in management?

A. Send blood for antinuclear antibody (ANA).
B. Send a repeat urinalysis.
C. Discontinue the trimethoprim-sulfamethoxazole.
D. Obtain HIV testing.
E. Administer intravenous immunoglobulin.

57.3 A 7-year-old boy has a rash on his lower extremities and pain in his right knee. He has had a low-grade fever and abdominal pain, and he has felt tired. He is nontoxic appearing, but he has palpable petechiae on his lower extremities and buttocks. His right knee is mildly edematous and he can bear weight on his right leg, but complains of pain. His prothrombin time (PT), partial thromboplastin time (PTT), and platelet counts are normal. Which of the following is the best next step in management?

A. Begin a course of systemic corticosteroids.
B. Begin empiric antimicrobial therapy for sepsis.
C. Obtain a urinalysis and provide supportive care.
D. Perform aspiration of the synovial fluid in his right knee.
E. Administer intravenous immunoglobulin.

57.4 A 3-year-old boy has pallor, lethargy, and decreased urine output. He was well until the preceding week, when he had fever, vomiting, and bloody diarrhea (now resolved). On examination, he is lethargic and has hepatosplenomegaly and scattered petechiae. Urinalysis reveals hematuria and proteinuria. Which of the following statements about his condition is accurate?

A. A complete blood (cell) count (CBC) is likely to reveal thrombocytosis.
B. Initial therapy includes systemic corticosteroids.
C. Empiric antimicrobial therapy for sepsis should be initiated.
D. An emergent oncology consultation for probable leukemia should be arranged.
E. Peripheral blood smear is likely to reveal helmet cells and burr cells.

## ANSWERS

57.1 **A.** This child has the classic ITP features of isolated thrombocytopenia in a well-appearing child. An examination and peripheral blood smear are necessary. If no lymphadenopathy or organomegaly is found and the peripheral blood smear is normal, initial management includes close observation and a protective environment.

57.2 **C.** The thrombocytopenia may be the result of the trimethoprim-sulfamethoxazole; the medicine is discontinued and her platelet count is monitored. If thrombocytopenia continues, she may have ITP and is followed for chronic ITP. Chronic ITP occurs in older children (female predominance); it may be seen with autoimmune disease such as systemic lupus erythematosus or with chronic infections including HIV.

57.3 **C.** This child has signs and symptoms of HSP, a vasculitis of the small vessels with renal, gastrointestinal, joint, and dermatologic involvement. Initial therapy consists of hydration and pain control. With renal involvement, urinalysis reveals red blood (cell) counts (RBCs), WBCs, casts, or protein. Gastrointestinal complications include hemorrhage, obstruction, and **intussusception**; abdominal pain requires careful evaluation.

57.4 **E.** This child has features of HUS, which frequently follows a bout of gastroenteritis; it has been associated with *E coli* 0157:H7, *Shigella*, and *Salmonella*. Patients have pallor, lethargy, and decreased urine output; some have hepatosplenomegaly, petechiae, and edema. Laboratory findings include hemolytic anemia and thrombocytopenia; peripheral blood smear demonstrates helmet cells, burr cells, and fragmented RBCs. Acute renal failure is manifested by hematuria, proteinuria, and an elevated serum creatinine level. Management is supportive with careful monitoring of renal and hematologic parameters; dialysis may be required.

## Clinical Pearls

- Idiopathic thrombocytopenic purpura is the most common cause of acute thrombocytopenia in a well young child.
- Approximately 70% to 80% of children with idiopathic thrombocytopenic purpura have spontaneous resolution within 6 months.
- Hemolytic-uremic syndrome consists of nephropathy, thrombocytopenia, and microangiopathic hemolytic anemia; it is associated with *E coli* 0157:H7, *Shigella*, and *Salmonella*.

## REFERENCES

Casalla JF, Pelidis MA, Takemoto CM. Disorders of platelets. In: McMillan JA, Feigin RD, DeAngelis CD, Jones MD, eds. *Oski's Pediatrics: Principles and Practice*. 4th ed. Philadelphia, PA: Lippincott Williams & Wilkins; 2006:1731-1736.

Davis ID, Avner ED. Hemolytic-uremic syndrome. In: Kliegman RM, Behrman RE, Jenson HB, Stanton BF, eds. *Nelson Textbook of Pediatrics*. 18th ed. Philadelphia, PA: WB Saunders; 2007:2181-2182.

de Inocencio J. Henoch-Schönlein purpura (anaphylactoid purpura). In: Rudolph CD, Rudolph AM, Hostetter MK, Lister G, Siegel NJ, eds. *Rudolph's Pediatrics*. 21st ed. New York, NY: McGraw-Hill; 2003:842-844.

Eddy AA. Hemolytic uremic syndrome. In: Rudolph CD, Rudolph AM, Hostetter MK, Lister G, Siegel NJ, eds. *Rudolph's Pediatrics*. 21st ed. New York, NY: McGraw-Hill; 2003:1696-1698.

Eddy AA. Henoch-Schönlein purpura nephritis. In: Rudolph CD, Rudolph AM, Hostetter MK, Lister G, Siegel NJ, eds. *Rudolph's Pediatrics*. 21st ed. New York, NY: McGraw-Hill; 2003:1688-1689.

Freedman MH. Disorders of platelets. In: Rudolph CD, Rudolph AM, Hostetter MK, Lister G, Siegel NJ, eds. *Rudolph's Pediatrics*. 21st ed. New York, NY: McGraw-Hill; 2003:1555-1557.

Higuchi LM, Sundel RP. Henoch-Schönlein syndrome. In: McMillan JA, Feigin RD, DeAngelis CD, Jones MD eds. *Oski's Pediatrics: Principles and Practice*. 4th ed. Philadelphia, PA: Lippincott Williams & Wilkins; 2006:2559-2562.

Scott JP, Montgomery RR. Idiopathic thrombocytopenic purpura and hemolytic-uremic syndrome. In: Behrman RE, Kliegman RM, Jenson HB, eds. *Nelson Textbook of Pediatrics*. 18th ed. Philadelphia, PA: WB Saunders; 2007:2082-2085.

Sheth RD. Hemolytic-uremic syndrome. In: McMillan JA, Feigin RD, DeAngelis CD, Jones MD, eds. *Oski's Pediatrics: Principles and Practice*. 4th ed. Philadelphia, PA: Lippincott Williams & Wilkins; 2006:2600-2602.

# Case 58

A 2-year-old boy presents with inability to walk for 2 days after falling from the bed onto a carpeted floor. He lives with his mother, 15-month-old sister, and 3-month-old brother. On physical examination, the child is apprehensive and has pain on right thigh palpation. Radiographs of the right lower extremity reveal a femur fracture.

- What is the most likely diagnosis?
- What is the next step in the management of this child?

# ANSWERS TO CASE 58:

# Child Abuse

*Summary:* A 2-year-old boy presents with a 2-day history of inability to walk. The only trauma noted is a fall from the bed. A metaphyseal femur fracture is present.

- **Most likely diagnosis:** Physical abuse.
- **Next step:** Obtain a skeletal survey.

## ANALYSIS

### Objectives

1. Understand the importance of reporting suspected child maltreatment.
2. Recognize that child abuse is suspected if significant inconsistencies exist between the physical injury and the trauma history.

### Considerations

The only trauma history for this child is a fall from a bed onto a carpeted floor; it is unlikely that a significant injury (femur fracture) would arise from a common, insignificant fall. The history seems incongruent with the injury. The mother's delay in seeking medical care for 2 days from symptom onset is concerning. Cases of suspected abuse are reported to Child Protective Services (CPS) or law enforcement. Thus, the next steps are to obtain a complete skeletal survey to detect other bony injuries and to report this child's possible abuse case to CPS.

# APPROACH TO

# Child Abuse

## DEFINITIONS

**CHILD PROTECTIVE SERVICES (CPS):** Local governmental agency responsible for investigating suspected child maltreatment cases.

**MUNCHAUSEN SYNDROME BY PROXY:** Abuse in which the caretaker falsifies symptoms or inflicts injury upon a child to necessitate medical intervention.

**ABUSIVE HEAD TRAUMA (SHAKEN BABY OR SHAKEN IMPACT SYNDROME):** Brain injury resulting from violent shaking of the infant or shaking the infant followed by collision of the head against a hard surface. Infants may present with seizures, respiratory arrest, a bulging fontanelle, or irritability. Intracranial injury is found with computerized tomography (CT) or magnetic resonance image (MRI), and **retinal hemorrhages** may be visualized on funduscopy. Skeletal injuries such as rib fractures may also be present.

## CLINICAL APPROACH

Child maltreatment is common, with approximately 1 million substantiated cases per year in the United States. Child maltreatment includes neglect and physical, sexual, and emotional abuse; children often suffer from more than one type. **Neglect is the most common form of child maltreatment and consists of failure to provide adequate nutrition, shelter, supervision, or medical care.** Physical abuse accounts for approximately 20% of cases, occurring when caregivers inflict excessive physical injury. Although the definition of "appropriate" corporal punishment is argued, physical abuse is considered when marks (eg, bruising, lacerations, burns, or fractures) result. Sexual abuse occurs in 10% of substantiated maltreatment cases (see Case 12).

Munchausen syndrome by proxy is a less common form of child abuse. Affected children are hospitalized repeatedly with undiagnosed or vague conditions. Children may also have underlying medical conditions with abnormally frequent or persistent symptoms. The hospitalization is remarkable for a caretaker who takes great interest in the medical staff and interventions and often times has some type of medical background. The caretaker forms relationships with health-care providers and is often noted to be an exemplary parent. Munchausen syndrome by proxy ranges from fabricating symptoms to actual poisoning or suffocations.

Reporting of cases of child maltreatment has been mandated since the 1960s, resulting in increased public and medical awareness. Health-care providers legally are required to report suspected abuse to CPS or law enforcement.

Medical evaluation of suspected child maltreatment cases includes obtaining a medical history and a family assessment, conducting a thorough physical examination, obtaining appropriate diagnostic testing, and interviewing the child and the family. Routine medical history includes information about illnesses, hospitalizations, injuries, and pertinent family history. History should be carefully documented within the medical record as discrepancies to different providers or by different caretakers may provide vital information. A **developmental history** helps determine if the events described by a family is a plausible explanation for injuries found (eg, a 10-month-old child is unable to climb into a bathtub, turn on the water, and sustain second-degree burns only to the buttocks). Documentation must include who lives in the home and who provides care for the child.

An examination is performed with attention to any skin lesions. Body charts (or photographs) assist in documenting the injuries. **A skeletal survey (skull, chest, spine, and limbs) assists in obtaining evidence of prior trauma in children younger than 3 years.** Recent fractures may not be detectable on plain radiographs for 1 to 2 weeks after an injury; if necessary, bone scans demonstrate fractures within 24 to 48 hours of injury. Children with bruising often are evaluated with a platelet count and coagulation studies to eliminate hematologic disorders as a cause.

Although bruises and lacerations are common abuse indicators, they also are common in nonabused children. **Accidental bruises are usually found over bony areas** (knees, shins, elbows, forehead) and are appropriate for the child's developmental milestones. **Abdomen, buttocks, thighs, and inner arm bruises occur less frequently in cases of accidental trauma.** Characteristic child abuse injury patterns include looped cord marks, belt buckle–shaped lesions, multiple bruises in various stages of healing, hand prints, bite marks, and circumferential cord marks around the neck from strangulation. Burn injuries may resemble the insulting object, such as a steam or curling iron. **Intentional hot water immersion usually leaves a sharply demarcated border; the "stocking glove" distribution is a classic pattern.** Cigarette burns are circular and appear similar to impetigo.

The differential diagnosis of multiple ecchymoses includes hemophilia, immune (idiopathic) thrombocytopenic purpura (ITP), Henoch-Schönlein purpura (or other vasculitis), and disseminated intravascular coagulation (DIC). Patterned injury can result from folk medicine practices, such as cupping (a heated cup applied to the skin leaves a circular injury) or coin rubbing (leaves linear red marks on the back). A history, physical examination, and a few screening tests can help eliminate these diagnostic considerations.

Skeletal injuries suspicious for abuse include long bone metaphyses injuries, rib or complex skull fractures, and multiple fractures (especially those in various stages of healing). Spiral or oblique long bone fractures can result from unintentional rotating force injuries; they are no longer considered diagnostic of abuse. Nursemaid's elbow (radial head subluxation) occurs accidentally when a toddler falls while walking and holding an adult's hand (elbow dislocation occurs as the limb is pulled and twisted). Osteogenesis imperfecta, scurvy, cortical hyperostosis, and Menkes kinky hair disease are rare pediatric conditions with increased risk of bony injury.

## Comprehension Questions

58.1 A 2-year-old boy presents 4 hours after a left arm injury. He tried to run into the street, and his mother held his left hand tightly and he fell. Since then he has not moved his arm. Now he holds the arm close to his body with the elbow flexed and the forearm pronated. The elbow is not erythematous or edematous. He cries when the elbow is touched. Which of the following is the best next step in management?

A. Obtain a radiograph of the left elbow.
B. Order a skeletal survey.
C. Place the left arm in a sling.
D. Supinate the child's forearm while applying pressure over the radial head.
E. Apply traction to the forearm while increasing the degree of pronation.

58.2 A 15-year-old adolescent female has 2 days of nasal congestion and cough. Upon auscultation of her back, you find the lesions noted (Figure 58–1). Which of the following is the most likely etiology for her condition?

A. Cupping
B. Physical abuse
C. Disseminated intravascular coagulation
D. Henoch-Schönlein purpura
E. Coining

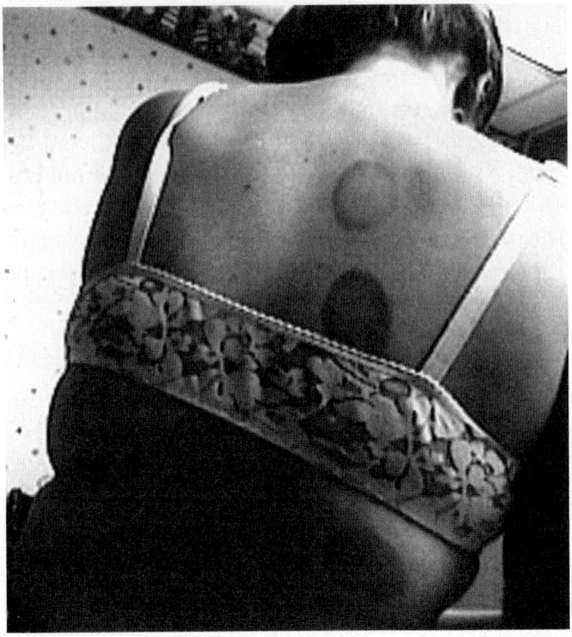

**Figure 58–1.** Picture of a child's back.

58.3 Which of the following describes the most common form of child maltreatment?

A. Sexual abuse
B. Physical abuse
C. Neglect
D. Emotional abuse
E. Munchausen syndrome by proxy

58.4 A 4-month-old girl is fussy, appears to have pain on palpation of the right leg, and has bluish sclerae. Radiographs reveal a right femur fracture. Her parents deny any severe trauma but report she had multiple fractures as a child. Family history is also likely to include which of the following?

A. Blindness
B. Hearing loss
C. Tall stature
D. Renal disease
E. Aortic aneurysm

## ANSWERS

58.1 **D.** This child's history is consistent with a traction injury involving an outstretched arm. The elbow is not swollen and the arm is held in a flexed and pronated position. The child likely has "nursemaid's elbow." To reduce the subluxation, apply radial head pressure while supinating the arm. If treatment is not delayed, he will usually begin using the arm promptly.

58.2 **A.** This adolescent has multiple perfectly circular lesions on her back consistent with cupping; when asked, she gives the history of cupping. Physical abuse injuries likely would not be identical in appearance. Patients with DIC will have significant systemic manifestation, and the pattern of ecchymoses would not be symmetrical. Coining causes ecchymosis in a linear pattern.

58.3 **C.** The most common form of child maltreatment is neglect (failure to provide adequate nutrition, shelter, supervision, or health care).

58.4 **B.** This infant has features of osteogenesis imperfecta, an autosomal dominant genetic disorder. Features include long bone fractures and vertebral injury with minimal trauma, short stature, deafness, and blue sclerae. Four types exist: type I is mild; type II is lethal (*in utero* or shortly thereafter); type III is the most severe; and type IV is moderately severe.

### Clinical Pearls

- All cases of suspected child maltreatment must be reported to Child Protective Services or law enforcement.
- If the history of trauma does not fit a patient's injury pattern, child abuse is suspected.
- If a child's development is inconsistent with the injury history, child abuse is suspected.

## REFERENCES

Carey JC, Bamshad MJ. Osteogenesis imperfecta. In: Rudolph CD, Rudolph AM, Hostetter MK, Lister G, Siegel NJ, eds. *Rudolph's Pediatrics*. 21st ed. New York, NY: McGraw-Hill; 2003:761-762.

Johnson CF. Abuse and neglect of children. In: Kliegman RM, Behrman RE, Jenson HB, Stanton BF, eds. *Nelson Textbook of Pediatrics*. 18th ed. Philadelphia, PA: WB Saunders; 2007:171-184.

Leventhal JM. Child maltreatment: neglect to abuse. In: Rudolph CD, Rudolph AM, Hostetter MK, Lister G, Siegel NJ, eds. *Rudolph's Pediatrics*. 21st ed. New York, NY: McGraw-Hill; 2003:463-470.

Marini JC. Osteogenesis imperfecta. In: Kliegman RM, Behrman RE, Jenson HB, Stanton BF, eds. *Nelson Textbook of Pediatrics*. 18th ed. Philadelphia, PA: WB Saunders; 2007:2887-2890.

Reece RM. Child maltreatment. In: McMillan JA, Feigin RD, DeAngelis CD, Jones MD, eds. *Oski's Pediatrics: Principles and Practice*. 4th ed. Philadelphia, PA: Lippincott Williams & Wilkins; 2006:174-181.

Sponseller PD. Bone, joint and muscle problems (osteogenesis imperfecta). In: McMillan JA, Feigin RD, DeAngelis CD, Jones MD, eds. *Oski's Pediatrics: Principles and Practice*. 4th ed. Philadelphia, PA: Lippincott Williams & Wilkins; 2006:2495.

# Case 59

A 2-year-old child suddenly develops inspiratory stridor, tachypnea, and chest retractions. He had been playing alone with his 6-year-old brother before this episode. He is afebrile. Apart from the stridor, his lung sounds are clear, and his physical examination is otherwise normal. A chest radiograph reveals no abnormalities.

- What is the most likely diagnosis?
- What is the next step in management of this patient?

# ANSWERS TO CASE 59:
## Foreign Body Aspiration

*Summary:* A 2-year-old child who was previously healthy experiences sudden onset of respiratory distress.

- **Most likely diagnosis:** Foreign body aspiration.
- **Next step in management:** The child's airway should be evaluated with bronchoscopy. Intravenous access should be established for administration of maintenance fluids and sedation for the procedure; the child should take nothing by mouth until his respiratory distress resolves. Oxygen saturation should be monitored closely.

## ANALYSIS

### Objectives

1. Recognize the signs and symptoms of childhood acute upper airway obstruction.
2. Know the differential diagnosis for childhood upper airway obstruction.
3. Know the principles of acute management of childhood upper airway obstruction.

### Considerations

This child's good health just prior to developing respiratory symptoms is a major clue to his diagnosis. Foreign body aspiration or anaphylactic responses to an allergen are the two most likely explanations for his sudden symptoms. The additional information that the child was playing alone with another child suggests a scenario whereby the older child may have "shared" a toy, a piece of candy, or another enticing object with our patient. Stridor may be easily confused for wheezing by less experienced clinicians, which might lead one to also consider lower respiratory etiologies in the differential diagnosis. Stridor, however, is characterized by its monophonic sound (ie, a single pitch) that is louder over the upper chest. In contrast, wheezing represents blockage of multiple small airways and is heard as a polyphonic sound (ie, multiple pitches), heard best with the stethoscope placed over the lung bases.

# APPROACH TO
# Suspected Foreign Body Aspiration

## DEFINITIONS

**STRIDOR:** A high-pitched, monophonic musical sound resulting from partial airway obstruction. The obstruction may be supraglottic (ie, above the vocal cords), glottic, and/or subglottic (ie, below the vocal cords).

**TACHYPNEA:** A respiratory rate that is faster than normal **for the person's age.** The resting respiratory rate for an infant or young child is faster than that of an older person. The average resting respiratory rate for an infant is 30 breaths/min, whereas an 8-year-old child breathes at 20 breaths/min, and an adult breathes at a rate of approximately 16 breaths/min.

**ATELECTASIS:** Collapse of a portion of the lung. Atelectasis may be due to intrinsic factors, such as blockage of the airway proximal to the atelectatic tissue, or extrinsic factors, such as a pneumothorax.

## CLINICAL APPROACH

**Foreign body aspiration is a common cause of respiratory distress in young children and is a major cause of morbidity and mortality in this age group.** Children younger than 3 years of age typically explore their environment by putting objects in their mouths. Commonly aspirated objects include nuts, popcorn, seeds, raw carrot and hot dog pieces, grapes, candies, small toys, and coins. Objects that lodge in the larynx or trachea can cause rapid asphyxia and death if not dislodged immediately. Objects that lodge in a bronchus may go undetected until granulation tissue and inflammation develop, which then results in atelectasis and pneumonia. Aspirated foreign bodies in the lungs may lead to chronic cough and wheezing that can be confused with asthma or other chronic obstructive pulmonary disorders. Foreign bodies in the esophagus may also induce respiratory symptoms via pressure exerted on the membranous trachea. A carefully obtained history describing the child's state just prior to the onset of symptoms and a complete review of systems often is key to making the correct diagnosis.

The general differential diagnosis for a child with stridor, tachypnea, and chest retractions includes infectious and other noninfectious etiologies. A child with fever, hoarseness, and a recent history of upper respiratory symptoms may have **croup (laryngotracheobronchitis)**. A variety of viral infections have been implicated, the most common being parainfluenza viruses; influenza, measles, respiratory syncytial virus, herpes simplex, adenovirus, enterovirus, mycoplasma, or parainfluenza type 3 also can cause croup. Diphtheria, once a common cause, is rarely seen today because of widespread vaccination. **Epiglottitis** (rare as a result of widespread *Haemophilus influenzae* b vaccination) is identified by its characteristic clinical signs: **drooling, a preference to sit in a tripod or upright position** ("sniffing" position), muffled vocalizations, inspiratory stridor, and absence of cough. Identification of epiglottitis is crucial because the high risk for sudden complete airway obstruction necessitates immediate care. **Bacterial tracheitis** caused by *Staphylococcus aureus* (or less commonly *Moraxella catarrhalis* or nontypeable *H influenzae*) can occur as a sequela to viral croup. Like epiglottitis, bacterial tracheitis can cause life-threatening airway obstruction and thus may require emergent intubation or tracheostomy. **Noninfectious causes** mimicking foreign body aspiration include **tracheomalacia, extrinsic airway compression (vascular ring, tumor), and intraluminal obstruction (papilloma, hemangioma).** The term *spasmodic croup* is used to describe the syndrome of sudden nighttime onset of hoarseness, "barky" cough, and inspiratory stridor in a previously healthy, afebrile child. Viral infections, respiratory allergies, gastroesophageal reflux, and psychosocial factors are implicated as possible etiologies for spasmodic croup.

Some aspirated objects (eg, a metal coin) are easily visualized on radiographs, and their appearance indicates their location. Coins lodged in the trachea appear as a line on the radiograph, because the cartilaginous rings on the anterior side of the trachea force the coin into this position. Coins in the esophagus result in dysphagia and milder respiratory symptoms; they appear as circles on radiograph. **Objects that are small enough to pass beyond the carina most typically lodge in the right mainstem bronchus**, because it is more vertical than the left bronchus. Objects made of plastic and other radiolucent materials are not visible on radiographs, although there may be other radiographic clues, such as a focal area of atelectasis or a shift of the mediastinum toward the unobstructed side on an expiratory film. Rigid bronchoscopy is diagnostic and therapeutic in cases of foreign body aspiration into an airway.

## Comprehension Questions

59.1 A 7-month-old boy with respiratory difficulty is brought to the emergency department at 3 AM. His mother reports that several family members have had "colds" over the past week. He first developed cough and coryza 3 days ago, and the cough has become "barky." On examination, he has an axillary temperature of 100.4°F (38°C), respiratory rate 55 breaths/min, and heart rate 140 bpm (beats/min). A moderately inflamed pharynx and inspiratory stridor are noted on physical examination. Which of the following is the next step in management of this patient?

A. Reassure the child's parents that his upper respiratory symptoms will resolve without antibiotics or other medication.
B. Obtain a chest radiograph.
C. Obtain a throat swab specimen for rapid testing for *Streptococcus pyogenes*.
D. Administer aerosolized racemic epinephrine and corticosteroids immediately.
E. Obtain blood, urine, and cerebrospinal cultures, and begin parenteral antibiotics.

59.2 A 14-month-old girl has a 6-hour history of fever to 102.6°F (39.2°C) and an increasingly ill appearance. She is anxious and does not want to leave her mother's arms, but she gives only a faint cry when approached. Her respiratory rate is 70 breaths/min and her neck is hyperextended. An area of moisture is noted on the shoulder of the mother's blouse. Which of the following is the next most appropriate step in management?

A. Perform a complete physical examination with particular emphasis on the mouth and upper airway.
B. Immediately secure the airway with an endotracheal tube in the emergency department.
C. Arrange for immediate transfer to the operating room to secure the airway via tracheal intubation or tracheostomy.
D. Administer aerosolized racemic epinephrine and nebulized steroids.
E. Obtain blood, urine, and cerebrospinal cultures, and begin parenteral antibiotics.

59.3 A 2-year-old boy is seen in your office after his parents report a "rough night." Following a few days of a mild upper respiratory symptoms but no fever, last night he had an episode of stridor and increased effort of breathing. He has done this twice previously in the last 2 months and was well before each episode. In the interim period he has been normal. Today, apart from some mild rhinorrhea, his physical examination is normal. Which of the following is the most likely etiology?

A. Spasmodic croup
B. Foreign body aspiration
C. Tracheomalacia
D. Extraluminal compression of the trachea by a tumor
E. *S pyogenes* pharyngitis

59.4 A 2-year-old boy with a 3-day history of upper respiratory congestion and cough now has inspiratory stridor, respiratory rate of 50 breaths/min, chest retractions, and a fever of 101°F (38.3°C). The next step in the management of his condition should be which of the following therapies?

A. Pseudoephedrine and dextromethorphan
B. Albuterol and cromolyn
C. Ampicillin and gentamicin
D. Cool mist and herbs
E. Aerosolized racemic epinephrine and steroids

## ANSWERS

59.1 **D.** This child's history and physical examination findings are typical of croup. Croup often presents at night when symptoms typically worsen. Cool mist is often used in an attempt to relieve laryngeal spasm; the evidence supporting its effectiveness is weak except in cases of allergic (spasmodic) croup. Aerosolized epinephrine and oral or aerosolized steroids are effective in reducing airway edema and relieving croup symptoms. Potentially irritating procedures (ie, use of tongue blades or needle sticks) are avoided unless necessary; agitation and crying aggravate the respiratory symptoms. Parenteral fluids rarely may be indicated if the child is not drinking well. Oxygen saturation should be monitored closely; a low saturation in croup indicates imminent airway obstruction.

59.2 **C.** This child's clinical picture is consistent with epiglottitis, a medical emergency. She is kept calm and is transported to an operating room where the airway is examined and secured by a surgeon and anesthesia team skilled in tracheal intubation and tracheostomy. Visualizing the pharynx in the emergency department may cause airway obstruction. Although rare in the United States, epiglottitis occasionally is seen in hypoimmunized children or as a result of infection with *S pyogenes*, *S pneumoniae*, or *S aureus*.

59.3 **A.** Children with spasmodic croup appear well during the daytime but develop nocturnal stridor and difficulty breathing; the cause is unknown. As this child's symptoms resolved during the daytime and he previously has had two similar episodes, foreign body aspiration is less likely (although always considered in a toddler with respiratory distress). Infants with mild tracheomalacia have stridor only intermittently (eg, with crying), but it is first noted in early infancy. A tumor compressing the trachea usually causes persistent or progressive symptoms but less likely intermittent stridor. Streptococcal laryngitis causes fever and throat pain but generally not significant stridor.

59.4 **E.** Aerosolized epinephrine and steroids are the only therapies that significantly improve symptoms of croup (in this case, likely viral). Systemic and nebulized steroids also reduce hospital admissions, length of hospital stay, and hospital reattendance.

## Clinical Pearls

- Foreign body aspiration should be considered in the differential diagnosis for a previously healthy young child with sudden onset of stridor and respiratory distress, as well as for a previously healthy child with chronic cough or wheezing.
- The differential diagnosis of foreign body aspiration also includes croup, epiglottitis, bacterial tracheitis, tracheomalacia, extrinsic airway compression, and other forms of intraluminal obstruction. Epiglottitis and bacterial tracheitis require stabilization in a calm environment by an expert skilled in airway management. Asthma and other forms of chronic obstructive pulmonary disease should be considered for the child with wheezing.
- Aspirated objects that pass beyond the carina usually lodge in the right mainstem bronchus.
- Rigid bronchoscopy is both diagnostic and therapeutic in cases of foreign body aspiration.

## REFERENCES


Cotton RT. Laryngotracheobronchitis or croup. In: Rudolph CD, Rudolph AM, Hostetter MK, Lister G, Siegel NJ, eds. *Rudolph's Pediatrics*. 21st ed. New York, NY: McGraw-Hill; 2003:1275-1276.

Rozenfeld RA. Atelectasis. In: Kliegman RM, Behrman RE, Jenson HB, Stanton BF, eds. *Nelson Textbook of Pediatrics*. 18th ed. Philadelphia, PA: WB Saunders; 2007:1831.

Schweich PJ. Airway obstruction. In: McMillan JA, Feigin RD, DeAngelis CD, Jones MD, eds. *Oski's Pediatrics: Principles and Practice*. 4th ed. Philadelphia, PA: Lippincott Williams & Wilkins; 2006:693-694.

Watts KD, Goodman DM. Wheezing in infants: bronchiolitis. In: Kliegman RM, Behrman RE, Jenson HB, Stanton BF, eds. *Nelson Textbook of Pediatrics*. 18th ed. Philadelphia, PA: WB Saunders; 2007:1775.

# Case 60

A 3-year-old boy presents for his second visit to see you. Two days ago he was seen with a 4-day history of intermittent fever spiking to 104°F (40°C) and irritability. His examination at that time was remarkable for bilateral conjunctivitis, oropharyngeal injection, and dry, cracked lips. He drank 4 oz of an electrolyte solution in the clinic and was sent home with instructions for symptomatic care. Today he returns with persistent fever and irritability. The physical findings noted previously are still present, but now he also has a maculopapular truncal rash, hand and foot edema, and an enlarged but nonsuppurative right anterior cervical lymph node.

- What is the most likely diagnosis?
- What is the best diagnostic test for this disorder?
- What is the treatment for this condition?

# ANSWERS TO CASE 60:
## Kawasaki Syndrome

*Summary:* A 3-year-old boy with high-spiking fevers and irritability of 6 days' duration. Conjunctivitis, an enlarged anterior cervical lymph node, oropharyngeal erythema, dry, cracked lips, a maculopapular rash, and edema of the hands and feet are present on examination.

- **Most likely diagnosis:** Kawasaki syndrome (KS; mucocutaneous lymph node syndrome).
- **Best diagnostic test:** No laboratory study is diagnostic. Echocardiography is used to monitor for coronary aneurysm development, the most serious potential disease complication. Elevated acute-phase reactants (erythrocyte sedimentation rate [ESR] and C-reactive protein [CRP]), normocytic anemia, and thrombocytosis support the diagnosis.
- **Treatment:** Early anti-inflammatory therapy with high-dose intravenous immunoglobulin (IVIG) and aspirin reduces the risk of coronary complications.

## ANALYSIS

### Objectives

1. Know the diagnostic criteria for KS.
2. Recognize the need for early diagnosis and treatment to prevent coronary complications.
3. Be familiar with other diagnostic possibilities in the differential diagnosis of KS.

### Considerations

Diagnosing KS can be difficult in the first few days of illness, when only a few classic clinical findings may be present. Adenoviral infection was perhaps the presumptive diagnosis at the first visit, although the intermittent fevers for 4 days and irritability might have prompted suspicions of another etiology. His diagnosis became more obvious on the sixth illness day when he manifested additional clinical signs, although other conditions still must be considered.

# APPROACH TO
# Fever and Rash

## DEFINITIONS

**POLYMORPHOUS RASH:** An exanthem that may take various forms among affected individuals, such as maculopapular, erythema multiforme, or scarlatiniform.

**STRAWBERRY TONGUE:** Erythema of the tongue with prominent papillae.

**THROMBOCYTOSIS:** Elevation of the platelet count above 450,000/$mm^3$. In KS this usually occurs after the 10th day of illness and may last for a few weeks.

## CLINICAL APPROACH

**Kawasaki syndrome is a generalized vasculitic disease of unknown etiology but is thought to be infectious.** The incidence is highest among **Asians**, but it is seen worldwide. It occurs most frequently in **children younger than 5 years** and slightly more frequently in boys than in girls.

The diagnosis of KS is based on finding the characteristic signs (Table 60–1), although children with fewer signs who later develop **coronary artery disease (CAD)** are recognized. Cervical adenopathy is seen less frequently than the other diagnostic criteria, occurring in 60% to 70% of patients. Incomplete disease occurs most frequently in infants, the group most likely to develop coronary complications. Although no test establishes the diagnosis, certain

**Table 60–1** DIAGNOSTIC CRITERIA FOR KAWASAKI DISEASE

Fever lasting for at least 5 d (or fewer days if defervescence occurs in response to early IVIG therapy) in a child without evidence of other more likely pathology, plus the presence of at least four of the following five signs:

1. Bilateral conjunctivitis, generally nonpurulent
2. Oropharyngeal mucosal changes including pharyngeal injection, injection or fissuring of the lips, and strawberry tongue
3. Polymorphous rash that is primarily truncal
4. Edema or erythema of the hands or feet in the acute phase; periungual desquamation in the subacute phase
5. Acute nonpurulent cervical lymphadenopathy

*Note: Patients with fever and three of these criteria can be diagnosed with Kawasaki disease when coronary aneurysm or dilatation is recognized by 2-D echocardiography or coronary angiography.*

laboratory findings are characteristic. The ESR and CRP are elevated, and normocytic anemia and leucocytosis are common. The platelet count is usually normal initially but often rises above normal by the 10th day; thrombocytopenia at illness presentation is rare and is a risk factor for development of coronary aneurysms. Sterile pyuria, cerebrospinal fluid pleocytosis, and mildly elevated hepatic transaminase level may be seen. Gastrointestinal (GI) symptoms may include diarrhea, vomiting, and hydrops of the gall bladder, and patients may have upper respiratory complaints and/or joint arthralgias. Cardiac echocardiography may identify abnormalities of the coronary arteries or other structures. The differential diagnosis of KS includes infectious and noninfectious conditions, such as streptococcal disease, staphylococcal toxin (toxic shock syndrome), rickettsial infection, measles, Epstein-Barr virus infection, drug hypersensitivity reactions, systemic-onset juvenile rheumatoid arthritis, and leptospirosis.

Successful treatment depends on rapidly **starting high-dose aspirin and IVIG.** Rapid defervescence generally occurs with this regimen. Aspirin therapy is later reduced from anti-inflammatory to antithrombotic doses and continued until 6 to 8 weeks after disease onset, when the ESR normalizes. Children with coronary artery disease require prolonged antithrombotic therapy.

**Even with treatment, approximately 5% of children develop coronary artery dilation, and 1% develop giant aneurysms.** Aneurysm risk factors include male gender, prolonged fever, age younger than 12 months, higher baseline neutrophil and band counts, lower hemoglobin level, and platelet count less than 350,000/mm$^3$. Children without known cardiac sequelae during the first month return to their normal state of health; those with persistent cardiac abnormalities may suffer significant morbidity. Death is rare and is caused by myocardial infarction or, less commonly, aneurysm rupture.

## Comprehension Questions

60.1 A 12-month-old child arrives for a well-child examination. He was hospitalized 2 months ago for KS and was taken off aspirin therapy 6 weeks prior to this visit. His most recent echocardiogram was normal. For this patient, special consideration should be paid to which of the following?

A. His developmental assessment
B. The abdominal examination
C. Live-vaccine administration
D. Serum hemoglobin evaluation
E. Assessment of possible lead toxicity

60.2 A 15-month-old child is on long-term aspirin therapy for coronary artery abnormalities that resulted from KS. In addition to his routine vaccinations required for school, he should receive which of the following?
A. Pneumococcal vaccine
B. Influenza vaccine
C. Meningococcal vaccine
D. Oral polio vaccine
E. Varicella vaccine

60.3 A 5-month-old irritable infant develops 3 days of high fever, a maculopapular diaper rash, and swollen, red lips. He has a mild normocytic anemia and a white blood cell count (WBC) of 15,000/mm$^3$ with a predominance of neutrophils and immature forms. Urinalysis is normal, but the cerebrospinal fluid shows a pleocytosis with a negative Gram stain. After 24 hours of ceftriaxone, he continues to have high fever and has developed foot edema. Subsequent management of this child should include which of the following?
A. Nystatin for the diaper rash
B. Repeat of the spinal tap
C. Addition of vancomycin to the antibiotic regimen
D. Pediatric cardiology consultation; beginning of IVIG infusions and oral high-dose aspirin
E. Continuing current management and following the culture results

60.4 Who of the following children with KS is at greatest risk for coronary artery disease?
A. A 5-year-old boy with 6 days of high fever, sterile pyuria, a truncal rash, and strawberry tongue
B. A 3-year-old girl with 5 days of high fever and cerebrospinal fluid pleocytosis
C. A 2-year-old girl with 5 days of high fever and an initial ESR of 80 mm/h
D. A 1-year-old boy with 6 days of high fever, a maculopapular rash, and mildly elevated hepatic transaminase levels
E. A 6-month-old boy with 11 days of high fever and a small pericardial effusion on initial echocardiogram

## ANSWERS

60.1 **C.** Live-virus vaccines (measles-mumps-rubella [MMR], varicella) are delayed for 11 months following high-dose IVIG administration; IVIG potentially interferes with the immune response. The measles vaccine, typically given as MMR at 12 months, is provided if the exposure risk is high, but reimmunization is required unless serologic testing indicates adequate antibody titers.

60.2 **B.** Children on prolonged aspirin therapy receive the influenza vaccine; they are at increased risk of Reye syndrome if they are infected and taking aspirin. While usually not required for day care or school attendance, the Centers for Disease Control and Prevention recommends that all children aged 6 months and older receive an annual influenza vaccine.

60.3 **D.** This child's initial presentation is consistent with, but not diagnostic of, KS (Table 60–1). His persistent fever and peripheral extremity edema increase the possibility of KS and should prompt further investigation and treatment.

60.4 **E.** Risk factors for development of coronary aneurysms include male gender, fever for more than 10 days, age younger than 12 months, low serum albumin or hemoglobin level, early cardiac findings (eg, mitral regurgitation or pericardial effusion), and thrombocytopenia.

## Clinical Pearls

- The diagnosis of Kawasaki syndrome (KS) is based on clinical criteria and should be strongly suspected in a young child with a combination of high fever for more than 5 days, oropharyngeal changes, conjunctivitis, extremity changes, rash, and cervical adenopathy.
- Children with incomplete disease ("atypical KS") can develop coronary artery abnormalities.
- The most important complication of KS is coronary artery disease. A pediatric cardiologist usually is involved in the care of these children.
- Early recognition and initiation of therapy for KS is key to preventing potential coronary complications.

## REFERENCES

American Academy of Pediatrics. Kawasaki disease. In: Pickering LK, ed. *2006 Red Book: Report of the Committee on Infectious Diseases*. 27th ed. Elk Grove Village, IL: American Academy of Pediatrics; 2006:412-415.

Ayusawa M, Sonobe T, Uemura S, et al. Revision of diagnostic guidelines for Kawasaki disease (the 5th revised edition). *Pediatr Int*. 2005;47:232-234.

de Inocencio J. Kawasaki disease. In: Rudolph CD, Rudolph AM, Hostetter MK, Lister G, Siegel NJ, eds. *Rudolph's Pediatrics*. 21st ed. New York, NY: McGraw-Hill; 2003: 844-845.

Feigin RD, Cecchin F, Wissman SD. Kawasaki disease. In: McMillan JA, Feigin RD, DeAngelis CD, Jones MD, eds. *Oski's Pediatrics: Principles and Practice*. 4th ed. Philadelphia, PA: Lippincott Williams & Wilkins; 2006:1015-1020.

Newburger JW, Takahashi M, Gerber MA, et al. Diagnosis, treatment, and long-term management of Kawasaki disease: a statement for health professionals from the Committee on Rheumatic Fever, Endocarditis and Kawasaki Disease, Council on Cardiovascular Disease in the Young, American Heart Association. *Pediatrics*. 2004; 114:1708-1733.

Rowley AH, Shulman ST. Kawasaki disease. In: Kliegman RM, Behrman RE, Jenson HB, Stanton BF, eds. *Nelson Textbook of Pediatrics*. 18th ed. Philadelphia, PA: WB Saunders; 2007:1036-1041.

SECTION III

# Listing of Cases

## Listing by Case Number

## Listing by Disorder (Alphabetical)

# INDEX

Page numbers followed by *f* or *t* indicate figures or tables, respectively.